THE ALPHA
SYLLABUS

THE ALPHA SYLLABUS

A Handbook of
Human EEG Alpha Activity

Edited by

BARBARA B. BROWN, Ph.D.

Chief, Experiential Physiology
Veterans Administration Hospital
Sepulveda, California
Lecturer, Department of Psychiatry
UCLA Medical Center
Los Angeles, California

and

JAY W. KLUG, A.B.

Research Associate
Experiential Physiology
Veterans Administration Hospital
Sepulveda, California

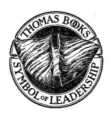

CHARLES C THOMAS · PUBLISHER
Springfield · *Illinois* · *U.S.A.*

Published and Distributed Throughout the World by
CHARLES C THOMAS • PUBLISHER
Bannerstone House
301-327 East Lawrence Avenue, Springfield, Illinois, U.S.A.

© *1974, by* CHARLES C THOMAS • PUBLISHER
ISBN 0-398-03020-0 (cloth)
ISBN 0-398-03021-9 (paper)
Library of Congress Catalog Card Number: 73-15547

With THOMAS BOOKS *careful attention is given to all details of manufacturing and design. It is the Publisher's desire to present books that are satisfactory as to their physical qualities and artistic possibilities and appropriate for their particular use.* THOMAS BOOKS *will be true to those laws of quality that assure a good name and good will.*

Printed in the United States of America
N-1

Library of Congress Cataloging in Publication Data

Brown, Barbara B
    The alpha syllabus.

    Bibliography: p.
    1. Electroencephalography. I. Klug, Jay W., joint author. II. Title. [DNLM: 1. Electroencephalography—abstracts. ZWL 150 B877a 1974]
RC349.E5B76   616.8'04'754   73-15547
ISBN 0-398-03020-0
ISBN 0-398-03021-9 (pbk.)

PREFACE

THIS HANDBOOK OF references and synopses of scientific publications on human EEG alpha activity has been prepared to facilitate searches of the scientific literature for the many aspects and attributes of EEG alpha that are reported in numerous scientific journals crossing many and varied disciplines.

The Alpha Syllabus is a compendium of recent reports containing significant information concerning EEG alpha. Scientific reports containing such information published prior to 1963 can be located in *A KWIC Index of EEG Literature,* published by Elsevier Publishing Company, 1965. For convenience, pre-1963 reports not contained in the *Syllabus* are listed alphabetically without abstracts in the Supplemental References.

Although an attempt was made to include as many publications as possible concerning EEG alpha, there are certain unavoidable omissions. These result from a variety of causes such as relative inaccessibility, unintentional oversights, and occasionally where the relationship of the report to alpha was obscure.

INTRODUCTION

A̲LL ABSTRACTS OF PUBLISHED reports which deal primarily with similar subjects are located according to topic headings indicated in the *Table of Contents*. The general headings in the *Table of Contents* indicate the principal emphasis of each article.

The headings classify characteristics and correlates of EEG alpha activity according to the basic nature of their physical, physiological, psychological or pathological relationship.

Since several attributes or correlates of alpha are generally reported on, a list of descriptors indicating other aspects importantly described or discussed is listed in the margin for each article abstracted. The descriptors either further define the particular characteristics reported on or indicate aspects of alpha correlated with the major characteristic. An index of descriptors is provided.

All major topics and descriptors refer to their relationship to EEG *alpha* unless specifically noted.

ACKNOWLEDGMENTS

The editors wish to thank the Korg Foundation and Silva Mind Control International, Inc. for their support of this project.

INSTRUCTIONS

To LOCATE ABSTRACT for special topics, refer to (a) the *Table of Contents* and (b) the *Descriptor Index*.

All abstracts relating predominantly to special topics are grouped together under the headings indicated in the Table of Contents.

For additional material, or to locate subtopics, refer to the Descriptor Index. In the Index all descriptors are given an identification by letter and number which identifies their location in the *Syllabus*. The letter refers to the section, and the number refers to the number of the abstract in the section indicated. Abstract numbers which appear in boldface type indicate articles which are grouped according to the Table of Contents as described above.

EXPLANATIONS ABOUT THE DESCRIPTORS

DESCRIPTORS INDICATING the major and minor topics dealt with in the research reports abstracted are listed in the margin for each abstract.

Each article is classified by its descriptors in a sequence indicating the relative order of significance of the variables or attributes or subjects described.

In addition to defining the major emphasis of the research reports, the descriptors serve two additional purposes: the identification of subtopics or secondary emphasis, and notations for cross-referencing.

In general and where appropriate for each abstracted report, the first two or three descriptors following definition of the major topic indicate the aspect of alpha or the condition in which alpha was studied and the variables correlated. For example, in abstract E21, the descriptors read: stress, mental tasks, EEG responses, alpha amplitude, data collection, telemetry. The first two descriptors indicate that the effect of *mental tasks* during *stress* were the conditions of the experiment. *Alpha amplitude* and *EEG responses* indicate the chief EEG parameters measured, and the variables correlated. The descriptor *data collection* indicates that a special technique for data collection was used, and the descriptor *telemetry* notes an additional qualifier of the data collection technique.

CONTENTS

THE ALPHA
SYLLABUS

SECTION A

NEUROPHYSIOLOGIC BACKGROUND

HISTORY

A 1.   Brazier, M.A.B.: Pioneers in the electrophysiology of the nervous system. *Electroencephalogr Clin Neurophysiol, 27:* 729, 1969.

The exhibit consists of several panels, each depicting the first public description of electrophysiologic discoveries and, where possible, the first published photograph of the results. The panels include: the first descriptions of the EEG (1875, 1890); the first DC studies of brain potentials (1875, 1883, 1890); the first reports of the effect of flicker on brain potentials (1887); the discovery of alpha blocking after sensory stimulation (1890). *history*

A 2.   Barnes, T.C.: Synopsis of electroencephalography. *Confin Neurol, 26:*532, 1965.

This is an index to electroencephalography and is an addendum to previous synopses. (*Confinia Neurologica, 8:*73, 1947 and 1948; *10:*394, 1950; *11:*40, 112, 177, 241, 368, 1951; *12:*65, 1952.) *history* *definitions*

A 3.   Brazier, M.A.B.: *A History of the Electrical Activity of the Brain: The First Half-Century.* New York, Macmillian, 1961, VII, pp. 119.

Describes the history of electroencephalography in terms of those who created it. The article begins with a short background summary leading to the discovery of electrical activity of the brain by Richard Canton. Beck, Horsley, Danilevsky, Kaufman etc. are among those mentioned. The article ends with a sketch of Hans Berger, the first person to record an EEG in man. *history*

THEORY

A 4.   Vorontsov, D.S.: What does the electroencephalogram ex-
        press? *Pavlov J Higher Nerv Activ, 10:42,* 1960.

        "Slow potentials" and outer cortex activity of apical den-   *theory*
        drites of pyramidal neurons are the main components of the
        EEG. Other neuronal activity is concealed by cortical ohmic
        and capacitive elements. Therefore, it can be said that the
        surface EEG shows only excitability of cortical neurons which
        are oriented in a vertical manner. The author suggests that
        intracortical leading off is required to make the surface EEG
        a valuable tool in the study of higher nervous activity.

A 5.   Brumlik, J., Richeson, W.B., and Arbit, J.: The origin of
        certain electrical cerebral rhythms. *Brain Res, 3:277,* 1966/
        1967.

        This paper reviews the literature on the origin of certain   *theory*
        electrical cerebral rhythms (alpha rhythms). Three cate-   *history*
        gories of theories are described: (1) neuronal, (2) mechanic- *origins*
        al, and (3) combination of neuronal and mechanical. Ac-
        cording to neuronal theories, neurones or astroglia of the
        brain generate the potentials which we call alpha rhythms.
        The neuronal group also includes dendritic potentials and
        reverberating circuit theories. The mechanical category re-
        lates these rhythms to cardiorespiratory foci which set the
        brain into mechanical motion. The third group contains
        combinations of the first two groups. The author presents
        both pros and cons on these topics and suggests that only
        experimentation can really uncover the true origins of these
        alpha rhythms.

A 6.   Nelson, G.K.: The measurement and significance of brain
        rhythms. *Trans South African Inst Electrical Engineers,*
        January 1960, p. 1.

        Describes the origins of research into EEG significance, con- *theory*
        temporary recording and analysis equipment, and results re-   *history*
        lating to psychological meanings of brain waves. It also ex- *instruments*
        plains the need for new display methods, specifically men-
        tioning toposocopy. Up-to-date information about psycho-
        physiological research laboratory equipment is presented.

A 7.   Dondey, M.: EEG terminology and semantics. *Electroenceph-alogr Clin Neurophysiol, 13*:612, 1961.

This article defines a semantic framework of EEG terminol-ogy for reading EEG records. Several examples of its use are also given.

*theory
definitions*

A 8.   Proler, M.L.: The alpha rhythm: Part I—Description and physiology. *Am J EEG Technol, 3*:65, 1963.

The report describes the alpha rhythm and some of its characteristics and physiological bases. The alpha rhythm is depicted as a smooth waxing and waning of the brain wave between 8 and 13 cps (varying 0 to 1 cps until senescence when it varies 1 to 2 cps) primarily originating from the occipital area with amplitude bounded between 5 and 110 μv. The alpha waves seem to be bilaterally similar in ampli-tude and frequency with synchrony being greater in the central regions than in the occipital area. If asymmetry is present, the hemisphere which is dominant is usually lower in voltage. It seems that any novel interest such as opening the eyes, concentration, etc., will cause alpha activity to dis-appear (blocking), while photic stimulation causes alpha to increase in frequency within bounds (driving). As the light flicker reaches the alpha frequency, the alpha will increase in frequency with the light until a critical frequency is reached. Then, the occipital waves either revert back to their regular rhythm, become subharmonic to the light stimulation, or disorganize into arrhythmic patterns. It is even possible to drive the contralateral occipital alpha only, which in addi-tion to other discoveries about multiple foci, etc., indicates that alpha activity is a function of several factors such as frequency, site and distance from the surface of the foci in-volved. Physiologically, five significant points were noted: (1) the intracortical feltwork of neurones seems to be the main energy source for alpha activity; (2) multiple foci pro-ducing an autorhythmic alpha element are present in both hemispheres but with some degree of frequency difference; (3) the symmetrical function of alpha is probably due to cortical generators; (4) midline structures of the thalamus have their own alpha which projects to cortical zones, regu-lates occipital rhythms, and aids in bilateral synchrony; and

*theory
definitions
criteria
alpha
  synchrony
alpha
  blocking
visual
  stimulation
generators
brain
  physiology*

(5) local autonomy is demonstrated by the intrinsic cortical rhythms which tend to asynchrony.

A 9. Mulholland, T.B.: Occipital alpha revisited. *Psychol Bull* (in press).

The alpha attenuation cycle, alpha or no-alpha alterations, describes the occipital EEG. The assumptions of singularity of the response of the EEG alpha rhythm and function equivalence of all alpha and all intervals of alpha attenuation upon which past occipital alpha rhythm descriptions have been based are evaluated against experimental evidence and a new interpretation is presented. Under this interpretation, the response of the occipital alpha rhythm is a time series, not a singular response. All alpha events are not functionally equivalent, nor are all no-alpha events; even their position in the time series is important.

theory
definitions
alpha
blocking

A 10. Zhadin, M.N.: Mechanisms involved in the emergence of synchronization of biopotentials in the cerebral cortex. *Biofizika, 14*:696, 1969.

The research examined the integrated potential in the surface layer of the cerebrospinal fluid created by the mutually independent activity of the cortical neurons. The effect of synchronization of the potential is shown mathematically to be more local when compared with the spatial distribution of EEG correlation. It does not depend on dipole source orientation. The integrated potential amplitude in this system is much less than that of the EEG and does not depend essentially on cellular orientation. Therefore, authors conclude that the EEG cannot be the mere summation of potentials of independent cells. The EEG must require a mutual connection in the cell activity.

theory
origins
EEG
synchrony

A 11. Zhadin, M.H.: Mechanisms for the emergence of biopotential synchronization in the cerebral cortex: II. A model of dependent sources. *Biofizika, 14*:897, 1969.

The part II experiment examines further the integrated potential on the surface of the cerebrospinal liquid layer, created by the mutually correlated activity of the cortical cells. The randomly orientated stellate and glial cells can-

theory
origins
EEG
synchrony

not create changes in potential, comparable in amplitude with the EEG. The EEG is said to be the result of weakly correlated activity of identically orientated pyramidal cells in the cortex. Amplitude of the integrated potential is found not to be a function of thickness and resistance of the cerebrospinal liquid layer. Strong and synchronized EEG features may arise at low levels of synchronization of cell activity. The author calls the EEG an "isolated general synchronized component" which emanates from many of the pyramidal cells. The EEG at each point, concludes the author, is created by practically the whole cortical volume.

A 12. Cooper, R., Winter, A.L., Crow, H.J., and Walter, W.G.: Comparison of subcortical, cortical, and scalp activity using chronically indwelling electrodes in man. *Electroencephalogr Clin Neurophysiol, 18:*217, 1965.

EEG records were taken from twelve patients to show that the scalp acts as spatial averager of brain electrical activity in humans and to evaluate the scalp EEG in the light of this information. Results showed that, since amplitude of cortical activity can be attenuated or not attenuated at different times and locations, amplitude may not be the only factor involved in scalp activity. Other factors might include cortical area involved and the degree of synchronous activity over this area. A very simple model described in detail indicates that signals can be recorded from the scalp only when large areas are involved in synchronous activity or when small areas are discharging very high voltage signals. It is suggested that characteristic fluctuations in alpha activity may be dependent on area of synchronous discharge rather than local amplitude variations. This theory may also explain other occurrences such as frontal beta activity from intercranial electrodes not being recordable on the scalp. Nonsynchronous waves would cause a greater canceling effect at these higher frequencies. The authors conclude that due to these discoveries scalp EEG's are very poor indicators of complex local cortical activity. They plead for higher working gains so that more information can be detected from the scalp and correlated with clinical conditions to make scalp recordings more significant.

theory
alpha
  amplitude
topography
alpha
  synchrony

A 13.   Stennett, R.G.: Alpha amplitude and arousal: A reply to
        Surwillo. *Psychophysiology, 2:*372, 1966.

        Arguments are presented in answer to W.W. Surwillo's   *theory*
        criticism of a statistical procedure used by R.G. Stennett to *alpha*
        test the hypothesis of an inverted U relationship between   *amplitude*
        alpha amplitude and palmar conductance. An attempt is   *arousal*
        made to: (1) clarify the rationale of the statistical technique *GSR*
        involved, (2) illustrate the fallacy of the conclusions to
        which Surwillo is drawn by his hypothetical data, and (3)
        point out certain methodological problems and pitfalls in-
        volved in studies along "the arousal continuum."

A 14.   Griesel, R.D.: The applicability of Wilder's law of initial
        value to changes in the alpha rhythm of the electroencephalo-
        gram. *Psychol Africana, 12:*122, 1968.

        By determining the regression slope of post-stimulus on pre-   *theory*
        stimulus alpha frequency and abundance scores, an attempt   *alpha*
        was made to establish whether changes in the alpha rhythm   *patterns*
        follow Wilder's law of initial value. Although it appeared
        that alpha activity is very sensitive to conditions of mild
        stress, this characteristic became apparent only when re-
        gression analysis was applied to the observations. The analy-
        sis also lent support to the hypothesis that alpha rhythm
        changes follow the law of initial value but more rigid con-
        trol observations will be needed to eliminate the "regression
        effect" before the hypothesis can be accepted without re-
        serve. The results also suggest that such regression scores may
        be useful indications of an individual's homeostatic function
        and/or susceptibility to stress.

A 15.   Joseph, J.P., Remond, A., Rieger, H., and Lesevre, N.: The
        alpha average: II. Quantitative study and the proposition of
        a theoretical model. *Electroencephalogr Clin Neurophysiol,*
        *26:*350, 1969.

        The alpha rhythm in its averaged form (Lairy et al., 1969;   *theory*
        Remond et al., 1969) results in configurations which depend   *alpha*
        upon a number of properties: mean frequency and its scatter,   *patterns*
        the mean amplitude, the interregional phase relationships   *data analysis*
        and the stability of these relationships. The article presents *definitions*
                                                                       origins

a physiomathematical model of such activity so that it can be simplified and, along with experimental information, help to explain such phenomena as the origin of the alpha rhythm. The model described is suggested by the typical and reproducible components of the alpha averager. The model's objectives are twofold: (1) to provide an explanation of the average alpha patterns in terms of underlying spontaneous activity (this is difficult with the conventional EEG) ; (2) to give an interpretation of the above model using the least number of mathematical concepts and the simplest hypothesis. An attempt is made to define the parameters of the alpha average through spatial symmetry, symmetry of amplitude, frequency stability, and global organization. The indices are derived from the theoretical model but are based on experimental data. An electrostatic model with a limited number of precisely located charges which evoke a sine wave is developed which satisfies the conditions. The model requires simply varying parameters to simulate both typical and atypical features of the alpha average. The author notes the oversimplification and approximation involved in the model, but he indicates that when applied to experimental data, it serves a useful purpose, particularly as applied to topography and chronology. The model goes beyond an analogy to partial interpretations of results and thereby is valuable in furthering the understanding of experimental and clinical observations.

A 16. Walter, W.G.: The functions of electrical rhythms in the brain. The twenty-fourth Maudsley Lecture. *J Ment Sci, 96:* 1, 1950.

This is a review of concepts and data concerning the relationship between electroencephalographic events and mental experience. It defines the magnitude of brain complexity underlying brain function. Models and data support the notion of plurality of alpha rhythms. The review uses photic flicker as a technique to distinguish real from imaginary mental experience, to explore mechanisms in epilepsy and various psychiatric problems and to relate EEG changes to emotion.

theory
alpha
  patterns
visual
  system
visual
  imagery
photic
  flicker
epilepsy

A 17.   Keidel, W.D., Engelen, S., and Rix, R.: Attempted explanation of alpha rhythm in human EEG by means of system theory. *Naturwissenschaften, 58*:91, 1971.

An hypothesis derived from the reafference principle was tested by presenting a crystal to one eye of a subject (the other eye being covered), first in stabilized and later in unstabilized form. The stabilized picture produced an alpha rhythm which vanished when an unstabilized picture was presented. The EEG spectra were analyzed by computer. The data emphasize the existence of an "internal clock" triggering eye movements as part of a complex closed-loop system as suggested by Norbert Wiener.

theory
visual
system
biorhythms

A 18.   Sherwood, S.L.: The abandonment of the absolute. *Ann NY Acad Sci, 138*:600, 1967.

Various theories of EEG wave production are considered. The properties of cells and cell networks are presented to support the proposition that "the EEG is the result of neuronal network activity, and the added or derived potential fluctuations caused by the chemical processes subserving their function."

theory
brain
physiology

A 19.   Darrow, C.W.: Psychological and psychophysiological significance of the electroencephalogram. *Psychol Rev, 54*:157, 1947.

Present evidence indicates that the EEG is not primarily a record of the integrative activities of the cortex but of facilitative and homeostatic regulatory processes which contribute to but are not essential to integrative cerebral function. The EEG is shown here to be a part of a regulatory mechanism which maintains varying degrees of equilibrium among alpha rhythms, cortical integrative activity, chemical condition and cerebral circulation with the autonomic nerves to the brain acting as an important influence. The article explains interrelations between these and how psychopathological effects develop as a consequence of an imbalance.

theory
brain
physiology
ANS

A 20.   Nigro, A.: The time in the electroencephalogram. *Riv Neurobiol, 15*:762, 1969.

The EEG may be examined in relation to the present/past components of the activity of consciousness. The present interpretative proposal regards the alternation of the two fundamental rhythms (alpha and beta) as an expression of present and past as a constant phenomenon of equilibrium for each phase of central nervous activity. It is proposed to consider the active condition of the organism as a moment of prevalence of the past component on a level with the consciousness of the structures, where the prevalence of the present leads to a state of higher reflection. An original graphical scheme is presented to illustrate this interpretative concept.

theory
consciousness
EEG
patterns

A 21. Needham, C.W., and Dila, C.J.: Synchronizing and desynchronizing systems of the old brain. *Brain Res, 11:285,* 1968.

This review of the experimental production of sleep and arousal is concerned with the formulation of an internally consistent concept of the various synchronizing and desynchronizing systems. It is difficult to imagine all the separate synchronizing and desynchronizing mechanisms as functionally discrete. Pathway analysis and frequency coding may relate portions of systems to one another. The "old brain" hypothesis, a structural and physiological substrate for a diversity of reports of sleep and arousal production, encompassing reticular, paleothalmic and limbic levels, has been presented.

theory
sleep
arousal
EEG
synchrony

ORIGINS

A 22. Miller, H.L.: Alpha waves-artifacts? *Psychol Bull, 69:279,* 1968. (Copyright 1968 by the American Psychological Association and reproduced by permission.)

Kennedy has argued that alpha rhythm recordings are artifacts caused by the mechanical pulsation (choroid plexus "pump") of a gel (the living brain) with different electrical potentials. This paper has been republished in a recent collection by Evans and Robertson. Kennedy's hypothesis seemed insufficiently supported and contradicted the consensus concerning the origin of alpha waves which existed at the time. Significant recent research is examined which provides strong, if not conclusive, evidence that alpha waves

origins
theory

represent a basic cellular process probably related to excitability. It is suggested that Kennedy's phenomenon be explored further to clarify any effect it may have on standard EEG recordings.

A 23.   Cohn, R.: The occipital alpha rhythm. A study of phase variations. *J Neurophysiol, 11:*31, 1948.

EEG recordings were obtained from nearly two hundred subjects under standard conditions to study voltage variations derived from homologous inter- and intrahemispheric brain regions. Results did not follow previous work by Adrian and Yamagiwa which was interpreted as indicating a wandering boundary of electric excitation as the prime determinant of the transient phase shifts observed. The basic idea of Adrian and Yamagiwa that the occipital region contains a junction area between two potential fields which gives rise to basic out-of-phase activity is confirmed. It seems that certain of the apparent out-of-phase activity recognized in simultaneous recordings from adjacent occipital regions is not due to shifting of the frequency variations of the separate oscillators developed around the calcarine fissure. A hypothetical model based on the assumption of four functional oscillators in the pericalcarme cortex is developed to account for the results obtained.

origins
theory
alpha phase

A 24.   Garoutte, B., and Aird, R.B.: Studies on the cortical pacemaker: Synchrony and asynchrony of bilaterally recorded alpha and beta activity. *Electroencephalogr Clin Neurophysiol, 10:*259, 1958.

Refined methods to study the bilateral synchrony of cortical spiking potentials, random or petit mal types, are described in this paper. The essentially synchronous character of homologous cerebral activity was confirmed in all patients studied, and this suggests the presence of a "central pacemaker" in the brainstem or thalmus to regulate cortical activity. Periods of up to fifteen seconds of clear alpha or beta activity were displayed on an oscilloscope and photographed on film allowing measurement of differences of phase to 2 msec with approximations to 1 msec sometimes possible. No consistent

origins
theory
alpha
synchrony
generators

time relationships between the waves from the two hemispheres was found. Alpha activity was lost in some cases due to deep lesions, and this was explained by a subcortical controlling center which is cut or disrupted by the lesions. A shifting asynchrony was explained by physiological characteristic of the cortex or pacemaker, that is, the idiocortical rhythms escape from the rhythmic influence from below and are then pulled back into synchrony again. As a point of definition, the idiothalamic rhythm according to Meyers, Shinners et al., 1949, is generally more rapid than the idiocortical rhythm, as required for control of the cortex by the thalmus. Another possible explanation for shifting asynchrony is anatomical shifting of function, as a result of physiological exhaustion of groups of neurons. Nevertheless, the authors reiterate that such a high percentage of synchronous activity in all patients strongly indicates a central pacemaker as a fundamental mechanism, under both normal and abnormal conditions.

A 25. Walsh, E.G.: Autonomy of alpha rhythm generators studied by multiple channel cross-correlations. *Electroencephalogr Clin Neurophysiol, 10:*121, 1958.

Ten subjects with an alpha rhythm that was attenuated with eyes open were recorded for EEG. In part one of the experiment, a sagittally disposed chain of electrodes from the frontal through parieto-occipital regions was used. After the parieto-occipital reversal of gradient was mapped, a transverse chain of electrodes was installed through the region where the gradient reversed. A special wave correlator with resonant chokes to tune EEG amplifiers was used to detect the polarity relationships. The device is fully described in the article. The results of this investigation are in agreement with past observations on generators but the cross-correlation provides additional information which leads to a different interpretation. Synchronized generators would be expected to cause the signals on either side of the region containing two phase reversals (the most common) to be in-phase. The cross-correlation showed that the currents either did not correlate or were in anti-phase. Therefore, it was concluded that there are at least two autonomous generators beating at the same rate.

origins
generators
instruments

A 26. Aird, R.B., and Garoutte, B.: Studies on the "cerebral pace-maker." *Neurology, 8:*581, 1958.

origins
generators
EEG
  synchrony

Simultaneous recordings from homologous sites from the two cerebral hemispheres were taken to measure the synchrony of brain waves including alpha, beta, spiking, slow and fast patterns. In excess of 50 percent of the brain waves studied were synchronous within the limits of accuracy of the technique ($\pm$ 1 msec for oscillographic measurements and $\pm$ 5 to 10 msec for paper recordings). Asynchrony of all brain waves varied from moment to moment in pseudo-rhythmic patterns about the point of perfect synchrony. These results lead to the postulation of a "cerebral pace-maker" located in the reticular substance of the upper brain-stem or the posterior bypothalamic area which operates via relay through the nonspecific diffuse projection nuclei of the thalamus and which serves to regulate the rhythms of both brain hemispheres at once. Modification of the function of this pacemaker through pathophysiologic influence or lesions is also discussed. Considerable value is seen in correlation of the electrophysiologic work with clinical findings in order to establish criteria to select patients for neurosurgery.

A 27. Tatsuno, J., Marsoner, H.J., and Wageneder, F.M.: Topography of accoustically evoked potentials triggered by alpha activity. *Acta Biol Med Ger, 25:*441, 1970.

origins
alpha
  abundance
auditory
  evoked
  responses
topography

Topographic differences of evoked potentials triggered by alpha activity were investigated on ten healthy volunteers. The late components of the potentials evoked by acoustic stimuli were obtained from wide areas of the cortex. The distance peaks (3 and 4) in successive tests were remarkably stable in the parietal region and gradually decreased towards the front occipital zone. These changes in stability and latency of the peaks suggest that a functional relation exists between the mechanism of the formation of the evoked potentials and the alpha generator.

A 28. Klijn, J.A.J.: The fine structure of the alpha rhythm in the EEG. *Pfluegers Arch, 328:*259, 1971.

origins
alpha
  frequency
  data analysis

A combination spectrum analyzer or inertialess EEG curve reader (acts as a slow read-in and fast repetitive read-out memory) and wave analyzer was used to demonstrate a fine structure in the occipital EEG which is most obvious in the delta and alpha bands. This structure is described as a composite of independent oscillators of variable strength and constant frequency spacing (0.4 cps) which demonstrate a highly related frequency drift (mean frequency drift 0.06 cps) tending to lower frequencies over the long term.

A 29.   Shiminke, G.A.: Alpha and beta waves in the human electroencephalogram. *Pavlov J Higher Nerv Activ, 11*:256, 1961.

This investigation deals with a possible relationship between alpha and beta activity. EEG's were recorded from the occipital lobe and filtered for 6 to 13 Hz and 15 to 30 Hz activity. It was found that eye closure increased alpha and beta amplitude while a light stimulus suppressed the amplitude of both alpha and beta. A debate as to the origin of these alpha and beta waves is offered. One possibility is that beta activity represents the second and third harmonics of alpha activity. On the other hand, it is possible that beta activity is produced first and that alpha results from special conditions of synchronization of this beta brain wave activity. Whether one of these theories is correct or not, it is clear to the author that, due to the similar reactions of alpha and beta seen in this experiment, alpha and beta activity originate from the same source and are related in a harmonic manner.

origins
harmonics
beta

A 30.   Jasper, H.H., and Andrews, L.: Electroencephalography III. Normal differentiation of occipital and precentral regions in man. *Arch Neurol Psychiatr, 39*:96, 1938.

A method for localized recording of autonomous bioelectric potentials of the normal human cortex through the unopen skull is described and a comparison of results from the occipital and precentral regions is presented. That occipital alpha is distinct in cortical origin from precentral alpha potentials is shown by the differential reaction to stimulation under different conditions and by spontaneous and independent occurrence in different regions. Usually, frequencies are the same, phase relations remain relatively constant, and

origins
topography
measurement
techniques
alpha
responses

effects of afferent stimulation are similar. Stimulus response relationships, on and off effects, etc., are also included.

A 31.   Lippold, O.: Origin of the alpha rhythm. *Nature, 226:*616, 1970.

This report argues against the commonly held view that the alpha rhythm originates in the occipital cortical neurons. Evidence is presented which suggests "that occipital alpha waves are generated by the standing potential across the eyes . . . (and) that the likely mechanism involves some form of modulation of this potential by oscillation in the extra-ocular muscles (tremor) at about 10 Hz when there is no sharply focused image on the retina." *origins visual system*

A 32.   Chapman, R.M., Cavonius, C.R., and Ernest, J.T.: Alpha and kappa electroencephalogram activity in eyeless subjects. *Science, 171:*1159, March 1971. (Copyright 1971 by the American Association for the Advancement of Science.)

Several reports have cast doubt on the cerebral origin of alpha and kappa electroencephalogram activity by charging that they are artifacts related to eye activity. Data are cited which eliminate the corneoretinal potential of the eyeball, tremor of the extraocular muscles, eye position, accommodation, and eye flutter as sources of alpha and kappa electroencephalogram activity. A subject with both eyes removed showed normal alpha and kappa electroencephalogram activity. Marked left-right differences in alpha activity were not found in one-eyed subjects whose eyes and extraocular muscles were completely removed on one side. *origins visual system kappa rhythm blindness*

A 33.   Ennever, J.A., Lippold, O.C.J., and Novotny, G.E.K.: The corneo-retinal potential as the generator of alpha rhythm in the human electroencephalogram. *Acta Psychol (Amst), 35:* 269, 1971.

A proposal is made that the alpha rhythm originates in the corneoretinal potential, which is modulated at 10 cps by extraocular muscle tremor. Anatomical arrangements of these muscles account for alpha waves existing mainly over *origins visual system* the occipital regions. The corneoretinal potential and the amplitude of alpha waves are shown to vary in direct proportion on the same side of the head. This relationship rules out the idea that nervous connections from the retina are responsible for the concordance since optic nerve fibers are distributed equally to both hemispheres.

A 34. Sato, K., Ozaki, T., Minura, K., Masuya, S., Honda, N., Nishikawa, T., and Sonoda, T.: On the physiological significance of the average time-and-frequency-patterns of the electroencephalogram. *Electroencephalogr Clin Neurophysiol, 13:*208, 1961.

The EEG response caused by photic and/or click stimulation can be seen in the power spectrum of the cross-correlation curve between EEG training and stimulation. An evaluation by peak height at the stimulation frequency will give average intensity of the response which is in turn proportional to the EEG generator activity with respect to stimulus frequency. Average frequency pattern of the EEG generator activity is determined from the frequency response (frequency characteristics) of the generator. This is an extension of the concept of excitability. The average time pattern is defined as the autocorrelogram of the generator response evoked by a single impulse with value unity. From the time pattern, the frequency response of the generator can be found and then expressed as a Fourier transform.

origins
perceptual
stimulation
spectral
analysis
cross-
correlation
auto-
correlation
generators

A 35. Barlow, J.S.: Rhythmic activity induced by photic stimulation in relation to intrinsic alpha activity of the brain in man. *Electroencephalogr Clin Neurophysiol, 12:*317, 1960.

The study employed autocorrelation analysis to determine the nature of the dominant rhymthic activity of the EEG and its persistence in time. Electronic averaging was used to determine the response in the EEG to photic stimulation. For example, 1 to 2 cps flashes give a first component occiput negative with a peak at 75 msec followed by an occiput negative at 120 msec. A rhythmic after-discharge (phase locked) to the flash was seen but was not a harmonic. Harmonics are also detected using these techniques and

origins
alpha
frequency
alpha
patterns

equipment. An intimate relationship between alpha activity
and sensory after-discharge as relates to frequency is indicated; the electrical activities must then stem from similar
neuronal mechanisms and are related to nonspecific rather
than specific sensory systems of the brain. These conclusions
conflict with other investigations; however, it has been
shown previously that drugs alter frequencies of alpha and
sensory after-discharge in different ways.

SECTION B

MEASUREMENTS

INSTRUMENTS

B 1. Saeba, P.J.: An alpha detection system for use with Grass model 7/78 polygraphs. *Electroencephalogr Clin Neurophysiol, 34*:105, 1973 (abstr).

An apparatus for biofeedback training experiments which can be used with Grass polygraphs is described and explained. This system includes: (1) a Grass 7P 5 ac preamplifier and 7DA driver amplifier to record occipital EEG activity; (2) a bandpass filter to filter alpha from the J6 output of (1) above; (3) a Grass 7P3 preamplifier to integrate the filter output; (4) a Grass 7DA driver amplifier to amplify the J34 output of the 7P3 preamplifier and display filtered and integrated alpha activity; and (5) a voltage comparator to detect voltages proportional to alpha amplitude at J6 of the last 7DA driver amplifier.

instruments
alpha
* frequency*
alpha
* amplitude*
biofeedback

B 2. Bickford, R.G., and Fortescue, P.: A pocket EEG diagnostic monitor for the neurologist. *Electroencephalogr Clin Neurophysiol, 31*:305, 1971 (abstr).

The device is about the size of a cigarette package and consists of a small amplifier and meter movement together with a switchable integrator circuit. The latter can be used to give a measure of alpha symmetry and will read directly in microvolts and amount of brain activity remaining in the case of suspected cerebral anoxic accident. The unit is constructed from integrated circuits, is self-contained with batteries and can be made very cheaply. The device will be useful in clinical practice for screening suitable patients before conventional EEG. It can be rapidly applied in the emergency room for making a quick estimate of cerebral function in cases undergoing resuscitation and for checking heart action (EKG) when the pulse is impalpable.

instruments
alpha
* symmetry*
EEG abnor-
* malities*

B 3.   Pasquali, E.: Alpha envelope detection and distortion. A polyphase rectifier circuit. *Electroencephalogr Clin Neurophysiol, 26:*106, 1969.

The extraction from a complex EEG signal of a wave form which follows the variations of alpha amplitude may be accomplished by filtering and detection. To avoid distortion of the original envelope the filter should have a low Q value and the detector smoothing circuit should not attenuate the components of the envelope wave form. A detector circuit that does not necessitate the use of a smoothing circuit is described. For the operation of this circuit the original EEG signal is phase shifted in identical successive steps. Each phase shifted signal is then rectified and combined with the others to give an output following closely the peaks of the signal (polyphase rectification). In this way the only distortion of the envelope is that due to the bandpass filter.

instruments
alpha
envelopes
alpha
amplitude

B 4.   Spunda, J., and Radil-Weiss, T.: A simple device for measuring the instantaneous frequency of the dominant EEG activity. *Electroencephalogr Clin Neurophysiol, 32:*434, 1972.

A device is described which converts instantaneous EEG frequency values into voltage levels for analysis. The device processes the EEG signal by amplifying and bandpass filtering the raw wave form and changing the state of a flip-flop at each positive-going zero crosspoint of the filtered signal. A series of waveform generators are activated by the flip-flop, eventually resulting in a voltage level corresponding to the frequency or wave period of the filtered signal.

instruments
EEG
frequency

B 5.   Hicks, R.G., and Angner, E.: Instrumental evaluation of EEG time relationships. *Psychophysiology, 6:*644, 1970 (abstr).

The instrument described is capable of analyzing minute time displacements of EEG waves from different cortical areas that are not affected by other components of the wave form, e.g. voltage. The instrument is modestly inexpensive, about two hundred dollars, and avails a technique to investigators who do not have a computer at their disposal. The

instruments
EEG phase

instrument can also be used for data reduction; therefore package computer programs can be used. Another advantage is the capability of immediate, wave-by-wave analysis, an on-line, real time analysis, a technique that most investigators with computer do not have. The technique described involves two basic applications of operational amplifiers, peak detection and a Schmitt trigger and standard logic circuits. The advantage of the instrument is its extreme stability, since once calibrated the circuit will remain in calibration for months, perhaps even years. Other advantages are modest ease of construction with the use of standard integrated circuits and ability to detect the large range of frequency responses found in biological potentials. In its present form this instrument does not give an index of phase measured in degrees; rather it provides an indication of rapidly shifting temporal relations between two different areas; for example, whether area A is in-phase, leading, lagging, or 180° out-of-phase with Area B. Voltage fluctuations in the input sinusoidal wave do not affect time displacement indications.

B 6. Huertas, J., and Westbrook, R.C.: A system for sensing and transmitting EEG. *Electroencephalogr Clin Neurophysiol,* *28*:90, 1970.

A single-channel EEG sensing and transmitting system has been developed which requires no special preparation of the subject's scalp or hair. Bipolar electrodes and a miniature biopotential transmitter are mounted on a head clip. The clip is placed over the subject's head, much like a set of earphones. The electrode consists of a silver-silver chloride pellet, a fritted glass disc and a sponge. The sponge and the porous glass disc are moistened with saline and a small cavity around the pellet is filled with a commercial electrode paste. The miniature biopotential FM telemetry system operated at approximately 90 mcps with a 100-foot range and a two-day operating life. It has a frequency response of 0.5 to 120 cps, an input impedance of 20 MΩ and an equivalent input noise of 1 μv RMS. EEG is displayed on an oscilloscope and an ink-pen recorder. Construction and circuit details are available from previous publications.

instruments
telemetry

B 7.   Vreeland, R.W., Yeager, C.L., and Henderson, J., Jr.: A compact six-channel integrated circuit EEG telemeter. *Electroencephalogr Clin Neurophysiol, 30:*240, 1971.

A lightweight, head-mounted telemeter for artifact-free EEG recording is described and demonstrated. Pulse position modulation and reduced battery voltages allow use of integrated circuits with slip-on rechargeable battery packs. Low noise pre-amplifiers with micro-pak transistors make telemetering of small amplitude EEG's practical; and, since the transmitter is crystal controlled, frequency drift is virtually zero. Needle, disc or depth electrodes (require external attenuation) can be used. Respiration, electrocardiogram and galvanic skin response can also be transmitted with additional external networks.

instruments
telemetry

B 8.   Paskewitz, D.A.: A hybrid circuit to indicate the presence of alpha activity. *Psychophysiology, 8:*107, 1971.

This report describes a circuit which, in conjunction with an analogue filter, greatly increases the accuracy of the identification of EEG alpha activity. With minor modifications, the same circuit may be used to identify other EEG frequency bands. Construction is simplified through the use of integrated circuits. A functional description and circuit details are given.

instruments
data
* collection*
alpha
* abundance*

B 9.   Boudrot, R.: An alpha detection and feedback control system. *Psychophysiology, 9:*461, 1972.

An alpha rhythm detecting and stimulus feedback display (visual and auditory) system is described. Parameters of the system can be chosen to match the psychological and behavioral processes with the EEG index in the time domain. Clocks, counters, computers, etc., are also controlled by the system which is designed for maximum flexibility.

instruments
biofeedback

B 10.   Pasquali, E.: A relay controlled by alpha rhythm. *Psychophysiology, 6:*207, 1969.

An electrical circuit energizing a relay is described, together with the response to a rectangular burst of alpha waves. This

instruments
biofeedback

circuit is useful when a certain amount of delay in de-energizing the relay was purposely introduced so that the relay might remain continuously energized by closely spaced alpha bursts. Fundamentally the circuit action is that of a leaky integrator whose output controls a relay with different energizing and de-energizing levels.

B 11. Pfeifer, E.A., and Usselman, L.: A versatile amplitude analyzer for EEG signals to provide feedback stimuli to the subject. *Med Biol Eng, 8:*209, 1970.

The technical note describes an amplitude analyzer which provides feedback cues to subjects in studies of EEG modification by feedback methods. This versatile device can be used with a variety of peripheral equipment such as bandpass filters, logic modules, displays, etc., and one can change the experiment easily without altering the electronic circuitry. The unit can be easily assembled since it is composed of commercially available circuit modules.

instruments
biofeedback

B 12. Misurec, J., and Chmelar, M.: Automatic quantification of EEG in the clinical psychopharmacology—a new type of interval analyzer. *Activ Nerv Sup (Praha), 14:*180, 1972.

A new type of interval analyzer for EEG's is described. Instrument uses zero crossings from output of an alpha filter.

instruments
data analysis
computer
analysis
drugs

DATA COLLECTION

B 13. Zhirmunskaya, E.A., and Makakova, G.V. Prolonged periodic fluctuations in the level of asymmetry of EEG wave fronts in various types of brain electrical activity. *Bull Exp Biol Med, 73:*102, 1972.

The investigation was conducted in order to determine the changes in the mean level of asymmetry of the ascending and descending forms of the EEG waves in time (sometimes called "G" waves) which are associated with normal, hypersynchronized and desynchronized EEG activity. Three types of EEG activity were analyzed: (1) regular alpha activity

data
collection
alpha
symmetry
psychopath-
ology
beta

with mean amplitude below 50 μv and well-marked zonal differences (9 subjects); (2) alpha activity almost without clear zonal differences between brain regions and with higher than normal amplitude and index (10 subjects); and (3) beta activity with regular slow waves (10 subjects). Six bipolar leads (occipitoparietal, occipitotemporal, interior parieto-interior frontal for each hemisphere) were analyzed by the manual method of A.A. Genkin. Correlation methods were performed and transverse of interhemispheric as well as longitudinal or intrahemispheric connections were evaluated. Results showed that changes in mean level of asymmetry actually form second-order waves in time with the period of fluctuation of these waves unstable and varied in a normal subject. In a patient with a pathologic problem the fluctuation pattern becomes more involved with the range of variations or amplitude of mean change value increasing sharply while the period or duration of change remains constant. A comparison of these results with those of correlation analysis of primary EEG recordings is given. The authors mention some possible functional connections of the "G" waves including a connection with orienting reflexes, facilitation and inhibition and spatial organization of brain electrical activity.

B 14.   Shaw, J.C.: A method for continuously recording characteristics of EEG topography. *Electroencephalogr Clin Neurophysiol, 29:*592, 1970.

A method for continuously recording EEG topography is described. Low-pass filters are used and signals from different sites are compared by correlation coefficient, regression coefficient, or time difference to a predetermined reference signal. Basically, the record is scanned with a window to produce a running estimate or moving average (experientially weighted) to get a continuous record of change in the chosen parameter. The method is demonstrated and shows that the topographical change in alpha activity during mental arithmetic differs from that due to eye opening. Alpha time asymmetry relationships in the hemispheres are discussed as well as the value of the technique in detection of pathological activity. The author feels that his method allows more full utilization of topographic information which in turn un-

*data
  collection
mental tasks
visual
  system
alpha
  symmetry
theory*

covers features not readily observable in primary records and which may be related to the functional organization of the cortex.

B 15. Walter, D.O., Muller, H.F., and Jell, R.M.: Semiautomatic quantification of sharpness of EEG phenomena. *IEE Trans Biomed Eng, 20:53,* January 1973.

> The article describes an inexpensive and easy method to automatically quantify the "sharpness" or "spikiness" of brain electrical activity using the rectified second derivative of the EEG tracing. A variety of phenomena can be distinguished using this method such as: (1) low amplitude rhythmic muscle potentials; (2) main peaks of each alpha wave; (3) responses to slow intermittent photic stimulation; and (4) spike discharges from epileptic patients. Further hand or electronic analysis may be desirable depending upon whether, for example, single phenomena or activity over time is of particular interest.

data collection spikiness

B 16. Shafer, W.A.: Telemetry on man without attached sensors. *NY J Med,* November 1, 1967, p. 2832.

> A biomedical monitoring system composed of a pair of sensing antennae placed near the subject, isolation amplifiers, a main amplifier, and recorders is proposed. The system would aid in evaluating cardiovascular functions, provide for long-term monitoring without skin damage from electrodes, monitoring a sleeping unconscious subject, monitoring animals, etc. Theoretically, the distortion effects created within the multiple electromagnetic fields of many frequencies within the environment are utilized. The distortion effects are created by minute changes in a volume conductor surrounded by variable fields. Only signals in the proper frequency spectrum are recognized and recorded. A unique waveform has resulted which is based on both obvious (size, weight, blood pressure, tissue density, position and subsurface) and unknown factors. It is felt that pathologic changes may be reflected in the waveform configuration.

data collection magnetic fields

B 17. Cohen, D.: Detection of magnetic fields outside the human head produced by alpha rhythm currents. *Electroencephalogr Clin Neurophysiol, 28:*102, 1970 (abstr) .

Excitable neural and muscle tissues produce changing electric currents in the surrounding volume conductor. It can be
shown that these changing currents must produce changing
magnetic fields both inside and outside the volume conductor. For example, the changing magnetic fields outside the
torso originating from the human heart have recently been
measured and studied with a sensitive detector in a highly
shielded chamber. The same equipment has now been modified and improved to search for the smaller magnetic fields
outside the human head produced by alpha rhythm currents.
The experiment consists of EEG leads from the scalp triggering a C.A.T. at each baseline crossover and also feeding one
channel; another channel is fed by a magnetic detector
placed in a different position around the head, at a distance
of about an inch. A weak magnetic signal is seen to grow out
of the noise, synchronous with the EEG crossovers. With
eyes open the crossover triggers are still present but the
magnetic signal vanishes; the signal also vanishes with increasing distance from the head, with eyes closed. Elaborate
and repeated precautions make it unlikely that the signal is
an artifact. A preliminary distribution of this magnetic alpha
field around the head is presented.

data
  collection
magnetic
  fields
alpha
  patterns

B 18.   Cohen, D.: Magnetoencephalography: Evidence of magnetic
fields produced by alpha-rhythm currents. *Science, 161*:784,
August 1968.

Four subjects with above-average alpha rhythms were recorded to investigate the possibility of the existence of magnetic fields around the head produced by alpha rhythm currents. The detecting device was a one-million-turn coil in a
thin-walled, brass electrostatic shield with a removable ferrite
rod core. Both the device and subject were housed in a
shielded enclosure and many experiments were done to verify the signal and to eliminate noise. A C.A.T. was used for
signal averaging and to extract the signal from the noise.
The recordings are referred to as magnetoencephalograms
(MEG) and results showed the maximum MEG to be approximately 1×10^{-9} gauss (p-p). A left-right symmetry
was found for the course distribution and technique used
here. No measurements with, for example, inion removed
have been done, but such changes are expected to alter the

data
  collection
magnetic
  fields
instruments
definitions

distribution significantly. The author suggests that the new distributions could reveal information about internal alpha rhythm sources and would represent a first step in evaluating the usefulness of the MEG.

B 19. Papakostopoulos, D., Cooper, R., and Walter, W.G.: A technique for the measurement of phase relationships of the EEG. *Electroencephalogr Clin Neurophysiol, 30:*562, 1971.

A method in which the sine and cosine components of the Fourier analysis of multichannel data are displayed as vectors for EEG phase/time relations measurement is described. Because of the interaction of amplitude and phase differences in bipolar montages, the use of common reference recordings is recommended. This technique has been demonstrated for alpha activity and flicker-evoked following responses, but the data is reported separately.

data collection EEG phase

B 20. Cohen, D.: Magnetoencephalography: Detection of the brain's electrical activity with a superconducting magnetometer. *Science, 175:*664, February 1972.

Magnetoencephalograms or MEG's (recordings of the magnetic fields around the head) are taken in this project with a superconducting magnetometer as an advance on the original method of an earlier article by Cohen (*Science, 161,* 784-786). These advances, including increased sensitivity, make MEG recording without noise averaging possible. The alpha rhythm can be seen in the normal MEG and in the EEG, with eyes closed, but the MEG shows that a higher detector sensitivity is necessary to see smaller brain events when the eyes are open. Abnormal MEG's, including direct-current component measurements, indicate that the MEG may provide new information which is different from that of the EEG.

data collection instruments definitions magnetic fields

B 21. Cooper, R.: An ambiguity of bipolar recording. *Electroencephalogr Clin Neurophysiol, 11:*819, 1959.

A case for the use of unipolar EEG recording systems as opposed to bipolar systems is presented. Examples of the ambiguity of time measurement which occurs whenever amplitude and time variant signals are compared using bipolar

data collection measurement techniques

techniques are also detailed. The average reference technique which is recommended does not need a large number of channels, but only a large number of electrodes connected to a common point through high resistances. Specific techniques recommended include unipolar systems where an indifferent electrode can be found and the Offner/Goldman (1950) technique in which the potential of an electrode is compared with the average of the potentials occurring at all electrodes. An example of this latter system is given.

B 22. Walter, W.G., and Parr, G.: Recording equipment and technique (Chapter II). In Hill, J.D.N., and Parr, G. (Eds.): *Electroencephalography*. London, McDonald, 1963, p. 25.

A review of methods for recording and measuring EEG records, including descriptions of instrumentation components and good recording practice.

data collection measurement techniques

B 23. Knott, J.R.: Concerning electrode arrays. *Am J EEG Technol, 1:3*, 1961.

A variety of EEG recording electrode placements is presented, each with its own theoretical basis. In many cases, the placement array utilized depends upon the particular project involved. This article describes some of the advantages and disadvantages of using some of these arrays.

data collection measurement techniques theory

B 24. Silverman, R.W., Jenden, D.J., and Fairchild, M.D.: A hybrid broad-band EEG frequency analyzer for use in long term experiments. *IEE Trans Biomed Eng, 20:*60, January 1973.

A system for broad-band EEG frequency analysis utilizing hybrid analog and digital techniques for long-term EEG frequency analysis is described. The digital output provides for efficient data collection. It is noted that subsequent data reduction can be conducted although such reduction is not explained here. The method is thought to be particularly effective in quantification of the effects of centrally active

data collection measurement techniques alpha frequency drugs

drugs on the EEG, and future clinical use of this technique is expected by the author.

B 25. Kaiser, E., and Petersen, I.: Bio-clock as reference in EEG analysis. *The Third International Conference on Medical Physics, 17:*728, 1972 (abstr).

A technique to correct the fluctuations in phase and frequency in the alpha rhythm of EEG activity which is disturbing in quantitative estimates of frequency spectral parameters is given. The alpha rhythm controls an adaptive digital delay line which allows the method to be referenced to alpha period. The output of this system appears at an almost constant rate, while a pilot light indicates frequency modulation complementary to that of the original alpha signal. Correlation, Fast Fourier Transform and other work with large time windows are especially important applications of this procedure.

data collection
spectral analysis
temporal stability

B 26. Estrin, T., and Uzgalis, R.: Computerized display of spatio-temporal EEG patterns. *IEE Trans Biomed Eng, 16:*192, July 1969.

A new technique to compute and display the electroencephalogram (EEG) as a spatio-temporal phenomenon is described. In this technique, position on a cathode ray tube is congruent with position in a recording array of electrodes on the head. The potential distribution over the area of the head covered by the array is computed and displayed as a contour map on the face of the tube. Succeeding displays represent distributions at successive instances of time and are photographed by a motion picture camera. The projected film recreates a time history of the potential field. Though this technique has been developed to investigate characteristic patterns of the electroencephalogram, it has application wherever it is necessary to investigate the time course of spatially distributed phenomena.

data collection
computer analysis
topography
spatio-temporal characteristics

B 27. Ellingson, R.J., Emde, J.W., and Shipton, H.W.: A correlator for EEG: Technical description and some preliminary findings. *Electroencephalogr Clin Neurophysiol, 34:*105, 1973 (abstr).

An inexpensive (circa two thousand dollars) instrument has been constructed which computes either the autocorrelogram of an EEG signal or the cross-correlation between two such signals. Data are accumulated continuously and the emerging correlation may be seen on an oscilloscope. Three time ranges (1.28, 2.56 and 5.12 sec) are provided and Δt is 5 msec. The output is decoded to provide an analog write-out either on an EEG channel or, more usually, on an x-y recorder. In the past, correlation studies have required either the recording of a limited time sample on a continuous tape loop or the availability of an on-line digital computer. Because of these and other technical requirements the technique has not been very widely used in clinical EEG. In preliminary studies now under way, early work has been duplicated.

data collection instruments auto-correlation cross-correlation

B 28.   Bectereva, N.P., and Zontov, V.V.: The relationship between certain forms of potentials and the variations in brain excitability (Based on EEG recorded during photic stimuli triggered by rhythmic brain potentials). *Electroencephalogr Clin Neurophysiol, 14:*320, 1962.

Using stimuli triggered by brain potential rhythms with varying stimulus to phase relations, the authors studied the exact nature of the relationship between timing of stimuli with reference to the phase of the brain waves and the pattern of activity. It has been previously shown that such activation enhances and brings out the changes in brain potentials due to pathological processes involving the brain stem and cerebral hemispheres which may be used in EEG investigations of brain tumors. In particular, augmentation of bursts of widespread high voltage activity occurs. Results indicate that within a single complete alpha cycle, there may be up to three-minute time zones during which stimuli evoke enhanced desynchronization of potentials. Moreover, various degrees of dependence of the EEG pattern on the relationship between stimulus and phase of brain wave as well as various degrees of stability of this relationship may exist. These may in turn change with the effects of drugs and patient condition. Results of this study are interpreted in terms of current views on the relations between brain waves and variations in brain excitability with consideration being

data collection visual stimulation phase of wave period brain damage given to Wedenski's concepts of the lability of neurodynamic structure.

B 29. Kohler, G.K., and Penin, H.: Demonstration of technical novelties in the field of clinical electroencephalography. *Electroencephalogr Clin Neurophysiol, 29:*219, 1970 (abstr).

A demonstration of synchronous television double-picture recording is given whereby the EEG or other physiological parameters are displayed on a divided screen with the subject. In addition to the camera, interval analyzers, tape recorders, etc., are also triggered by the EEG at the critical time. The technique may have wide use in patient monitoring, polygraphic recording, teaching and in other areas.

data
  collection
television

DATA ANALYSIS

B 30. Lesevre, N., Rieger, H., and Rémond, A.: Definitions and value of average alpha rhythm and topography. *Electroencephalogr Clin Neurophysiol, 23:*384, 1967.

This article presents the concept of the alpha average as an explanatory model to reduce the complexity of data provided by the spontaneous alpha rhythm. Eight bipolar pairs of electrodes located in both a median longitudinal and a transverse posterior montage were used. From these data, a computer gave chronograms, topograms or spatio-temporal maps. The chronotopographical organization of the alpha average demonstrated certain characteristics of spontaneous alpha activity including general structure and frequency stability, the latter being measured by the slope of decrease of alpha wave amplitude. While these effects were demonstrated on both montages, the transverse montage also yielded information about the degree of inter-regional liaison of the alpha rhythm. Phase reversals appeared to be random between hemispheres and suggested synchrony of frequency and of phase. Also, a midline axis of symmetry was seen at the points where phase reversal of the gradients and therefore the maximum of the alpha potential occurred. Other less typical examples such as no phase reversals were noted and it is suggested that these problems may mean that alpha activity explanatory models must be studied in new terms.

data analysis
topography
definitions
variability
phase
EEG
  synchrony

B 31.   Hjorth, B., and Berglund, K.: Quantitative description of an
         EEG trace as a function of time. *Electroencephalogr Clin
         Neurophysiol, 31:529*, 1971 (abstr).

Three descriptive parameters have been derived in order to *data analysis*
quantify the general characteristics of an EEG trace. These *time*
parameters, named activity, mobility and complexity, are *domain*
based on fundamental properties of each point in the wave *sleep*
curve: the distance to the mean of the curve, the slope of the
curve and the radius of curvature. Activity and mobility refer to amplitude and time scales respectively, whereas complexity refers to irregularity of the curve shape. Apart from
the descriptive aspect of the parameters, their statistical
nature offers interpretations related to models for generation of the EEG. If the curve is assumed to be the result of,
for example, superposition of a large number of individual
elements, activity—defined as the amplitude variance of the
curve—will correspond to the average rate of such elements,
proportional to it or only correlated, depending on the degree of interdependence between the elements. Mobility of
the curve—defined as the ratio between the standard deviations of the first derivative and the amplitude—describes the
average slope of the average element and thus may indicate
the influence of a physiological variable upon the average element. Complexity—defined as the Pythagorean difference between the mobilities of the derivative and the curve itself—is
transferred in the same way from the average element to the
composite curve. The relevance of the model may be investigated by means of a correlation analysis concerning the parameters and fundamental physiological variables. The parameters have been applied for data reduction of sleep recordings, thereby giving concentrated sleep profiles. Although the sine shape has probably no relevance in neurophysiological processes, the parameters can be expressed also
in terms of frequency. Mobility then corresponds to an
average frequency derived by means of frequency squared as
a weighting function. Complexity corresponds to a measure
of the frequency spread.

B 32.   Lehmann, D.: EEG analysis and psychological functions.
         Electroencephalogr Clin Neurophysiol, 30:270, 1971 (abstr).

The EEG can be analyzed in time and space. Machine analysis is desirable because of the large number of data typically collected in EEG recordings. Spatial analysis of field distributions of the human scalp EEG was performed on data collected by a multi-channel recording system. Sequences of equipotential maps were reduced to orbits of the location of maximum values of the electrical fields, which may reflect underlying generators, and to average field values per electrode, indicating the amount of relief. Further approaches to machine diagnosis of EEG in different experimental conditions are reviewed. These methods may lead to automated diagnosis of clinical EEG's. In addition, various aspects of the relation between psychological functions and EEG parameters are discussed; e.g. EEG reactivity as a function of the activation level, proportionate and nonproportionate EEG responses, the necessity for loading tests when perception or performance is compared with EEG characteristics, and the EEG as indicator of gating of brain functions. The relationship between EEG patterns and quality of memory storage in humans illustrates the expression of a gating function in the EEG. EEG period analysis in the time domain during learning shows that decrease of slow wave frequencies and increase of fast frequencies is systematically correlated with better quality of memory. In this study, the shapes of EEG frequency spectra were represented by their distribution means ($\times$ centroids) for statistical comparisons. Improved control of experiments and sophisticated numerical analysis of EEG records promise further insight into the relation of psychological to electrical aspects of brain activity.

data analysis
topography
spatio-
temporal
character-
istics
EEG
patterns
EEG
responses

B 33. Rémond, A., et al.: The alpha average: I. Methodology and description. *Electroencephalogr Clin Neurophysiol, 26*:245, 1969.

Studied the characteristics of alpha average activity of twenty normal subjects (8 adults and 12 children) and a few patients without cerebral involvement. Three successive montages were used, each one of eight bipolar derivations joined in a rectilinear chain. Despite imperfections in the method, which are explained, the alpha average appears as a reduced and simplified version capable of measuring, in their differ-

data analysis
topography
EEG
patterns

ent aspects: topography, chronology, phase relations and symmetry. This method makes it possible to characterize individuals from the EEG point of view and consequently to make valid comparisons between them.

B 34.   Glaser, E.M.: Comments on "Semiautomatic Quantification of Sharpness of EEG Phenomena." *IEE Trans Biomed Eng, 20:55,* January 1973.

It is suggested that the sharpness measure of EEG phe-   *data analysis*
nomena as described by Walter et al. (Semiautomatic quanti-   *spikiness*
fication of sharpness of EEG phenomena. *IEE Trans Biomed
Eng, 20:53,* January 1973) should be used cautiously because
of its dependence on signal strength as well as sharpness.
This problem is attributed to the use of the unnormalized
second derivative in Walter's method.

B 35.   Pechstein, J., and Dolansky, J.: Technique of visual frequency analysis of the waking EEG of young children. *EEG
EMG (Stuttg), 1:35,* 1970.

A clinically applicable interpretational method of wave   *data analysis*
counting which also considers the overlying waves of differ- *EEG*
ent lengths is presented. The change in the frequency spec-   *frequency*
trum in the waking EEG of young children and the accelera-   *children*
tion of the occipital background activity from the theta band   *EEG*
to the alpha band with age is a criterion of CNS bioelectric   *maturation*
development and the method is presented in contrast to that   *awake*
of Fujimori et al. Considerations of difficulties while recording EEGs and standardization of behavioral states are given.
Validation of the technique involved ten seconds of occipital
EEG from a six-month-old and an eighteen-month-old child
analyzed by two investigators, each ten times. Frequencies
of 5 cps (6-month-old) and 8 cps (18-month-old) were
dominant and the theta-alpha frequency spectra corresponded well between researchers.

B 36.   Frost, J.D., Jr., and Elazar, Z.: Three-dimensional selective
amplitude histograms: A statistical approach to EEG-single
neuron relationships. *Electroencephalogr Clin Neurophysiol,
25:499,* 1968.

Describes a statistical method for analyzing relationships between EEG activity and neuronal spike discharges. A three-dimensional selective amplitude histogram is produced which shows the frequency of occurrence of EEG amplitudes as a function of neuronal discharge time. This graph and related statistical derivations permit detection and quantification of nonrandom EEG-single unit correlations.

data analysis
EEG
  amplitude
neuronal
  activity

B 37. Visser, S.L.: Time interval histogram mode data processing of the alpha rhythm output integration. *Electroencephalogr Clin Neurophysiol, 27:668*, 1969 (abstr).

One hundred random EEG's were recorded for the output integration type experiment originated by Drohocki. According to the procedure, the number of pulses is a measure of the amount of energy under the curve. The data is processed in two ways: (1) the number of pulses per ten-second segment is counted and the mean (m) and standard deviation (SD) are calculated; (2) all time intervals between pulses are measured and m and SD are calculated for these. In this procedure, two analysis parameters, the coefficients of variance for both the number of pulses per ten seconds and the time intervals, were used and found to vary similarly for normal subjects with 10 cps alpha activity. In other subjects with slow or fast background patterns or fast or slow alpha activity, the parameters seemed to indicate a variety of different influences.

data analysis
EEG
  integration

B 38. Maynard, D.E.: A note on the nature of the nonrhythmic components of the electroencephalogram. *Activ Nerv Sup (Praha), 11:238*, 1969.

Previous work on spectral EEG analysis in the occipital region of drowsy subjects showed that the parts of the spectra contributed by alpha and beta activity were superimposed on a background component of 1.5 to 30 cps which decreased at about 12 dB/decade. This pattern persisted even in persons with little alpha and in general was a consistent feature in all records. This article attempts to formulate a rating scale for EEG frequency analysis of drowsiness and light sleep using a five-point scale. The author describes a mathe-

data analysis
EEG
  patterns
drowsiness
sleep
theta
beta

matical synthesis of the spectrum of this background activity from Poissonian random occurrence of specific waveforms and exponential waveforms.

B 39. Rosadini, G., and Rossi, G.F.: Spectral power analysis of the electroencephalogram during physiological sleep in man. *Activ Nerv Sup (Praha), 11:*106, 1969.

Preliminary results of a spectral analysis of cerebral electrical activity during waking and nocturnal sleep in healthy subjects are reported. The occurrence and characteristics of rhythmicity are considered. Rhythmicity (i.e. periodic oscillating potentials phase locked in time) is present during relaxed wakefulness and during sleep. However, frequency and topographical distribution of rhythms are different in the two conditions. Rhythmicity is evident in certain sleep phases and not in others. The different quantity, frequency and spatial distribution of electrical rhythms observed in wakefulness and in the several sleep phases indicate that these functional states may be mediated by different brain systems or mechanisms.

data analysis
sleep
wakefulness
EEG
 rhythmicity
EEG
 frequency
topography
theory

B 40. Itil, T., Gannon, P., Akpinar, S., and Hsu, W.: Quantitative EEG analysis of electro-sleep using frequency analyzer and digital computer methods. *Electroencephalogr Clin Neurophysiol, 31:*294, 1971 (abstr) .

Owing to the fact that no previous study has been carried out with the use of quantitative EEG, we designed a control study to investigate physiological correlates of electro-sleep. Ten male volunteers were recorded on four different days after an adaptation EEG. Two of the recordings were made while the electro-sleep machine (Electrosone 50®) was on, and two other recordings when the machine was off. In each session ten-minute EEG recordings were carried out during resting time and another ten-minute recording was taken when the patient was given a task (reaction time measurement) . The right occipital to right ear EEG lead was analyzed using digital computer period analysis as well as an analog frequency analyzer. Patients who exhibited no changes of vigilance in their EEG's (decrease of vigilance)

data analysis
electro-sleep
vigilance
EEG
 patterns

when the machine was off also showed no significant changes when the machine was on. On the other hand, any subject who exhibited a slight-to-moderate drowsiness pattern during the off recording did show a slight-to-moderate sleep pattern when the machine was on. In the total group, both computer analysis and analog frequency analyzer data demonstrated no significant EEG differences between the on and off sessions recorded during resting time. However, the EEG data obtained during reaction time measurements demonstrated an increase in 5-10 cps activity and a decrease in fast alpha and beta activity when the electro-sleep machine was on as compared with the off recordings. These findings are discussed from the clinical and neurophysiological points of view.

B 41. Bickford, R.G.: Physiology and drug action: An electroencephalographic analysis. *Fed Proc, 19:*619, 1960.

An explanation of physiologic and drug effects on the EEG is presented. The author theorizes reasons why the EEG does not directly reflect physiologic and drug effects and cites certain oversights of past research. The author notes that the psychologic setting influences the EEG and must be controlled at some level, and that physiologic influences importantly affect the EEG. EEG quantification methods must also be considered. A general survey of the effect of drugs on the EEG is given. It is pointed out that French and associates have shown that the multisynaptic reticular system is sensitive to drugs in contrast to the lateral sensory systems and that this is regarded as an important mechanism underlying the behavioral manifestations of the anesthetic state. Other drug types, states and effects are considered.

data analysis
drugs
alpha
  frequency
smoking
hyperventilation

B 42. Saltzberg, B., and Burch, N.R.: Period analytic estimates of movements of the power spectrum: A simplified EEG time domain procedure. *Electroencephalogr Clin Neurophysiol, 30:*568, 1971.

The relationships between zero crossing descriptors (period analytic descriptors) are mathematically described in this article. Evidence is presented showing that counting zero

data analysis
frequency
  analysis

crossings over an epoch is equivalent to computing the auto-correlation function and taking its derivatives at zero lag or squaring and integrating derivatives of the EEG time trace over each epoch.

B 43.   Matousek, M.: Frequency analysis in routine electroence-phalography. *Electronecephalogr Clin Neurophysiol, 24:365,* 1968.

This study was initiated to develop an automatic method to partially substitute for visual evaluation of background activity in the EEG. Frequency analysis output has proved to be too variable to be utilized directly in this application. Results of frequency analysis of fifteen-second epochs of EEG activity indicated the theta/alpha + 2t ratio, where t is the epoch length, to be approximately equal to visual estimates of the amount of theta activity. Amount of theta activity was presumed from past experience with visual evaluations of EEG background activity to be an indicator of abnormality. It must be noted that the theta/alpha + 2t ratio is a purely operational indicator and has no necessary physiological significance. This method can be used along with visual evaluation techniques. In some applications such as patient screening it could even stand alone, and an instrument to automatically output theta/alpha +2t measurement results was constructed to this end.

data analysis
frequency
  analysis
alpha
  abundance
theta

B 44.   Walter, W.G., and Shipton, J.: Alpha characteristics. *Electro-encephalogr Clin Neurophysiol, 6:177,* 1957.

No ideal method for alpha rhythm analysis, for example a seven-dimensional continuum, exists; however a combination of the A-scale frequency analysis and toposcopy contains much of the basic information and is presented here. The disadvantage is that the data must be processed further to relate it to spontaneous or planned changes during an experiment. Also, all analyses require statistical assumptions about how brain activity can be sampled which are necessary due to the inability to record and display all available information. Experiments must thus be conducted to evaluate the validity of these assumptions. An application of such princi-

data analysis
frequency
  analysis
topography
alpha
  patterns

ples to alpha rhythms showed alpha rhythms to be plural and with components usually distinguishable by frequency, phase relations, domains and relationships to mental changes. Results can be displayed on a single diagram by condensing the time scale and plotting time versus the desired parameter such as the six frequency components in 8 to 13 cps activity. Preliminary results indicate that such a transformation and display can show relationships between brain physiology and psychological factors which may prove difficult to detect by conventional methods.

B 45. Lettich, E., and Margerison, J.H.: Presentation of data from low frequency analysis to illustrate serial changes in the electroencephalogram. *Electroencephalogr Clin Neurophysiol, 13*:606, 1961.

A technique of superimposition of data from a BNI Low Frequency Wave Analyzer allows serial EEG investigations to show actual changes or to discover correlates without information loss. In some cases this treatment will determine whether additional statistical analysis may be valuable.

data analysis
frequency analysis
temporal stability

B 46. Kaiser, E.K., Pétersen, I., Selldén, U., and Kagawa, N.: EEG data representation in broad-band frequency analysis. *Electroencephalogr Clin Neurophysiol, 17*:76, 1964.

Possibilities of simplifying data from EEG frequency analysis are discussed. A six-filter system is specified. The advantages of analog to frequency inversion and pulsed readout are stressed. A three-component frequency profile display system similar to the color triangle is demonstrated. The effects of electrode placement, sleep and hyperventilation are shown.

data analysis
frequency analysis
sleep
hyperventilation

B 47. Dumermuth, G., Huber, P.J., Kleiner, B., and Gasser, T.: Analysis of the interrelations between frequency bands of the EEG by means of the bispectrum. *Electroencephalogr Clin Neurophysiol, 31*:137, 1971.

The more or less random character of spontaneous EEG activity justifies the application of mathematical models developed in time series analysis. Among the methods numeri-

data analysis
bispectral analysis

cal spectral analysis has proved to be a powerful tool for analyzing and quantifying EEG data, especially background activity. The spectral decomposition of an EEG sample into its frequency components, giving (after appropriate smoothing) the power spectrum, provides complete information about the statistical properties of an EEG sample only under the assumption that the underlying process is stationary and Gaussian. If this assumption is violated, only partial information is obtained and higher order moments should be investigated. Whereas by the power spectrum the second central moment is analyzed in detail, the bispectrum allows a detailed analysis of the third central moment, which is influenced either by interrelations between frequency components or by nonstationarity of the signal. The bispectrum may therefore display important additional information about the properties of a stochastic signal like the EEG. In the stationary case this information is of great value in the investigation of phase-locking between different frequency bands, e.g. between alpha and beta activities. In addition, some new insights into the nonlinear aspects of the EEG generating process might be expected. Bispectra of artificial signals are shown in order to explain the basic aspects of this extension of spectral analysis, and selected examples of EEG bispectra demonstrate the interesting possibilities which this method offers in the field of EEG analysis.

SPECTRAL ANALYSIS

B 48.   Pfurtscheller, G., and Haring, G.: The use of an EEG autoregressive model for the time-saving calculation of spectral power density distributions with a digital computer. *Electroencephalogr Clin Neurophysiol, 33:*113, 1972.

This article presents a method for EEG analysis using an autoregressive model to calculate autocorrelation functions and power density distributions which saves 30 percent of the time required for such calculations using other means. If used in conjunction with the Fast Fourier Transform, the technique can save 95 percent of execution time over usual power density distribution calculation procedures. Further mathematical considerations and factors affecting the time saved in particular cases are also discussed.

spectral analysis computer data analysis analysis

B 49. Dumermuth, G.: Spectral analysis of the EEG. *Epilepsia, 13:* 473, 1972.

Spectral analysis is defined as a statistical method for investigating the variance of an EEG signal or the covariance between one or more EEG channels. The power spectrum is a decomposition of the total variance of an EEG signal into the contributions from different frequency bands, while the cross spectrum is a similar decomposition of covariance between EEG signals. Normalization of this gives coherence spectrum or a measure of mutual correlation between equal frequency bands (near 1 for strong phase locking; near 0 for weak phase locking). The mutual phase relationship between coherent frequency components is given by the phase spectrum. Compared with other methods, spectral analysis is superior because of its mathematical-statistical basis. Nevertheless, cost and time consumption cause its use to be restricted.

data analysis
spectral analysis
computer analysis
coherence
variability

B 50. Walter, D.O., et al.: Remote spectral and discriminant analysis of EEG's. *Electroencephalogr Clin Neurophysiol,* *24:*732, 1969.

Packaged solid state amplifiers and studio band FM modulators were used to transmit EEG's over standard telephone circuits to a central computer system and to retransmit analytic results back to the source. If the computer system is that of the Space Biology Laboratory, a small, time-shared general purpose computer (Scientific Data Systems 930®) will acquire the data and transmit it to a special purpose frequency domain computer (Time/Data 100) for Fourier transformation; the transformed data is converted to spectra and cross-spectral derivatives such as coherence. Spectra and coherence will be collected by the 930 for several adjacent epochs. When collection is complete, the 930 will calculate contours of spectral intensity or of coherence and transmit these maps back to the point of acquisition for presentation on a storage oscilloscope; the maps can also be plotted on paper for later reference. If the computer system is that of the Data Processing Laboratory, a medium-sized time-shared general purpose computer (SDS 9300®) will acquire the

data analysis
spectral analysis
computer analysis
telemetry
coherence

data and transmit it to a large time-shared general purpose machine (IBM 360/91®) in the Health Sciences Computing Facility, where it will be spectrally analyzed as above. This system can also retransmit contour maps, or the results of other forms of analysis.

B 51. Walter, D.O.: Spectral analysis for electroencephalograms: Mathematical determination of neurophysiological relationships from records of limited duration. *Exp Neurol, 8:*155, 1963.

Spectral analysis is a mathematical method which contains and generalizes frequency analysis. The form of spectral analysis most applicable to EEG is tutorially presented, using both algebraic formulae and four simplified illustrative examples. The examples are each converted into an auto-correlogram and autospectrogram, functions whose graphic presentation clarifies the structure of each example partly by emphasizing regular at the expense of irregular components, partly by analyzing the intensity of regular activity into components at each frequency. The formulae for cross-correlograms and cross-spectrograms are presented and are illustrated by converting pairs of examples into functions which clarify their interrelationships. Not only are the advantages of autospectrograms retained by cross-spectrograms, but they also emphasize activity shared between two traces, and include the mean phase angle relating such shared activity, at each frequency. The coherence function is applied not only to calculate the quantity of interdependence between pairs of illustrative examples, but also to supply probable bounds on the other calculated relationships. Finally, discussion of the assumptions underlying spectral analysis prepares the method for application to actual EEG, given in preceding papers.

data analysis
spectral analysis
computer analysis
autocorrelation
cross-correlation
coherence

B 52. Kleiner, B., Fluhler, H., Huber, P.J., and Dumermuth, G.: Spectrum analysis of the electroencephalogram. *Comput Programs Biomed, 1:*183, 1970.

Digital auto and cross spectral analysis has become an important method for quantifying and analyzing electroencephalographic data. This paper presents a set of four procedures written in ALGOL, which perform spectrum analysis of up to fourteen simultaneously recorded EEG channels on a medium- to large-size computer. The first procedure reduces the data after smoothing by a digital low-pass filter with variable cutoff frequency. By the elimination of the higher frequency components of no interest, aliasing is prevented. The reduced but still interleaved data are then rearranged by channels. The third procedure performs the Fast Fourier Transformation. Finally, the spectral quantities as power spectrum, cross spectral amplitude, phase, coherence and gain are computed for preselected channel combinations. Smoothing in the frequency domain is performed either by a rectangular or truncated normal spectral window of variable width.

data analysis
spectral analysis
computer analysis
autocorrelation
cross correlation
coherence

B 53. Hjorth, B.: EEG analysis based on time domain properties. *Electroencephalogr Clin Neurophysiol, 29:306, 1970.*

A method to describe the general characteristics of an EEG trace in a few quantitative terms is introduced. Its descriptive parameters are entirely based on time, but they can also be derived from the statistical moments of the power spectrum. Thus the method provides a bridge between a physical time domain interpretation and the conventional frequency domain description. Further, the parameters are based on the concept of variance, giving them an additive property so that the measured values pertain also to any basic elements from which a complex curve may be composed by superposition. The proposed method offers a way to on-line measurement of basic signal properties by means of a time-based calculation, requiring less complex equipment compared to conventional frequency analysis. The data-reducing capability of the parameters was experimentally demonstrated in the recording of sleep profiles.

data analysis
spectral analysis
computer analysis
time domain

B 54. Walter, D.O., Rhodes, J.M., Brown, D., and Adey, W.R.: Comprehensive spectral analysis of human EEG generators in posterior cerebral regions. *Electroencephalogr Clin Neurophysiol, 20:*224, 1966.

Using the bilateral centro-parietal (C3-P3-C4-P4), parieto-occipital (P3-01, P4-02), and left-to-right occipital (01-02) placements of the 10-20 electrode system for recording, subjects were presented with twenty minutes of flashes, clicks and other physical stimuli delivered by an automatic device with pretaped instructions. A button was to be pressed after hearing three tones, with some third tones delayed or manipulated. Spectral analysis by computer gave graphic forms such as contour maps, and the parameters used included spectral intensity (power spectra density) and coherence, a quality showing strength of relationships between brain areas. Results included the possibility of two independent generators functioning in the same frequency band but orthogonally polarized, and the article contained mathematical details for such a condition. Also, wider than usual (2 to 5 cps instead of 0.5 to 1.0 cps) alpha peaks were seen and could suggest shared sidebands of the alpha wave.

data analysis
spectral analysis
computer analysis
visual stimulation
auditory stimulation
generators
coherence
spatio-temporal characteristics

COMPUTER ANALYSIS

B 55. Hjorth, B.: The physical significance of time domain descriptors in EEG analysis. *Electroencephalogr Clin Neurophysiol, 34:*321, 1973.

A method of quantifying EEG characteristics which was proposed by the author earlier is developed further here to show that it gives information comparable to that derivable from conventional frequency analysis. Superimposed responses of general physical systems analyzed using these time domain descriptor techniques yield much information about the generating systems involved. Therefore, in addition to simplifying quantification of curve characteristics, the method can also be used for interpretation in terms of physical models. In this way the descriptors may directly or indirectly have physiological correlates, a fact which is substantiated by clinical findings.

data analysis
computer analysis
time domain

B 56. Leader, H.S., Cohn, R., and Broome, P.: Digital computer reading of the human EEG. *Electroencephalogr Clin Neurophysiol, 31:*294, 1971 (abstr).

The report presents the achievement of the recording and the digital computer processing and reading of 8 simultaneous channels of EEG data. The basic instrumentation consists of eight amplifiers, an A/D converter (400/sec for each channel), a scanner and formatter. These operate into a nine-track digital magnetic tape recorder. The peak selecting logic is fundamentally similar to that described earlier. The presently programmed patterns comprise over thirty categories of descriptors, in terms of modern EEG usage. To date, the criteria for the descriptors are established a priori (from clinical experience), but as data accumulate, the criteria are being determined statistically from the computer-derived data. Diagnosis, or the counting and correlation of the various descriptors recognized, is also established on an experiential basis; but again, as the library of computer-based data keeps accumulating, the correlations will result directly from the computer measurements.

data analysis
computer analysis
definitions
EEG patterns

B 57. Wennberg, A., and Zetterberg, L.H.: Application of a computer-based model for EEG analysis. *Electroencephalogr Clin Neurophysiol, 31:457*, 1971.

The parameter analysis of EEG is based upon a model that describes its spectral properties in parametric form. The spectrum is divided into several components of two general types, I and II. A component of Type I has its greatest spectral density at zero frequency and is described by one frequency parameter, the band width, and one power parameter, the power content. A component of Type II is described by two frequency parameters, the center frequency and the band width, and by two power parameters: the power content and a parameter describing spectral asymmetry around the center frequency. A computer program is available for estimating the EEG parameters and for calculating the statistical uncertainty in these parameters. This study is a first attempt to apply the analysis in practice. In twenty-five healthy young men, EEG's classified as normal on visual evaluation were selected for analysis. The physiological interpretation of these parameters is discussed. The analysis permits an exact determination of the parameters and their relationships. The hypothesis that beta activity is a harmonic of

data analysis
computer analysis
spectral analysis
EEG patterns
alpha harmonics

alpha activity is discussed. The relationship between the band widths for delta and alpha components is investigated. Detailed studies are made for alpha activity: a comparison of the power content in different regions of the brain, the relationship between band width and power content and a comparison of the center frequency and power content for recordings taken symmetrically on the skull. Variations with time in the center frequency of the alpha activity were also studied.

B 58.   Sklar, B., Hanley, J., and Simmons, W.W.: A computer analysis of EEG spectral signatures from normal and dyslexic children. *IEE Trans Biomed Eng, 20*:20, January 1973.

It is possible to differentiate between twelve dyslexic children and thirteen normal age- and sex-matched children on the basis of spectral estimates of their electroencephalograms (EEG's). The children were monitored during various mental tasks and rest situations. Data dimensionality was reduced by banding various spectral components and eliminating others. The reduced spectral vectors were used as an input to a stepwise discriminant analysis program which, in effect, selected the variables most disparate between the two groups (dyslexic and normal). The most prominent spectral differences appeared in the parieto-occipital region during the rest, eyes-closed phase. The dyslexic children on the average had more energy in the 3 to 7 Hz band and the 16 to 32 Hz band, and normals in the 9 to 14 Hz band. During the reading tasks, the autospectral disparity between the two sample populations was reversed at 16 to 32 Hz; normals tended to have greater energy. The coherences of all activity between various scalp leads displayed a particular pattern and were used as the most prominent discriminating feature during reading. Within the same hemisphere, coherences between leads were higher in dyslexics than in normals on the average, and, between symmetrical regions across the midline of the head, coherence tended to be higher in normals. Statistics are given, however, since the discriminating variables were gleaned from a search technique; other techniques are employed for providing confidence in the findings.

data analysis
computer analysis
spectral analysis
adolescents
dyslexia

B 59. Bickford, R.G., Fleming, N.I., and Billinger, T.W.: Compression of EEG data by isometric power spectral plots. *Electroencephalogr Clin Neurophysiol, 31*:630, 1971 (abstr).

The problem of the large volume of data to be analyzed in both clinical and research EEG work is solved here by using a computer graphic technique to compress the data by about 1 to 1000. A PDP-12 computer, for example, calculates the frequency spectrum of the EEG on eight-second segments, and the line representing the spectral calculation after smoothing is graphed as a sequence in a three-dimensional plot (100 lines per inch). Activity at any frequency is seen as a mountain. A forty-five-minute recording can then be compressed to a 3 × 1.5 inch per channel size and all channels can be shown on half a page. This method allows assessment of a patient's or subject's EEG recording quickly; it displays frequency variable states like sleep stages, photic stimulation responses, spike wave discharges, coma state variation and progressive deterioration in brain death; and it clearly shows shifts in the alpha spectrum during mental tasks or feedback. In general, any significant changes or trends in EEG activity can be easily detected.

data analysis
computer analysis
spectral analysis
EEG responses

B 60. Timsit-Berthier, M., Koninckx, N., Timsit, M., and Dongier, M.: Use of electronic calculators in psychiatric EEG: electroclinical correlations in classical EEG and study of cerebral slow potentials. *Electroencephalogr Clin Neurophysiol, 31*: 412, 1971 (abstr).

The systematic employment of electronic calculators (computers and averagers) since 1965 has made it possible to see more completely and more precisely the significant correlations between the electrical activity of the brain and various disturbances of behavior. A first technique consisted in the statistical treatment, with the help of the computers of the "Centre de Calcul" of the University of Liege (IBM 7040 and 360-44), of the data resulting from the analysis of EEG reports and the clinical histories of 733 subjects, including 46 psychopathic personalities, 66 psychotics, 64 psychosomatics, 375 neurotics and 95 control subjects. The results con-

data analysis
computer analysis
CNV
psychopath- ology

firm in essence the findings from the literature but some remain controversial, particularly the excess of theta activity, slowing of the alpha rhythm and the presence of delta activity during overbreathing in hysteropsychopathic subjects. On the other hand, the rolandic rhythms were seen more easily in the obsessional series. A poor arrest reaction had a pejorative value without, however, any specificity. A second technique, carried out with the aid of an averager (Enhancetron®), aimed, by summation, to show the slow cerebral potential changes which are invisible in the basic record. Used in 850 subjects, it has made it possible to show in psychotics, and to a lesser extent in neurotics, the presence of a general change in the negative slow potential, prolongation of the contingent negative variation (CNV), appearance of negative slow deflections after imperative sensory stimulation (thus independent of the CNV proper) and persistence of the motor readiness potential after completion of movement (Kornhuber phenomenon). These characteristics are sufficiently constant to have semiological value of practical usefulness to the clinician (unusual in psychiatric EEG), in particular for the diagnosis of early schizophrenia in which the curves are abnormal in 97 percent of cases so that the discovery of a normal curve in a suspect subject almost formally excludes this diagnosis. It results from this double approach that the hysteropsychopathic disturbances of behavior show themselves more readily in the classical EEG records, while those of the psychotic group express themselves by abnormalities in the negative slow potentials.

B 61. Walter, D.O., Kado, R.T., Rhodes, J.M., and Adey, W.R.: EEG baselines in astronaut candidates estimated by computation and pattern recognition techniques. *Aerosp Med, 38:* 371, 1967.

Data from the electrophysiologic records of fifty astronaut candidates were analyzed to establish baselines during varying states of sleep and wakefulness. Spectral analysis revealed characteristic patterns for each condition despite wide differences among subjects.

data analysis
computer analysis
EEG patterns
wakefulness

B 62. Daniel, R.S.: Electroencephalographic correlogram ratios and their stability. *Science, 145:*721, August 1964. (Copyright

1964 by the American Association for the Advancement of Science).

Autocorrelations of electroencephalograms can be reduced to ratios of estimated power among distinguishable parameters of typical tracings: the dominant rhythm, background activity, abundance and total power. These data reduction methods permit statistical evaluation of differences among experimental conditions, thus extending the usefulness of graphic correlograms in research. Ratios discriminate between two experimental conditions and two subjects, while showing stability over days.

data analysis
autocorrelation
alpha
patterns
stability

SECTION C

PHYSICAL ATTRIBUTES

ABUNDANCE

C 1.   Behrendt, T., and Duane, T.D.: Coincidence of EEG alpha patterns in humans. *Electroencephalogr Clin Neurophysiol, 31*:418, 1971 (abstr).

Results from an earlier study reported evidence for the hypothesis that alpha activity in one subject modifies the incidence of alpha in another. This project pursues this idea further by using hybrid analog-digital methods to study alpha patterns and to measure incidence of coincidental appearance of the alpha waves. The experiment required simultaneous EEG recording of three subjects; two identical twins and one unrelated person. Mathematical analysis, including 2×2 contingency table techniques, showed higher than random occurrences of alpha and also seemed to confirm the hypothesis that in some cases the alpha patterns of one subject may have influenced the appearance in another.

alpha abundance
alpha patterns
alpha symmetry
social interaction

C 2.   Johnson, L.C., and Ulett, G.A.: Quantitative study of pattern and stability of resting EEG activity in a young adult group. *Electroencephalogr Clin Neurophysiol, 11*:233, 1959.

Bipolar and monopolar EEG activity of 182 young male adults was recorded using an electronic analyzer presented here to be reliable and valid for EEG activity quantification. Findings include: (1) an EEG pattern similar to that observed visually including greatest activity in the alpha range with marked individual differences for all comparisons; (2) the observation that the occipital area contributes most to the parieto-occipital activity; (3) EEG activity profile shapes over twenty-four frequencies which were stable over a nine-month period but which showed smaller amounts of activity in the initial recordings; (4) comparisons within individual subjects revealing that 50 percent of the profiles were stable but exhibited marked individual differences with high alpha

alpha abundance
alpha patterns
EEG patterns
stability
topography

activity subjects showing the least change over time; (5) parieto-occipital activity similar to the distribution of monopolar activity in the occipital, parietal and frontal areas with the alpha range showing the greatest activity in all areas; (6) stability of monopolar and parieto-occipital activity of similar degree; and (7) a relation between poor organization of brain waves from three monopolar leads and instability of EEG activity over time. It was also noted that four subject groups with respect to cortical organization were found: (1) sixteen with high occipital and well-organized brain electrical activity; (2) seventeen with organized cortical patterns but no prominent occipital alpha activity; (3) eight with predominent slow activity and general disorganization and (4) five with multipeaks of activity and general disorganization.

C 3.   Armington, J.C., and Chapman, R.M.: Temporal potentials and eye movements. *Electroencephalogr Clin Neurophysiol,* 2:346, 1959.

Two subjects were simultaneously recorded from temporal electrodes and electrodes located close to the eyes. It was concluded that the so-called "kappa" rhythm and eyelid flutter are independent.

alpha
  abundance
kappa
  rhythm
eye
  movements

C 4.   Takahashi, T., and Ushirobata, H.: Diffuse sigma rhythm—correlation with diffuse alpha rhythm. *Folia Psychiatr Neurol Jap,* 24:109, 1970.

Four hundred six patients having diffuse alpha in their waking EEG's and one hundred control patients without the waking diffuse alpha were recorded for EEG during sleep to determine the relative incidence of diffuse sigma. A total of 341 subjects had diffuse sigma in their sleep EEG's. Significantly more of the subjects with diffuse alpha had the diffuse sigma. The authors concluded that the phenomena were tied togehter and that sigma and alpha may be caused by analogous mechanisms.

alpha
  abundance
diffuse
  alpha
sigma
  rhythm
sleep
  theory

C 5.   Gale, A., Harpham, B., and Lucas, B.: Time of day and the EEG: Some negative results. *Psychon Sci,* 28:269, 1972.

Twenty subjects were studied on four occasions at four times of day, on a random schedule. The times of day were 0700, 1100, 1500 and 2000 hours. The resting EEG was recorded on each occasion during eyes-open and eyes-closed trials. The results were: (1) there were no general effects for the time of day nor any indication of an interaction between time of day and personality (extroversion-introversion and neuroticism); (2) the subjects maintained rank order for alpha abundance, within the group, over the four visits $(p < .01)$; (3) extroversion was directly related to degree of variability across sessions $(p < .05)$; and (4) alpha abundance was greater on the first visit than on the last visit $(p < .05)$. These results demonstrate the within-subject stability of the EEG and show that, for simple tasks of this nature, time of day has no effect on the EEG.

alpha
  abundance
biorhythms
stability
personality

C 6.   Paskewitz, D.A., and Orne, M.T.: On the reliability of baseline EEG alpha activity. *Psychophysiology, 10:*202, 1973 (abstr).

The study observed alpha baseline levels over several days. Analysis revealed most deviations from a subject's modal alpha tended toward increased activity which was associated with independent evidence of drowsiness. Increased slow rolling eye movements, as with early sleep onset, were clearly associated with diminished alpha density. The report discussed the implications of the results in studies of alpha activity.

alpha
  abundance
variability

C 7.   Mulholland, T.B.: Occurrence of the electroencephalographic alpha rhythm with eyes open. *Nature, 206:*746, 1965.

In this experiment, nonsense syllables were projected on a screen in a dark room for 0.2 second whenever alpha occurred. It was expected that such alternating alpha and non-alpha periods would cause activation. Alpha activity was not reduced greatly as expected and it was the atypical subject who could not participate due to insufficient alpha with eyes open. Under similar conditions with eyes open in an illuminated room during feed-back, subjects had no trouble producing enough alpha to continue the experiment. Thus

alpha
  abundance
eye opening
EEG
  activation

alpha feedback and attention experiments with pattern stimuli with eyes open are feasible according to these results.

C 8. Pisani, D., Ardizzone, E.C., Di Stefano, M., and Nigro, A.: The variations of the alpha percentage of the EEG in neurotic and epileptic patients during memorizing. *Neopsichiatria, 33:1*, 1967.

Findings of an experiment studying changes in percentage of alpha activity in neurotic, epileptic and other neurological patients in relation to position and memorizing are presented and discussed. Lower percentages of alpha at the time of memorization were seen in the neurotics.

alpha
* abundance*
memory
neurotic
* tendency*
epilepsy

FREQUENCY

C 9. Hoefer, P.F.A., deNapoli, R.A., and Lesse, S.: Perodicity and hypsarrhythmia in the EEG. *Arch Neurol, 9:*424, 1963.

The investigation assumed that a distinctive EEG abnormality (periodic synchronous bursts) occurred in conditions other than those of organic mental changes, seizures, etc., and that the abnormality could be produced experimentally. Findings were reported on fifty-four patients and nine primates. Etiologic mechanisms are discussed. The wide distribution of the abnormality suggests it may be a release phenomenon.

alpha
frequency

C 10. Burdick, J.A.: Relation of alpha frequency to amplitude variability. *Percept Mot Skills, 26:*216, 1968.

EEG recordings were taken of fifty males (17 to 62 years) for fifteen minutes with eyes closed to investigate the possible link between alpha frequency and amplitude variation in the normal wakeful state. The electrodes were placed in the left occipital region with reference to both ears. Artifacts were manually deleted and an integrator summed every twenty seconds of EEG record. Using thirty successive twenty-second periods, mean integrated amplitude (MIA), standard deviation (SD) and coefficients of variance (CV = SD/MIA)

alpha
frequency
alpha
* amplitude*
variability

were calculated. Chi-square analyses between CV and alpha frequency and MIA and alpha frequency were run. The statistical results showed no significant correlation between alpha frequency and amplitude variation in the experiment, even though these parameters are being used in practice and seem to be showing results.

C 11.   Carrie, J.R.G.: The modal alpha wavelength. *Electroencephalogr Clin Neurophysiol, 27:*703, 1969 (abstr) .

Under standard experimental conditions occipital EEG recordings were taken on sixty-seven subjects. Frequency of occurrence of waves of different duration in a sample of one thousand consecutive waves in a band pass including alpha activity were shown in histograms (profiles) derived using the technique of Frost. Results showed a significant positive correlation (+ 0.80) between mode location and alpha frequency as assessed by written record measurement and visual inspection. Modal alpha representation ranged from 16.6 percent of the one thousand samples to 2.5 percent. Modal height and wave length at the mode locations proved not to be correlated. All EEG records were evaluated verbally by experienced electroencephalographers and five categories according to alpha activity stability were described. It was found that the average magnitudes of modes in the corresponding histogram profiles differed from one another. These differences proved significant when the group with poor alpha rhythms as assessed visually were statistically compared with those having alpha frequency simply stated without mention of wave form stability.

alpha frequency
alpha amplitude
stability
data analysis

C 12.   Gaarder, K., and Speck, L.B.: The quasi-harmonic relations of alpha and beta peaks in the power spectrum. *Brain Res, 4:*110, 1967.

EEG recordings were made on twenty-four control subjects, twelve alcoholics, and fourteen psychopaths with eyes closed to investigate quasi-harmonic relations between peaks of activity in the EEG power spectra. Electrodes were placed from left occipital to vertex and left anterior temporal to vertex and one-minute recordings were used to generate the power spectra. Harmonics produced by artifacts were deleted by close monitoring and checkout. The spectra were examined

alpha frequency
theory
spectral analysis
psychopathology
beta harmonics

for two clearly defined peaks between 7.5 and 29 cps, the peaks being arbitrarily referred to as alpha and beta peaks. Four controls, four alcoholics and four psychopaths met this requirement in their occipital-vertex record and, in addition, the second peak was nearly twice the frequency of the first in all cases. Some subjects also satisfied the criteria in their anterior temporal-vertex leads with the same double frequency phenomena observed above. Similar peak relations occurred during random interval stimulation except for frequency variation. The authors admit possible varying interpretation of these results but suggest the quasi-harmonic peaks represent fundamental timing properties of the nervous system. Synchrony of neuronal firing with a period of approximately 50 msec is found in some individuals and indicates a power spectrum peak near 20 cps. Alpha occurs when every other cycle is suppressed. A lack of alpha or beta peaks would then, under this theory, be accounted for by a rapidly shifting basic periodicity or desynchronization (lack of redundancy) accompanying, for example, data processing.

C 13.   Frost, J.D.: Wave length analysis of the EEG—The alpha profile. *Electroencephalogr Clin Neurophysiol, 27*:702, 1969 (abstr) .

An on-line computer method which automatically quantifies alpha frequency and its constancy or stability is described in this article. EEG frequency is treated independently of amplitude, but the method differs from that of Tecce and Mirsky since it makes a precise wavelength measurement and only alpha activity is included. Occipital activity is filtered (6 to 14 cps) and wavelengths are measured by the interval between successive positive going baseline crosses (zero cross method) . One thousand consecutive alpha waves are measured and counted with 2 msec resolution. Total time of the analysis process is also recorded since it depends upon percentage time and average frequency of alpha activity. Histograms are plotted with the abscissa representing wavelength and the ordinate the number of waves per category. Mode, then, correlates to the electroencephalographer's alpha frequency and the distribution spread is a quantitative measure of alpha variability.

alpha frequency variability measurement techniques data analysis

C 14. Olsen, P.Z., Stoier, M., Siersbaek-Nielsen, K., Hansen, J.M., Schioler, M., and Kristensen, M.: Electroencephalographic findings in hyperthyroidism. *Electroencephalogr Clin Neurophysiol, 32:*171, 1972.

alpha frequency thyroid levels

Twenty-six of thirty-two patients with untreated thyrotoxicosis had an abnormal EEG. The severity of the hyperthyroidism evaluated by several thyroid function tests was correlated with the degree of diffuse paroxysmal activity and fast activity above 15 μv, but no correlation was found with the alpha frequency. After two to six weeks of treatment the EEG's showed a decrease in the alpha frequency parallel to the normalization of the thyroid function tests. The paroxysmal and fast activities subsided gradually and incompletely but significantly, while the slow activity did not show any significant decrease after two to three years. At the end of the observation period more than half of the patients still had EEG's which were abnormal, although less pronounced. Six patients with relapses of hyperthyroidism had aggravation of the EEG abnormalities, which again subsided after treatment was reinstituted. It is concluded that hyperthyroidism causes a characteristic pattern of severe EEG changes which may only subside gradually and incompletely, indicating persisting cerebral dysfunction in spite of an otherwise successful treatment of the hyperthyroidism.

C 15. Obal, F., Szabon, J., Borcsok, E., and Foldi, M.: Effect of tonsillectomy on the EEG. *Acta Med Acad Sci Hung, 26:*317, 1969.

alpha frequency physical illness beta

Twelve subjects were recorded for EEG prior to and two to five days following tonsillectomy to determine the effects on the EEG. The incidence of frequencies from 1 to 30 Hz were analyzed in the two recordings. The EEG was found to be slower overall following the surgery. The overall incidence of beta activity was reduced and the frequency of the alpha rhythm was reduced. Specifically, 30 Hz, 25 Hz and 11 Hz were significantly reduced and 20 Hz, 12 Hz and 9 Hz incidences were significantly increased.

C 16. Poole, E.W., Taylor, J.M., Sowerby, J.E., and Poole, B.G.: Relationship between frequency of EEG and tremor rhythms in health and disease: preliminary results from assessment of finger tremor in routine EEG examinations. *Electroencephalogr Clin Neurophysiol, 21:*617, 1966 (abstr).

Three groups of subjects (less than 25 years, 25 to 54 years, and greater than 54 years) consisting of 100 nonpatients and 350 EEG referrals were recorded for EEG in this experiment. Contralateral EEG's were done from electrodes (P_3-O_1) and analyzed with tremor using a B.N.I. frequency analyzer. A simple light strain gauge accelerometer was used to measure the tremor. For analysis purposes, abundance of each frequency between 2 and 16 cps (excluding 13 and 15 cps) was measured from four ten-second epochs with eyes closed and one with eyes open. Significant positive correlations were found, especially between the mean and 6 to 12 cps dominants. These findings were not universal to all age and clinical groups and therefore further study on the particular circumstances of occurrence of these correlation and maturation effects is recommended. Nevertheless, these results suggest that EEG and tremor outputs can be related.

alpha frequency motor performance maturation eye opening data collection

C 17. Poole, E.W., and Taylor, J.M.: Preferred and non-preferred EEG frequency components in post-central areas. Observations with particular reference to 3-7 c/sec. *Electroencephalogr Clin Neurophysiol, 28:*211, 1970 (abstr).

EEG recordings were taken of 100 nonpatients and 350 EEG referrals, as well as 500 prison inmates. The frequency components of the post-central area (P_3-O_1) were assessed by summing abundances during four ten-second epochs using a wave form analyzer. Dominant and minimum abundances in the 3 to 7 cps range seemed to have significant associations with dominant frequencies. It was also found that predictions could be made in the 3 to 7 and 6 to 12 cps ranges from such things as slow (2 to 3 cps) or fast (14 to 16, 22 to 24 cps) abundances. Although the experimenter admits his results may depend on arbitrary frequency limits and methodology, he feels that at least the frequency content of the EEG at rest has been proved by this research to derive, in part, from a range of inter-related frequencies rather than a narrow band and totally independent variables and frequency components.

EEG frequency alpha frequency

C 18. Hawkes, C.H., and Prescott, R.J.: EEG variation in healthy subjects. *Electroencephalogr Clin Neurophysiol, 34*:197, 1973.

Twenty-seven healthy subjects were recorded for EEG activity while performing simple visual procedures to maintain a constant level of attention. EEG indices were analyzed by analysis of variance. Age, sex and menstruation did not significantly affect the variance of the indices. In general, fluctuations during a session indicated continued fluctuations from day to day. It should be noted that the data did not fit normal distributions, a fact that resulted in the use of an *ad hoc* method for describing these EEG indices of variability.

EEG frequency
EEG amplitude variability
attention
aging
sex differences

C 19. Boddy, J.: A re-examination of the relationship between reaction time and EEG wave period. *Electroencephalogr Clin Neurophysiol, 30*:367, 1971 (abstr).

Attempts were made to replicate Surwillo's finding (*Electroencephalogr Clin Neurophysiol, 15*:105, 1963) using other methods of period analysis. In the first experiment a mean EEG period was obtained for each subject using an automated power spectrum-based frequency analysis system. Seventeen subjects were used and the EEG from derivations P_3-O_1 and P_4-O_2 was analyzed for about a minute while subjects had their eyes closed. EEG recording and RT sessions were successive. The inter-individual correlation between visual RT and mean EEG period was 0.05, clearly nonsignificant. In the second experiment mean values of the EEG period were determined by making linear measurements, on the EEG chart, of EEG samples with between five and ten clearly identifiable successive waves. The EEG was sampled in the period of one second immediately preceeding each RT stimulus. The auditory and visual RT's of twenty subjects were measured during conditions of high incentive, but while they had their eyes closed. EEG recording was from the dominant hemisphere, the temporal derivation T_3-T_5 during auditory RT's and the occipital derivation T_5-O_1 during visual RT's. The inter- and intra-individual correlation coefficients between EEG period and RT were 0.21 (r[N = 20] > 0.36, $P < 0.10$) and 0.10 for auditory RT and 0.26 and 0.10 for visual RT. Thus, there was a failure to replicate the

EEG frequency
reaction time
phase of wave period

findings of Surwillo in both experiments. Possible sources of the discrepant findings will be discussed.

AMPLITUDE

C 20.   Berkhout, J.: Comparative frequency distributions of large and small amplitude rhythms of the human electroencephalogram. *Electroencephalogr Clin Neurophysiol, 19:*598, 1965.

Thirty-two patients with organic brain damage and thirty-eight normal subjects were studied. Rhythmic events between 7 and 15 cps from the left occipital bipolar leads were counted by frequency from one hundred seconds of awake resting EEG recordings for each subject. Rhythmic events were defined as sequences of ten equidistant ($\pm$ 10%) baseline crossings, and two amplitude ranges were delineated, a low range of less than 20 μv and a high range of greater than 50 μv peak to peak. Frequency histograms for each subject group, amplitude range and eye condition showed a larger small amplitude band width for both groups and slower large amplitude activity for the pathological group. Similar histogram shapes and individual mean frequency deviations between groups suggest that this slowing of large amplitude activity was indeed a shift in the distribution rather than additional slow frequency EEG material. Small amplitude activity showed no differences between groups but did peak at 12 to 13 cps as opposed to 10 cps for large activity during eyes closed. During eyes open, there was no large alpha and no change from eyes-closed activity for slow alpha. Also, near zero statistical correlations were found between the amplitude ranges. Viewing this evidence as proof of independent sources for the two amplitude ranges and remembering the unresponsiveness of the small amplitude activity to group, eye condition, etc., some type of threshold restriction for routine frequency analysis is suggested since significant shifts in one level of activity may be masked by allowing different activity levels into the analysis.

alpha
  amplitude
alpha
  frequency
generators
eye opening
brain
  damage
criteria

C 21.   Leissner, P., Lindholm, L.E., and Petersen, I.: Alpha amplitude dependence on skull thickness as measured by ultrasound technique. *Electroencephalogr Clin Neurophysiol, 29:*392, 1970.

Utilizing the temporal and parietal electrode positions of the   *alpha*
10-20 system, twenty-seven subjects were compared for skull   *amplitude*
thickness and EEG amplitude. The method involved ultra-   *skull*
sound beams passed through the skull at various angles caus-   *thickness*
ing echoes from the inner and outer skull surfaces which ap-   *data*
peared on a screen and were photographed. Using thirty one-   *collection*
second sequences of good alpha recording, peak-to-peak   *ultrasound*
amplitudes were measured and mean values determined for
each lead. Assuming cortical alpha amplitude, cerebrospinal
fluid and soft tissue attenuation to be equal, the method used
can give attenuation differences for each millimeter difference of bone and be accurate on skull thickness to ± 3 mm.
Operation and autopsy cases were used as verification. Nine
persons had bone asymmetry of 33 percent or more, with
alpha amplitude decreases of 20 to 70 percent on the thinner
sides. Also, skull thickness was greater on the left side. The
authors suggest that CSF and soft tissue, etc., which were assumed equal, could be a source of error. Nevertheless, they
feel that thickness measures could be of value in cases of
distinct alpha asymmetry with no apparent explanation.

C 22.   Glass, A.: Factors influencing changes in the amplitude histo-
         gram of the normal EEG during eye opening and mental
         arithmetic. *Electroencephalogr Clin Neurophysiol, 28:423,*
         1970.

The amplitude histogram mode of time-series analysis with   *EEG*
graphs, magnetic tape and a fixed program averaging com-   *amplitude*
puter was used to study factors influencing EEG amplitude   *data analysis*
changes (considered in isolation). Standard deviations about   *eye opening*
the mean of the normally distributed amplitude for each   *mental tasks*
condition and subject and analysis of variance revealed a
significant but different reduction in the standard duration
of the amplitude for both eye opening and mental arithmetic
as well as an interaction of these effects (i.e. greater effects
due to calculation when eyes closed). The amplitude decrement appears to be linear to the amplitude of the less active
condition. That is, greater amplitude during eyes-closed im-
plies a greater decrease caused by arithmetic or eye opening.
Eye-opening causes a larger rate of decrement than mental
arithmetic. Also, an amplitude level of the less active condi-

tion below a certain threshold may indicate an increment rather than a decrement during the "stimulus" condition. The results agree with other findings in related fields and a neuronal (dendritic) hypothesis of cortical activity.

PHASE

C 23.   Zhirmunskaya, E.A., and Makarova, G.V.: Distribution of the average level of asymmetry of the phases of the EEG waves over the human brain surface. *Fiziol Zh SSSR, 56:* 1321, 1970.

The distribution of the average level of asymmetry of the phase of ascending and descending EEG waves, one of the parameters used in quantitative analysis of the EEG, was studied while the twenty-two subjects were in states of (1) physiological quiet but still awake, (2) photic stimulation and (3) exposure to other functional tests. The average level of asymmetry was found to be distributed along longitudinal and latitudinal gradients on the surface of the cortex. It was also discovered that this parameter varied with different patterns of EEG activity. Absolute magnitudes decreased from occiput to forehead and from left to right temple and the sign of asymmetry changed from negative to positive during physiological quiet. During reactive changes in EEG structure the average level of asymmetry increased. Positive signs of asymmetrical level were associated with desynchronized EEG's while negative signs were linked to hypersynchronized EEG activity.

alpha phase
alpha
symmetry
data analysis

C 24.   Hori, H., Hayasaka, K., Sato, K., Harada, O., and Iwata, H.: A study on phase relationship in human alpha activity. Correlation of different regions. *Electroencephalogr Clin Neurophysiol, 26:*19, 1969.

This study used six normal male adults (27 to 35 years) with a well-organized alpha rhythm and three patterns of monopolar leads with reference to the nose. The EEG was displayed on a cathode ray oscilloscope through the decatron toposcope and recorded on film. Data analysis was performed by using the correlation coefficient (r) and shows the topo-

alpha phase
topography
origins
theory

graphical phase relationships of alpha waves between the regions of the brain. According to the r's, the scalp could be divided into three blocks: (1) the frontal region—r approaches to 1 (0.91 to 0.98—highest values of r); (2) the parietal and occipital regions along the parasagittal line—r between 0.65 and 0.87 (moderate values of r); (3) the temporal region and adjacent occipital and parietal areas—r is 0.52 to 0.65 (lowest values). The author also offers a discussion of the various theories on the origin of alpha and functional relationships between regions of the brain in light of his findings.

C 25. Martinius, J., Hoovey, Z., Heinemann, U., and Weinmann, H.M.: The inter-hemispheric phase relations of the occipital alpha rhythm in childhood. *Electroencephalogr Clin Neurophysiol, 30:*248, 1971.

The EEG's of children (6 to 16 years) were studied for phase relations between alpha activity from both occipital regions to assess irregularity in the developing EEG. The analogue material was transformed to digital form and analysis showed age-related and inter-individual differences in the inter-hemispheric alpha phase relations variability. As in adults, occipital alpha peaks of less than 5 msec showed a definite phase difference. The author hopes to extend this technique to neurological and psychiatric disorders in children.

alpha phase
children
EEG
maturation
hemispheric
dominance

C 26. Barlow, J.S., and Estrin, T.: Comparative phase characteristics of induced and intrinsic alpha activity. *Electroencephalogr Clin Neurophysiol, 30:*1, 1971.

Twenty-two subjects were recorded with eyes closed from a midline array of five electrodes between occiput and vertex to study phase characteristics of intrinsic alpha activity and alpha activity induced by use of slowly repeated flashes. Only eleven subjects had sufficiently developed rhythmic after-waves from intermediate flash intensities to be examined and nine of these were carried through the full range of flash intensities. Using the stimuli for induced alpha and the background occipital alpha for intrinsic alpha activity to trigger the computer, an analysis by averaging showed no

alpha phase
visual
stimulation
alpha
synchrony
alpha
amplitude
generators

close parallel between induced and intrinsic alpha. The flash-induced alpha waves did appear more synchronous than the intrinsic alpha activity and were generally of larger amplitude for intermediate flash intensities. The authors speculate about generator mechanisms and functions such as the possibility of "reverberating circuits" causing the rhythmic after-waves, an idea long suggested as a basis for immediate and short-term memory.

C 27. Goldstein, S.: Phase coherence of the alpha rhythm during photic blocking. *Electroencephalogr Clin Neurophysiol, 29:* 127, 1970.

The pre- to post-blocked phase angle relationship of the photically blocked alpha rhythm is examined in light of a pacemaker model. The question is asked whether this pacemaker is in continuous operation during photic blocking even though, within this period, the detected alpha oscillation may vanish. The analysis of the data shows first, a post-blocked alpha rhythm coherence and second, a mean zero phase angle between the post-blocked and pre-blocked wave trains. These results are consistent with the idea of a basic pacemaking system, but because of conservation of phase information during the photic block, they are at variance with the concept that photically induced desynchronization must take place at the pacemaker level. The results are discussed further in terms of a visual information intake model used by Gaarder et al.

alpha phase
photic
flicker
alpha
blocking

C 28. Magnus, O., and Ponsen, L.: The influence of the phase of the alpha rhythm on the cortical evoked response to photic stimulation. *Electroencephalogr Clin Neurophysiol, 18:428,* 1965 (abstr).

The cortical evoked response to photic stimulation was recorded from fourteen healthy young adult subjects with a neon stroboscope triggered on a pre-set phase of the alpha rhythm allowing at least 2 sec between flashes. An average of spontaneous activity was also obtained with the stroboscope covered. This was subtracted from the average response to light at the same phase and analysis was performed on this parameter as well as the original response. Several

alpha phase
phase of
wave
period
visual
evoked
response
photic
flicker

preliminary conclusions were reached. Responses obtained in this way are more easily reproduced than those to random flashes. Alpha rhythms continue for about 50 msec unchanged until the gradual, sometimes partial, extinction of the spontaneous activity. After 200 to 250 msec a new rhythmic response begins which resembles, as regards frequency, symmetry and changes with vigilance, the spontaneous alpha rhythm. A better insight into the origin of the so-called "ringing" or rhythmic response to photic stimulation is allowed by this method.

SYNCHRONY

C 29. Strobos, R.J.: Significance of amplitude asymmetry in the electroencephalogram. *Neurology (Minneap), 10:799, 1960.*

Four hundred EEG's, half with amplitude asymmetry as the only abnormality and half completely normal, were analyzed for localization of amplitude asymmetry in relation to clinical data. Results showed that amplitude asymmetry as well as depressed amplitude in the occipital area and in some cases other areas in the dominant hemisphere may occur in normals. It was also found that amplitude asymmetry in a region other than the dominant occipital lobe usually indicates a lesion and that the continuation of asymmetrical activity during sleep serves to increase its localizing value. Most often, but not always, the lesion is located in the same hemisphere as the activity of depressed amplitude.

*alpha
synchrony
alpha
amplitude*

C 30. Hoovey, Z.B., Heinemann, U., and Creutzfeldt, O.D.: Inter-hemispheric "synchrony" of alpha waves. *Electroencephalogr Clin Neurophysiol, 32:337, 1972.*

The inter-hemispheric synchronization of alpha waves recorded monopolarly from two homologous occipital points was measured by determining the intervals between peaks of simultaneously recorded right and left alpha waves. The data are supported by classical cross-correlation of short (0.32 sec) successive recording periods. The mean values of inter-hemispheric peak differences were between ± 2.5 msec, but the values for individual bilateral alpha pairs varied con-

*alpha
synchrony
variability
alpha
amplitude*

siderably (range above ± 20 msec). The standard deviations of the mean interhemispheric alpha intervals can be taken as a measure of synchrony between the two hemispheres. They showed large variations between individuals. In subjects with good alpha synchrony (small standard deviation), the amplitude correlation between simultaneously recorded right and left alpha waves was high, and vice versa. On the time axis, right-left peak intervals of alpha pairs varied continually, with one side leading for a time and then the other leading. Such periods were of the order of some seconds (3 to 5 sec).

C 31.   Runnals, S., and Mulholland, T.: A method for the study of bilateral asymmetry of cortical activation. *Am J EEG Technol, 4*:15, 1964.

Using a stimulus-brain response feedback loop (Mulholland and Runnals, 1962), cortical activation responses (alpha blocking, desynchronization, or reduction of alpha amplitude) were obtained from homologous brain regions in order to detect brain pathology. Two cases are presented as examples and it is concluded that according to these preliminary results dissimilarities of cortical activation in homologous regions can be observed with this feedback method allowing fast convenient comparisons of regions of the cortex with respect to initiation and habituation of activation by a sensory stimulus.

alpha synchrony brain damage alpha blocking

C 32.   Roth, N., and Klingberg, F.: The occurrence of alpha burst activity in connection with the respiratory phase with reference to the activity level. *Acta Biol Med Ger, 25*:185, 1970.

The transformation of the EEG in the sense of increasing synchronization is regarded as an electrophysiological expression of decreasing vigilance. In this stage, characterized by synchronization, the CNS can perform only simple, largely automatized performances, not requiring a high degree of activation. In the transition to lower vigilance a phase was found where some physiological parameters vary synchronously with respiration. Very probably these variations are attributable to the changes in the brain stem activity due to respiratory regulation. The conclusion is drawn that acti-

alpha synchrony vigilance respiration

vating factors in the respiratory regulation (inspirium) causes a shift in the vigilance in the sense of activation. During the more passive part of the respiratory cycle the reduced vigilance is expressed in an increase in EEG synchronization.

C 33. Martinius, J.W., and Hoovey, Z.B.: Bilateral synchrony of occipital alpha waves, oculomotor activity and "attention" in children. *Electroencephalogr Clin Neurophysiol, 32:*349, 1972.

Thirteen children (8 to 11 years old) with normal intelligence were recorded for EEG to determine the relationship of bilateral alpha synchrony to concentration. Ten children were dyslexic, ten had reported learning problems related to inability to concentrate, and ten were normal control subjects. The subjects were required to discriminate between 500 Hz and 1500 Hz tones and to recall tone sequences. The phase lag between alpha in the two hemispheres ranged between 1 and 30 msec in the resting condition with 78 percent falling between 1 and 10 msec. During the tasks, some of the children showed increased alpha pair activity which was associated with a decrease in large phase differences, an increase in synchrony of the two hemispheres and better performance in discrimination and memory. Significantly more of the control subjects showed this type of change than other groups.

*alpha
synchrony
attention
children
auditory
stimulation
learning
memory
dyslexia*

C 34. Liske, E., Hughes, H.M., and Stowe, D.E.: Cross-correlation of human alpha activity: Normative data. *Electroencephalogr Clin Neurophysiol, 22:*429, 1967.

Forty-two asymptomatic adult males were studied by history, physical examination and EEG. Cross-correlograms were generated from the EEG data derived from P_3-O_1 and P_4-O_2. Twenty-four subjects exhibited phase lead to the right and eighteen to the left. None was exactly in zero phase. Average-phase shift for the group was 0.83 msec to the right. The range of the phase shifts was from 4 msec left to 7 msec right. This report emphasizes that not all normal subjects are essentially synchronized with respect to their alpha activity, although in most normals there is clearly some imperfect

*EEG
synchrony
alpha
synchrony
alpha
phase
hemispheric
dominance*

neurological mechanism operating to phase align the alpha activity. In a number of normal subjects a surprising degree of right-sided alpha phase leading was seen; a degree not approached in those subjects in which left-sided alpha activity was phase leading. These findings tend to support textbook statements that cerebral dominance for alpha rhythm more often resides in the right hemisphere of normal humans in the sense that it more often exerts an average phase lead over the alpha activity generated in the left hemisphere.

C 35. Bruck, M.A.: Average voltage as a measure of phase synchrony in the EEG. *Electroencephalogr Clin Neurophysiol, 19*:601, 1965.

This article describes a method for determining phase synchrony in the EEG using the voltage levels obtained from brain wave records from two regions to be compared for phase synchrony with referential and bipolar leads simultaneously. Equal voltages indicated complete phase synchrony. A complete relationship between voltage and synchrony was found and various techniques were used to establish a correlation. The resulting regression equation was used in conjunction with a nomogram to calculate the synchrony ratio. Synchrony ratios and voltages have proved important as an aid in diagnosis. Previous work has shown that the mean of the combined synchrony ratios and voltage values is higher in controls than in schizophrenics if the EEG's are normal upon conventional inspection. Also, 26 percent of the controls had higher values than the schizophrenics.

*EEG
  synchrony
voltage
phase*

C 36. Aird, R.B., and Gastaut, Y.: Occipital and posterior electroencephalographic rhythms. *Electroencephalogr Clin Neurophysiol, 11*:637, 1959.

Occipital waves evoked by jerky eye movements which were first referred to as "lambda waves" by Evans in 1952 are described in this article. A slow alpha variant rhythm showing a two to one frequency relationship to the underlying occipital alpha rhythm was found in a small percentage of the subjects. A correlation between this variant and emotional instability and a dysfunction in the diencephalon or deeper

*EEG
  synchrony
eye
  movements
emotion
lambda
  waves*

structure was suggested, but no correlation with convulsive susceptability was indicated. Further details on this and other slow posterior rhythms are also presented.

TOPOGRAPHY

C 37. Perez-Borja, C., Chatrian, G.E., Tyce, F.A., and Rivers, M.H.: Electrographic patterns of the occipital lobe in man: A topographic study based on use of implanted electrodes. *Electroencephalogr Clin Neurophysiol, 14:*171, 1962.

Twenty-six patients with various mental disorders were recorded for EEG to study the topographical distribution of electrographic pattern in the occipital lobe. For each pattern, the electrode of maximal activity was located according to such criteria as persistence, voltage (referential recordings) and phase reversals (bipolar tracings). By plotting these positions on the sagittal and coronal planes of the Yoss atlas, composite maps were made. Alpha rhythms (8 to 16 cps) and the fast rhythms (25 to 30 cps) were widely distributed within the occipital lobe and extended to the parietal and temporal lobes. The alpha activity seemed to originate from multiple occipital and extra-occipital foci which overlap in influence but are under the relative control of a central pacemaker. The fast activity was previously reported by Gastaut but no support of his suggestion of origins remote from the occipital electrodes was found. No significant patterns could be found for the slow spontaneous activity which was only recorded occasionally. The light-induced activity was recorded from discrete areas of the occipital lobe medial portions in or near the calcarine region. The response to patterned visual stimulation (lambda waves) also came from the superolateral part of the occipital lobe. The variety of patterns correlates with the complex and diverse visual functions in man. It is suggested that in his opinion surface electrograms just cannot present the entire, true picture.

topography
generators
origins
visual
stimulation
theory

C 38. Lehmann, D.: Topographical assessment of the EEG. *Electroencephalogr Clin Neurophysiol, 32:*713, 1972 (abstr).

Methods for assessment of electrical EEG fields on the human
scalp are described using forty to fifty recording points and
equipotential maps. Data reduction techniques are presented
which allow compressed representations of data derived from
the map series. Maximal field values and degree of belief of
the field (average absolute amplitude per electrode) permit
selection of pronounced distributions and uncover dominant
frequencies in the temporal EEG. Successive maps are averaged during a dominant EEG frequency, and the standard
deviations of the mean field values across maps indicate distribution of EEG activity. It is felt by the authors that three
stationary generators may account for the main characteristics of human alpha EEG fields. To this end they hope to
present a model of scalp EEG fields utilizing a minimal number of generators, the strength and location of which is described as a function of time.

topography
alpha
 frequency
generators

C 39.   Lehmann, D.: Topography of spontaneous alpha EEG fields
in humans. *Electroencephalogr Clin Neurophysiol, 30*:161,
1971 (abstr).

Spontaneous EEG activity was recorded simultaneously from
many points on the scalp of normal human subjects, using
a forty-eight-channel amplifying and recording system. The
data were transformed into sequences of equipotential maps,
constructed in short intervals (e.g. 1, 4 or 8 msec). These
maps show the distribution of potential fields on the scalp.
The location of the positive and negative maximal values of
each map were plotted to study changes of the spatial distribution of the potential fields. Further, the average amplitude
per electrode in each map was plotted. The average amplitude increases when the maps have a pronounced relief and
decrease when there is a flat field distribution. During 10/sec
alpha EEG spindles, the average amplitude exhibits periodic
fluctuations of 20 cps. At about the peak time of one cycle,
the positive maximum resides in the precentral-central area,
and the negative maximum is occipital; the next cycle shows
inverted polarities, and so on. A common spatial pattern of
sequential field distributions during EEG alpha spindles
shows three preferred scalp areas for the location of EEG

topography
alpha
 amplitude
alpha phase
variability
generators

field maxima; left occipital, right occipital and precentral-central. The field maxima step clockwise or counterclockwise from area to area. Typically, the map relief is pronounced when the field maxima reside within the preferred areas; relief is flat when the maxima are between preferred areas. The value of the potential field oscillates at 10 cps in each of the three areas with phase lags; the smallest phase lag usually exists between the two occipital areas. This sequence of EEG field distribution during spontaneous alpha spindles may be compared with fields produced by three coupled oscillators.

C 40.   Sorel, L.: A comparative study of basal rhythms in man using bipolar and vertical montages. *Electroencephalogr Clin Neurophysiol, 30:*248, 1971.

The author used a twenty-four-channel EEG machine to record cerebral electrical activity simultaneously from classical bipolar montages and from unipolar vertical montages with reference to an indifferent electrode placed on the neck. Some three hundred normal subjects, and 7,700 patients with a variety of diseases, were studied by this means, and three categories emerged from those who had a basal rhythm of alpha type at a rate of 8 to 12 cps and responding normally to eye-opening. Results: (1) the records obtained by the two methods were obviously similar; (2) a difference was caused by the presence of a rhythm recordable from the reference electrode on the neck; (3) a further apparent difference existed because of the presence in some cases of a basal rhythm in the anterior and middle regions of the head on vertical montage which was not seen on conventional bipolar recordings because of the frequent areas of isopotentiality found with this technique. It thus appears that the alpha rhythm is in fact confined to the posterior head regions in only 25 percent of cases. In the majority, the basal rhythm has a "skullcap" distribution, predominant in the central and even anterior regions, and is reactive in all areas to eye-opening. This idea, which had a purely technical basis (amplitude gradients, phase reversal of sine waves) was confirmed by four groups of tests. The basal rhythm, in normal physiological conditions, seems to be predominant in parieto-cen-

topography
alpha phase
psychopathology
brain damage
epilepsy
physical illness

tral regions. An occipital or occipital-neck localization is not apparently pathological although it is less common. On the contrary, a forward spread of the basal rhythm, which at the same time continues to react normally to eye-opening, is found (if the basal rhythm is of normal frequency) in psychopathological disturbances and (if the basal rhythm is slowed) in inter-ictal epileptic dysfunction and various organic diseases.

C 41. Otto, E., and Kobryn, U.: Asymmetry of the quantity and maximum voltage level of 8/s to 13/s waves in homologous derivations of the electroencephalogram of healthy probands. *Psychiatr Neurol Med Psychol (Leipz), 21:287, 1969.*

Under standard conditions the EEG's of one hundred healthy subjects were recorded using four electrode montages. Histograms of the percentage quantity of 8 to 13 cps waves were made. Two subjects showed the greatest alpha activity over the precentral region in the monopolar derivations. Statistically significant asymmetry of the alpha waves was found in sixteen cases. (Wilcoxon's test at 5% level). Dominance of the right to left was 13.3 and there was no relation to handedness. The maximum alpha wave voltage was significantly higher in the right hemisphere in nineteen cases and higher in the left hemisphere in three cases. (Wilcoxon—P ⩽ 5%).

topography
alpha
symmetry
hemispheric
dominance

C 42. Shaw, J.C.: Measuring and recording EEG topography. *Electroencephalogr Clin Neurophysiol, 29:107, 1970 (abstr).*

The amplitude and pattern of EEG signals depend on the electrode sites from which they are derived. The measurement of this spatial dependence or topography has two important applications. The first is the detection of localized brain damage or dysfunction. The second is the study of the association between normal rhythms and mental activity. Because of the topographical organization of function in the cortex, it is reasonable to expect the spatial distribution of EEG activity to be related to mental activity, particularly when this requires direction of attention to one sensory or perceptual modality. The method described uses the activity recorded at one electrode site as a reference or template

topography
data
collection
mental tasks
hemispheric
dominance

signal and examines its distribution at the other sites. Three measures are used: the correlation coefficient, regression co-efficient and time difference. A small analogue computer has been programmed to compute running estimates of these measures for two channels at a time. Changes in these para-meters can then be monitored and related to other events. An EEG focus can be detected in the presence of generalized activity (noise) provided that the signal is available noise free as a template in at least one channel. The association between alpha rhythm distribution and mental activity is being studied, and it has been demonstrated that the change in alpha distribution produced by a mental arithmetic task differs from that caused by opening the eyes. Hemisphere differences in alpha rhythm timing relationships have also been confirmed. One development of the technique will be to measure the residual variance of activity at a test signal electrode when the contribution from surrounding reference signals has been partialled out. The residual activity may possibly represent the activity from the underlying cortex more closely. Another will be simultaneous multi-channel analysis to replace the present system which analyzes two channels at a time replayed from magnetic tape.

C 43.   Lippold, O.: Bilateral separation in alpha rhythm recording. *Nature, 226:459*, 1970.

When recorded at different locations on the scalp with the conventional systems of electrode placement, the waves of alpha rhythm tend to show a fairly high degree of correlation in their phase. It would be useful to know whether this correlation represents a true neuronal synchronization or whether it results from the inability to record separately the activity of different foci of alpha waves, because the po-tentials due to these foci are conducted for some distance over the scalp. Alpha waves have two main loci of phase reversal, bilaterally symmetrical over the occipital regions. A pair of electrodes moved in any line to pass through one of these loci will show such a phase reversal. In most individ-uals, the apparent foci of origin of alpha waves are about 5 cm lateral to the midsagittal plane and about 5 cm above

topography
measure-
ment
techniques
alpha
symmetry
phase

the inion. Two electrodes can be placed on any line struck from one of these two and thus should not record any activity from it. If the radius of the arc is 10 cm, the pair of electrodes can be placed across the field due to the opposite focus and will record maximally from this. It can be seen that, although a general correspondence exists in the onset and termination of the trains of potentials, waves can be present on either side of the head and not necessarily accompanied by waves on the opposite side. It is also clear that there is not any constant phase relation between the waves on the two sides and that the frequency is slightly different (usually by less than 0.5 Hz). The extent of the differences between the two sides varies among subjects; often the amplitude is consistently larger on one side (by a factor of 2 or 3) and in many cases the onset of the bursts of waves is always earlier on the one side.

C 44. Lehmann, D.: Multichannel topography of human alpha EEG fields. *Electroencephalogr Clin Neurophysiol, 31:439,* 1971.

For each of five adult subjects, at least thirty minutes of spontaneous resting EEG recording with eyes closed was taken (artifacts, etc., were edited before processing). Alpha wave epochs of 500 to 1000 msec were analyzed with a total of 2 to 7 sec of alpha activity for each subject. The data were transformed into equipotential field maps and the resultant field distributions were simple and showed one or two positive and negative maximal values per map. These values were located in three preferred areas: pre-vertex to parietal, left occipital and right occipital. Maximal values stepped clockwise or counterclockwise from area to area. Field values near ears were often discontinuous with surrounding areas but were similar at both ears. Relief waxed and waned twenty times per second, and with successive peak values of the relief, the maximal field values alternated between anterior and posterior locations. The data seems to suggest that the assumption of three semi-independent, stationary generators, each oscillating at about 10 cps, can account for the major properties of the alpha fields observed here.

topography
data analysis
generators

C 45. Lehmann, D.: Scalp EEG field topography in humans. *Electroencephalogr Clin Neurophysiol, 31:*288, 1971 (abstr).

EEG data were transformed into equipotential maps of field distributions. Orbits of positive and negative field maxima were plotted demonstrating continuous or stepwise location changes. General rules for analysis were: underlying generators are easily located for simple concentric fields as under the maximum field value and average field value per electrode indicates relief for equidistant electrodes. Using these ideas, it was seen that one central and two occipital field maxima were present during alpha activity with the maxima stepping clockwise or counterclockwise between locations. In averaged visual responses, simultaneous, bilateral maxima were observed occipitally, indicating activity in both hemispheres. After 150 msec, evoked distributions resembled spontaneous fields. Concentric fields were found for regular spike and wave patterns. Field distributions during sleep slow waves were complex and asymmetrical.

topography
data
 analysis
generators

C 46. Cooper, R., and Mundy-Castle, A.C.: Spatial and temporal characteristics of the alpha rhythm: A toposcopic analysis. *Electroencephalogr Clin Neurophysiol, 12:*153, 1960.

A twenty-two-year-old male with a 9.75 cps stable alpha rhythm of medium voltage of about 20 μv from the parieto-occipital area was used to investigate relations between initiation of voluntary movement and phase of the alpha rhythm. A six-channel EEG, Walter automatic frequency analyzer and a B.N.I. helical scan toposcope were used during all experiments. Although no significant relations between movements and phase were found, two main categories of antero-posterior spato-temporal distributions were found. In one, the instant of maximal amplitude of alpha waves became progressively later or earlier depending upon nearness of the electrode to the occiput. In the other, maximal amplitude occurred simultaneously in all channels but usually with a sign change over occipital areas. Extra interhemispheric synchrony was seldom seen. An overall explanatory theory of the nature and generation of alpha activity is also presented.

topography
motor per-
 formance
alpha
 synchrony
instruments
theory
generators

SECTION D

DEVELOPMENT

GENETICS

D 1. Dieker, H., and Lauschner, E.: Studies on the genetics of particularly regular alpha waves of high amplitude in the EEG of man. *Humangenetik, 4*:189, 1967.

Four monozygotic and two dizygotic pairs of twins who carried this EEG pattern were examined. The brain wave patterns of thirty-five families, consisting of 146 persons, were analyzed. These families had been chosen from an unselected series of propositi. The Motokawa method for the quantitative determination of the regularity of the alpha waves was modified for the interpretation. This method offered the possibility of showing a positive correlation between the average amplitude of the EEG and its regularity. The monozygotic pairs of twins proved to be concordant, the dizygotic were discordant. Hence, a genetic basis of this characteristic is assumed. The results of the family investigations gave some indications for an autosomal dominant mode of inheritance; at least one parent of each propositus had also an unusually regular, high-voltaged alpha EEG, about half of the siblings showed the trait and there was no sex difference. No correlation was found between the EEG trait and somatic or constitutional properties. On the other hand, a correlation with personality is possible, as marriages between persons with the EEG trait were more frequent than expected.

genetics
alpha
   amplitude

D 2. Young, J.P.R., Lader, M.H., and Fenton, G.W.: A twin study of the genetic influences on the electroencephalogram. *J Med Genet, 9*:13, 1972.

Thirty-two male twin pairs (17 monozygotic and 15 dizygotic; 19 to 40 years old) were recorded for EEG to determine the similarity of EEG patterns between twins and the extent to which genetic characteristics influence the EEG. Alpha index, alpha amplitude, amplitudes of activity in frequency

genetics
alpha
   patterns
EEG
   patterns

bands ranging from 2.3 to 4.0 Hz to 13.5 to 26.0 Hz, the duration of the alpha blocking response, and the latency of the visual evoked response were measured to determine EEG similarities. Correlations between monozygotic twins were significant for all variables except the amplitude of the 2.3 to 4.0 Hz activity. Only two of the correlations reached significance for the dizygotic group; amplitude of 13.5 to 26.0 Hz activity and evoked response latency. The authors concluded that there is a significant genetic contribution to EEG pattern.

D 3.   Vogel, F.: The genetic basis of the normal human electroencephalogram. *Humangenetik, 10:*91, 1970.

The genetic basis of the normal human electroencephalogram (EEG) was analyzed. Twin investigations showed complete concordance for most EEG characteristics in monozygotic twins of all age groups. Differences in high age include focal abnormalities and dysrhythmic groups. These differences failed to show a relation to mental performance. For a number of special EEG variants, population frequencies were determined, and the mode of inheritance was established. The following variants were analyzed: (1) variants of the alpha rhythm including low voltage EEG (simple autosomal dominance), borderline cases of the low voltage EEG (mixed genetic basis), quick (16 to 19/sec) alpha variants (simple autosomal dominance), slow (4 to 5/sec) alpha variants (mode of inheritance still unknown; behavioral abnormalities), and monotonous alpha waves (probably simple autosomal dominance) and (2) the EEG with beta waves including differences in relation to age and sex (beta waves are especially frequent in elderly women), certain types of beta groups in frontal and precentral leads showing simple autosomal dominant mode of inheritance, and diffuse beta waves, the general model of multifactorial inheritance in combination with a threshold effect seemed to be appropriate. Difficulties of the analysis are mentioned, and some theoretical and practical aspects of the results are discussed.

genetics
alpha
  patterns
beta

D 4.   Dumermuth, G.: The use of variance spectra for a quantitative comparison of the EEG in twins. *Helv Paediatr Acta,* *24:*45, 1969.

Numerical spectrum analysis provides a powerful modern tool for analyzing and quantifying EEG data, especially background activity. This paper presents digitally computed variance spectra of the resting EEG of a small series of monozygotic and dizygotic juvenile twins. The study shows that the statistical properties of the background activity in the centroparietal and parieto-occipital regions in the waking state may be considered as genetically determined.

genetics
EEG
 patterns

MATURATION

D 5.   Churchill, J.A., Grisell, J., and Darnley, J.D.: Rhythmic activity in the EEG of newborns. *Electroencephalogr Clin Neurophysiol, 21*:131, 1966.

Rhythmic 7 to 12/sec activities, in several ways simulating alpha activity of adults, was observed in 313 out of 717 EEG's of newborns. Newborns delivered with their heads positioned right occiput anterior, transverse, or posterior showed greatest amounts of alpha-like activity in right hemisphere leads, whereas infants born left occiput transverse or posterior showed greatest activity on the left. Compression of one hemisphere during birth may depress the electrical activity, the hemisphere at risk being determined by the position of the head. Infants born under circumstances which were potentially brain injuring, such as breech or cesarean section during labor, less often showed this alpha-like activity than infants born by uncomplicated vertex delivery or cesarean section performed before labor. No relationship between the Apgar index for asphyxia, or predelivery sedation given the mother, and alpha-like activity was observed. The Shepovalnikov hypothesis that a larval alpha rhythm already exists at birth deserves consideration although further work is required to prove conclusively that the newborn alpha-like activity is not an artifact.

maturation
origins
brain
 damage

D 6.   Berhard, C.G., and Skoglund, C.R.: On the alpha frequency of human brain potentials as a function of age. *Skand Arch Physiol, 82*:178, 1939.

The EEG's of two hundred subjects from four months to *maturation*
thirty years were investigated for alpha frequency. Numer- *alpha*
ous plots and graphs are presented, but the general finding *frequency*
was a continuous increase in frequency with increasing age.
A mathematical interpretation was attempted and Brody's
growth curve proved best suited. Observations seem to indicate different phases in the development process, and the
authors warn against attaching undue significance to their
mathematical correlations. It is suggested that further correlations of this data to anatomical and physiological data of
development would be useful, remembering that some cortex
layers necessary to produce alpha activity are not fully developed histologically until ages eighteen to twenty years.

D 7.   Olofsson, O., and Petersén, I.: The development of the EEG
        in childhood. *Electroencephalogr Clin Neurophysiol, 32:*
        710, 1972 (abstr).

It was the aim of this study to describe the development of *maturation*
the EEG in relation to age and sex in normal children. EEG *alpha*
data were collected which can be used for the evaluation of *frequency*
normal values within the framework of different states of *alpha*
illness in children. The investigation was carried out in the *responses*
form of a cross section and is based on EEG records of 743
children (389 girls and 354 boys) and 185 adolescents (94
females and 91 males). The probands were not related. In
selecting them, thirteen criteria were used for normality.
The history of all probands was checked three times. Besides the waking EEG at rest, in at least 80 percent of the
children and 100 percent of the adolescents the EEG was
recorded during hyperventilation, photic stimulation and
sleep. From the point of view of development, the following
patterns were especially interesting: alpha rhythm, nonrhythmic activity of low frequency, rhythmic 2.5 to 4.5 cps
posterior activity, rhythmic 6 to 7 cps anterior activity, mu
rhythm, 14 and 6/sec positive sharp waves, and paroxysmal
EEG activity in general. Also reactions to hyperventilation
and photic stimulation of a nonparoxysmal kind showed a
clear dependence on development. Compared with normal
children, normal adolescents showed less sex difference and
no age differences. This is possibly the expression of a

maturation process coming to an end. Before final assessments can be made as to whether the recorded EEG findings can be regarded as normal findings of healthy individuals, longitudinal investigations should be carried out in healthy individuals with repeated EEG records and psychological tests.

D 8. Mizuno, T., Yamauchi, N., Watanabe, A., et al.: Maturation patterns of EEG basic waves of healthy infants under 12 months of age. *Tohoku J Exp Med, 102:*91, 1970.

A simplified method for an evaluation of maturation patterns of the EEG waves of healthy infants under twelve months of age is reported. The EEG basic waves were divided into ten bands according to frequency ranges (I-X bands). An averaged integrated voltage was calculated at each of the frequency bands (I-E%, II-E%, I-E%). When R = (E% of VIII + E% of IX) / (E% of II + E% of III) was calculated and plotted against the age in months, a linear figure was obtained which demonstrated a maturation pattern of the EEG basic waves of infants with advance in age.

EEG
maturation
frequency

D 9. Zislina, N.N., and Tyukov, V.L.: Age-specific changes in the frequency-spectrum of the electroencephalogram in 3-8 yr. old children. *Zh Vyssh Nerv Deiat, 18:*293, 1968.

One hundred and sixty-four subjects (twenty-three 3- to 4-year-olds, sixty-six 5- to 6-year-olds, seventy-five 7- to 8-year-olds) were used to develop criteria to assess EEG's of children in the course of histographic analysis of changes with increasing age over the entire EEG frequency range. Histographic analysis of the occipital, central and frontal areas reveals a quantitative picture of the changes observed. The dominant rhythm in the occipital region varied from 7.5 cps at three to four years to 9 cps at seven to eight years. A drop of four to five times was seen in the number of oscillations between 4 and 7 cps by eight years. A similar drop was not observed in the anterior cortical areas. Two separate foci of rhythmic activity were seen: (1) occipital alpha activity from 7 cps at three to four years to 9 cps at eight years; and (2)

maturation
EEG
frequency
theta

theta waves in the central cortical areas from 4 cps at 3 to 4 years to 7 cps at eight years.

D 10.   Metcalf, D.R.: Some critical points in normal EEG ontogenesis. *Electroencephalogr Clin Neurophysiol, 30:*163, 1971.

During normal EEG ontogenesis, there are "nodal points" which interlock with other aspects of development. The discontinuous EEG of immaturity, best seen in sleep and NREM sleep, usually disappears by one month. Associated sharp and slow bursts, normal to age three weeks, are attenuated by five weeks. Vertex dominant 12 to 14/sec sleep spindles appear by five to seven weeks, preceded by continuous small amplitude 16 to 18 cps rudimentary spindles. Spindles often are sharp, large amplitude and prolonged at two to four months; eight to ten second duration spindle bursts are rare after five months. After approximately three months, infants fall asleep directly into NREM sleep, rather than REM sleep, as is the case earlier. Sleep and awake behaviors become predictably associated with physiological measures (EEG, EOG, EMG and Resp.) at this time. Stage 3-4 sleep becomes separately differentiated after approximately four months. Spontaneous K complexes first appear at five months and develop rapidly until one year, after which development slows. At three years, K complexes, spindles and sleep rhythms are orderly. From three to nine years, "distortions" of spindles and K complexes normally occur. Distortions include intermingled K's and spindles, vertex spikes, spikes intermingled with K's and spindles; all may occur as generalized paroxysms. Maximal incidence is at five to seven years. "Distortions" may resemble "epileptiform" discharges. They are rare under age two and over age twelve years. Distorted sleep patterns are best evaluated with scalp-to-scalp montages which differentiate vertex from temporal or occipital activity.

maturation
EEG
patterns

D 11.   Pond, D.A.: The development of normal rhythms. In Hill, J.D.N., and Parr, G. (Eds.) : *Electroencephalography.* London, MacDonald, 1963, p. 193.

This article recounts and summarizes the research which has *maturation*
been done concerning the development or brain electrical *EEG*
activity. It is concluded that very little is presently known *patterns*
about the physiological basis and psychophysiological effects
of this area of development.

D 12.   Pechstein, J.: Konstanz des theta-alpha-medianwertes (TAM-
Wertes) im kindlichen EEG-frequenzspektrum bei geöffne-
ten und geschlossenen augen. *EEG-EMG (Stuttg), 1:*107,
1970.

The theta-alpha-median (TAM value) has been demon- *maturation*
strated as an important measure of the dominant occipital *children*
background EEG activity in infants of less than two years. *alpha*
The present study was made to determine the value of the *frequency*
TAM measure in children between four and twelve years. *theta*
Visual frequency analysis was made of the waking-EEG
under both eyes-open and eyes-closed conditions. Although
both behavior and spectral values changed considerably,
TAM values remained about the same for each child under
the conditions. The authors suggest that there may be a
check system of vigilance and this could control the balance
of theta-alpha wave production.

D 13.   Pechstein, J., and Dolansky, J.: Zur methodik der visuellen
frequenzanalyse des Wach-EEG im fruhen Kindesalter. *EEG-
EMG (Stuttg), 1:*35, 1970.

Although the increasing frequency of occipital rhythm from *maturation*
theta to alpha frequencies during childhood represents a *data analysis*
criterion of bioelectric development of the CNS, no standard, *alpha*
reproducible numeric limits of the frequency variation of *frequency*
this development exists. A new technique of interpretational *theta*
wave counting is described which also considers overlying
waves of different lengths. Records of two infants of different ages were evaluated by two different investigators ten
different times. Results showed the small error of the technique as well as the significance of the theta-alpha frequency
spectra (TAM value) in infants.

D 14. Pechstein, J.: Development of baseline activity of the EEG in early childhood. The theta alpha median value (TAM value) as a serviceable parameter of dominance in the waking EEG of the first 2 years of life. *Fortschr Med, 88:*1170, 1970.

A study was made of the frequency distribution in fifty-one EEG curves of healthy children below the age of two years, by means of a method of interpreting wave length measurements specially devised to overcome the difficulties in the evaluation of the mixed activity in the EEG of early childhood. In spite of considerable individual variability of particular frequencies, the different age groups showed frequent distribution patterns which could be adequately characterized and determined quantitatively by introduction of the TAM value. Subdivision into five age groups—three, six, twelve, eighteen and twenty-four months—showed a distinct age specificity of the TAM value with surprisingly little variability in each age group. The form of the age curve of the TAM values corresponds with that of the special development curve of the brain weight and may be regarded as a functional correlate of the morphological development of the CNS. It is concluded that the TAM value gives a development specific criterion suitable for comparative statistical studies of a stage of bioelectric development in the waking EEG of the young child. Further, the TAM value may be used as a new parameter of reference for the dominance of the baseline activity in the EEG. As early as eighteen months, the TAM value reaches the alpha sector of the frequency spectrum.

maturation data analysis EEG frequency theta

D 15. Pechstein, J.: The theta-alpha median value as a reliable measure of dominance in the waking EEG during early infancy. *Electroencephalogr Clin Neurophysiol, 30:*167, 1971 (abstr).

A special method was developed for the measurement and interpretation of wave lengths which paid special regard to the difficulties in dealing with mixed activity of the EEG in early infancy. With this technique fifty-eight EEG records of children of healthy families in the first two years were made

maturation data analysis theta

with respect to the distribution of frequencies. Although there was considerable individual scatter, it was noted that some frequencies showed recurrent patterns of distribution in the different age groups. These could be well characterized and given numerical values by the introduction of the theta-alpha median value ("TAM value"). By putting them into five age groups of three, five, twelve, eighteen and twenty-four months, one found a marked specificity for age of the TAM values and surprisingly little scatter in each age group. The curve of the TAM values corresponds in shape to the specific development curve of brain weight. There is no doubt that it can be regarded as functionally correlated with the morphological development of the CNS. The TAM value gives a specific numerical measure for comparative statistical investigations regarding the bioelectrical state of development in the waking EEG of young children. It also seems suitable for the determination of the dominant basic EEG frequency. The TAM value reaches at eighteen months the alpha range of the frequency spectrum. The application of TAM values will probably also be an advantage when methods of data processing become available by which an automatic frequency analysis of the EEG can be performed.

D 16. Schulte, F.J., and Bell, E.F.: Bioelectric brain development: An atlas of EEG power spectra in infants and young children. *Neuropädiatric, 4:*30, 1973.

Sequences of bioelectric brain development were followed in infants by frequency spectral analysis during different states and stages of sleep. Three sequences occurred regularly: (1) decreased spectral power over 5 Hz during the last few weeks before term; (2) occurrence of 12 to 14 Hz sleep spindle activity with high interhemispheric coherence at about ten weeks, increasing to peak power at 6 to 8 months, then decreasing; and (3) occurrence of hypnogogic theta with high interhemispheric coherence toward the end of the first year.

maturation
spectral
 analysis
sleep
alpha
 frequency
theta

D 17. Petersén, I., and Matousek, M.: EEG frequency analysis in healthy children (1-16 years) and adolescents (16-22 years). *Electroencephalogr Clin Neurophysiol, 32:*714, 1972 (abstr).

This study deals with EEG findings in normal children and adolescents (1 to 22 years) obtained by means of broad-band frequency analysis. All subjects were carefully selected. Besides the automatic analysis, the EEG records have been repeatedly evaluated by visual inspection. Age-dependent decrease of amplitudes in delta, theta and lower alpha frequency bands, together with increase of faster alpha activity, is described quantitatively. Statistically significant changes of total amplitudes (i.e. summated amplitudes of all frequency bands) and changes in amount of beta activity have been found only in younger age groups (1 to 16 years). Substantial differences may be obtained if the results are expressed in absolute values (i.e. as mean amplitudes in microvolts) or in relative values (i.e. in percentage). For instance, the amount of alpha (7.5 to 9.5 cps) activity decreases significantly with age, but its percentage increases simultaneously. The development of EEG activity proceeds faster in posterior areas and is slower in central areas. In general, age-dependent changes occur nearly linearly in children and almost logarithmically in adolescents. Inter-individual variability, asymmetry and anteroposterior differences tend to increase during maturation. Intra-individual variability (i.e. second-to-second fluctuations of amplitude as measured during the same examination) decreases with age. The dominating activity is characterized not only by larger amplitudes, but also by relatively higher intra-individual variability. This may be demonstrated even for theta activity but not for dominant delta activity in the youngest age group. Sex differences, larger amounts of beta activity in girls, have been statistically confirmed in the group of adolescents. Some well-defined differences between immature and mature but abnormal EEG's have been found. Theoretically, it may be possible to diagnose so-called maturation defects in this way. The correlation coefficient with age is highest in a theta/alpha quotient, where an empirically stated constant value is added to the denominator. The correlation is highest when compared with other studied parameters, independent of the EEG derivation used and of age category. Such a single parameter, or a proper combination of more parameters, seems to be useful for quantitative evaluation of the EEG.

maturation
children
adolescents
alpha
  frequency
alpha
  amplitude
alpha
  abundance
topography
variability
EEG
  patterns

D 18.   Eeg-Olofsson, O., and Petersen, I.: Sex differences in the

EEG of normal children and young persons aged 1 to 21 years. *Acta Paediatr Scand (Suppl), 206:95, 1970.*

The experiment involved 928 individuals—483 females and 445 males—in the ages of one to twenty-one years without mutual kinship. Sex differences were mainly found in childhood. A statistically significant positive correlation for girls was found with alpha frequency (1 to 15 years), rhythmic 2.5 to 4.5 cps activity in posterior derivations (2 to 7 years), and mu rhythm (2 to 14 years). In the case of boys, a statistically significant positive correlation was found with rhythmic 4 to 5 cps activity with posterior accentuation during drowsiness (1 to 2 years) and rhythmic 6 cps activity in anterior derivations also during drowsiness (4 to 14 years). The amount of more or less conspicuously asymmetrical theta activity with no clear relation to drowsiness was found statistically significantly more in boys than in girls in the ages one to eight years. In the ages nine to thirteen years there was no sex difference, while from fourteen to twenty-one years there was a statistical significant preponderance for girls. From eight years on girls showed significantly more paroxysmal responses to intermittent photic stimulation compared to boys. In these ages activation by intermittent photic stimulation was discontinued because of resulting effects significantly more in girls.

*maturation
children
adolescents
sex
differences
EEG
patterns*

D 19. Eeg-Olofsson, O.: The development of the electroencephalogram in normal children and adolescents from the age 1 through 21 years. *Acta Paediatr Scand (Suppl), 208:46, 1971.*

The present investigation has shown the significance of the fact that age and also, to a certain degree, sex must have primary consideration in the judgment of the EEG in children and adolescents.

*maturation
children
adolescents
EEG
responses*

D 20. Eeg-Olofsson, O.: The development of the electroencephalogram in normal adolescents from the age of 16 through 21 years. *Neuropädiatrie, 3:11, 1971.*

The age period investigated was sixteen through twenty-one years. The investigation was carried out as a transverse study and comprises EEG examinations on 185 adolescents—ninety-four females and ninety-one males. The material is described

*maturation
adolescents
EEG
patterns*

with regard to start of puberty, birth order and social family data. EEG was recorded at rest, during hyperventilation, and intermittent photic stimulation in all subjects. Sleep activation was successful in all but one female, who, however, attained deep drowsiness. The amount of nonrhythmic, low-frequency activity was estimated in the resting records, which were classified as having "minute" ("supernormal" EEG), "normal" ("normal" EEG), "slightly increased," and "moderately increased" amount of low frequency activity. The two last-mentioned findings occurred at 4.9 percent and significantly more often in females than in males. Observed rhythmic patterns at rest were slow alpha variant, polyphasic potentials, 5 to 6 Hz activity in (temporo-) occipital derivations, 6 to 7 Hz activity in anterior derivations during drowsiness, and mu rhythm.

D 21. Surwillo, W.W.: Human reaction time and period of the EEG in relation to development. *Psychophysiology, 8:*468, 1971.

Simple auditory reaction time (RT) and an auditory RT task requiring a disjunctive reaction were investigated in a group of 110 boys aged 46 to 207 months. Electroencephalograms (EEG's) were recorded during actual performance of these tasks to determine the extent to which differences in RT associated with development could be accounted for by developmental changes in the EEG. Measures of average EEG period were derived from peaks and troughs of all waves recorded in the time interval between stimulus and response of each trial. Results confirmed previous findings of a significant relationship between RT, auditory reaction time and development RT. Auditory reaction time followed a reciprocal power-law function with age, and hence both measures decreased more rapidly in the earlier years. Choice RT showed a more rapid decline with increasing age than simple RT. Correlations were high, with log simple RT versus log Age $= -.874$, and log choice RT versus log Age $= -.861$. Developmental changes in EEG period could account for only a small fraction of these high correlations. The possible role of EEG half waves as time quanta in information processing was discussed in relation to development.

maturation
reaction
time
EEG
frequency

HEMISPHERIC DOMINANCE

D 22.   Giannitrapani, D.: Attenuation of EEG in left and right-preferent subjects. *Proc of the 74th Ann of the APA,* 1966, p. 127.

Twelve left-preferent and twelve right-preferent subjects (mean age—25 years; 6 male and 6 female) were recorded for EEG's to relate laterality preference to brain hemisphere dominance. Eight equidistant anterioposterior comparisons were taken in each hemisphere as well as nine left-right comparisons between homologous scalp areas. Using devices developed by Darrow, no difference between left and right drawing conditions (eyes closed) was noted. Therefore, the average scores of these conditions were further analyzed by subtraction from the control (resting—eyes closed) scores and factorial analyses of variance. The resulting scores showed greater depression of EEG activity on the left side under all conditions (rest and drawing—both eyes closed), although attenuation scores between hemispheres for left-preferents were smaller in general. There was no mirror effect found. It is concluded that attenuation scores are not enough to determine and measure dominance, but that separate values for all EEG components may pin down brain area responsibility and uncover differential attenuation values among translateral comparisons which were masked in this experiment.

hemispheric dominance EEG symmetry

D 23.   Galin, D., and Ornstein, R.: Lateral specialization of cognitive mode: An EEG study. *Psychophysiology, 9:*412, 1972.

EEG asymmetry was studied in normal subjects during verbal and spatial tasks. Recordings were made from the left and right temporal and parietal areas, and the ratios of average power (1 to 35 Hz) in homologous leads T_4/T_3 and P_4/P_3 were computed. This ratio (right over left) was greater in the verbal tasks than in the spatial tasks. With this measure authors were able to distinguish between these two cognitive modes as they occur in normal subjects, using simple scalp recording.

hemispheric dominance EEG symmetry cognition

D 24.   Smyk, K., and Darwaj, B.: Dominance of a cerebral hemi-

sphere in electroencephalographic record. *Acta Physiol Pol,*
*23:*407, 1972.

Thirty-four of 166 people tested for dominance of cerebral *hemispheric*
hemisphere were also given EEG examinations to investigate *dominance*
the possible relationship between hemispheric dominance *alpha*
and asymmetry of alpha amplitude. Recordings from the *amplitude*
parieto-occipital area showed that the dominant hemisphere
exhibits a decrease in alpha amplitude. Results also showed
the EEG evaluation to be a much better indicator of cerebral
or hemispheric dominance when compared with the other
test methods applied.

AGING

D 25.   Otomo, E.: Electroencephalography in old age: Dominant
alpha pattern. *Electroencephalogr Clin Neurophysiol, 21:*
489, 1966.

EEG's of 1007 subjects and patients sixty years and over were *aging*
analyzed with special reference to the pattern of the domi- *alpha*
nant alpha waves. The difference in mean value of the fre- *frequency*
quencies of the dominant alpha waves in normal subjects
(9.47 + 1.73 cps) and in neurological patients (8.65 + 1.64
cps) was statistically significant. The mean values of frequencies of the dominant alpha waves tend to decrease significantly with increasing decade after the seventh decade.
No significant difference in mean values and in the distribution curves of the frequencies of the dominant alpha waves
were noted in normotensive and in the hypertensive subjects.

D 26.   Morozova, T.V.: A correlational analysis of the frequency of
alpha rhythms in the EEG of normal aging individuals and
in patients with geriatric psychoses. *Zh Nevropatol Psikhiatr,*
*70:*1667, 1970.

EEG analysis of eighty-five normal subjects and ninety-eight *aging*
patients over sixty years of age and suffering from various *alpha*
psychoses of old age revealed that alpha frequency decreased *frequency*
with age. Whether young or old, Early schizophrenia showed *psychoses*
no significant difference in alpha rhythm frequency from

normal subjects. Also alpha and duration of the disease did not seem to be related. Patients suffering from vascular psychosis did exhibit a lower frequency of alpha activity than the controls when ages were similar. A negative connection between alpha frequency with age and duration of disease was found in this latter group.

D 27. Kanowski, S.: EEG and geriatric psychiatry. *Electroencephalogr Clin Neurophysiol, 30:*268, 1971 (abstr).

The literature on the relationship between aging and EEG patterns was reviewed. After fifty years the EEG tends to become more variable, beta activity increases, alpha slows and there is an increase in the intermixture of theta and delta frequencies. In severely disturbed patients there appears to be a correlation between slowing of alpha, generalized theta and delta waves and the degree of intellectual capacities along with certain affective-emotional disturbances.

aging
EEG
frequency

D 28. Matousek, M., Volavka, J., Roubicek, J., and Roth, Z.: EEG frequency analysis related to age in normal adults. *Electroencephalogr Clin Neurophysiol, 23:*162, 1967.

The EEG's of 106 normal subjects were recorded to study the relation between EEG frequency and age in the adult population. The recordings were checked visually, and activity from two frontal and two temporoparietal leads was analyzed by a broad-band frequency analyzer. Coefficients of correlation and regression between frequency analysis outputs and age were derived. It was found that while delta, theta and alpha activity decreased significantly in quantity with age, the quantity of beta activity increased but not significantly. Thus, the beta/alpha ratio also increased significantly with age, and due to the divergent behavior of the numerator and denominator described above this ratio seems to be a somewhat constant and reliable indicator of age changes. No significant difference was seen between correlation coefficients for the frontal versus the temporoparietal recordings. It is felt that results of this study could be of value in clinical electroencephalography.

aging
data analysis
EEG
frequency
theta
beta

D 29. Gerson, I.M., and Chat, E.: Electroenchephalographic studies on the aging process: Psychometric correlates. *J Am Geriatr Soc, 15*:185, 1967.

Based on the literature and a study on 493 subjects, this paper presents tentative generalizations about the EEG in elderly people. These generalizations include: (1) slow-wave foci are found mainly over temporal areas (principally on the left side) in both the intellectually impaired with physical disease and the intellectually normal with physical disease, but slow-wave foci in combination with diffuse EEG abnormalities were seen chiefly in intellectually impaired people; (2) the alpha waves decrease in frequency in the aged and tend toward decreased amplitude and percent time present; (3) fast beta activity is prominent to age eighty, after which it decreases; and (4) 6 cps or less diffuse slow-wave activity is rare in the aged, but a 7 to 8 cps alpha rhythm is more common. It is recommended that deteriorative forces such as neurohormonal and general metabolic diseases should be considered in future aging process studies. Cerebral arteriosclerosis among psychiatric patients was mentioned here as a possible source of diffuse slow-wave abnormalities. However, it is cautioned that these deteriorative relationships do not apply to all EEG findings in elderly persons, and that in some cases such diffuse slow activity may be insignificant.

aging
EEG
patterns
alpha
frequency
physical illness
theta
beta

D 30.   Wang, H.S., and Busse, E.W.: EEG of healthy old persons—A longitudinal study. I. Dominant background activity and occipital rhythm. *J Gerontol, 24*:419, 1969.

Fifty-five elderly volunteers leading active lives and free from illness were recorded for EEG over a three- to four-year period to investigate changes in dominant background activity and occipital rhythms with respect to age, sex, race and socioeconomic factors. Results showed: (1) fast activity was more common in early than in late senescence; (2) age and occipital rhythm frequency are negatively correlated; (3) occipital rhythm in females tended to a faster frequency and higher amplitude than in males, and (4) low socioeconomic status related to more beta activity. In some cases two demographic factors were seen to interact and cause

aging
EEG
patterns
alpha
frequency
beta

greater effects than either alone. No EEG variable proved to be significantly related to race, and percent-time of occipital rhythm was independent of age, sex, race and socioeconomics. The authors feel that control of demographic factors and health states in studies of senescent EEG's is required.

D 31. Surwillo, W.W.: The relation of response time variability to age and the influence of brain wave frequency. *Electroencephalogr Clin Neurophysiol, 15:*1029, 1963.

One hundred subjects were monitored for response time variability and average EEG frequency during the time between stimulus and response in order to investigate the possible influence of brain wave frequency on increased variability of response time with age. Earlier reports of a positive correlation between reaction time variability and age were paralleled but no basis involving within-subject period variability could be found. However, this correlation disappeared when the average brain wave period was held constant by partial correlation. Assuming that the brain wave cycle is the basic unit of time in the organization of simple behavior, differences in response time variability are seen as natural results of differences in brain wave period.

aging
reaction
time
EEG
frequency

D 32. Obrist, W.D., et al.: Relation of the EEG to intellectual function in senescence. *J Gerontol, 17:*197, 1962.

The relationship between EEG and intelligence scores was explored in a community of elderly subjects. No significant relationships were found in volunteer subjects, but in old-age-home residents and hospital elderly, low intelligence scores tended to be associated with diffuse slowing of the EEG and a slow alpha rhythm. Performance test results correlated better with the EEG than did results of verbal tests. State of health was felt to be another important factor.

aging
intelligence
EEG
patterns

D 33. Otomo, E., and Tsubaki, T.: Electroencephalography in subjects 60 years and over. *Electroencephalogr Clin Neurophysiol, 20:*77, 1966.

Six hundred and fifty EEG's were examined in 466 normal subjects and patients over sixty years old. Abnormal EEG's were observed in 32.7 percent of normal subjects and in 44.5 percent of neurologically normal cases. The incidence of EEG abnormalities tended to augment with increasing decades in neurologically normal cases. The existence of high blood pressure did not seem to influence the incidence of EEG abnormalities either in neurological or non-neurological cases. In hemiplegic and hemiparetic patients who had survived more than one year after the apoplectic attack, EEG's were normal in 14.5 percent and 27 percent respectively. No difference in the incidence of abnormal EEG was noted between right and left side paralysis; however, the correlation of the side showing more prominent EEG changes with the clinically paralyzed side was significantly higher in right-sided than in left-sided paralysis in right-handed subjects. Alpha blocking was noted in 57.6 percent of neurologically normal subjects, decreasing significantly with increasing decade after the sixth, and was significantly lower in neurological patients than in subjects with no neurological manifestations. "Flat" EEG's were found in 8.6 percent of neurologically normal subjects and their incidence tended to decrease with increasing decade after the sixth. No significant difference was noted between neurologically normal and abnormal cases. The buildup after hyperventilation was poor in general, and was absent in 73 percent of 401 cases.

aging
EEG abnormalities
alpha blocking
neurologic problems

PHYSIOLOGIC INFLUENCES

ANS

E 1.   Surwillo, W.W.: The relation of amplitude of alpha rhythm to heart rate. *Psychophysiology, 1:*247, 1965.

Ninety-nine male subjects were used as subjects in an analysis of the relationship between heart rate and alpha amplitude in a reaction time response situation. A low arousal condition was defined as one in which a subject was told to press a key whenever a 250 Hz tone was presented. A high arousal condition was defined as one in which subjects were told to respond as quickly as possible. Under these conditions the author reported no inverted U functional relation between heart rate and alpha amplitude. Individual data presented appear to show some relationship but no statistical analysis was presented.

ANS
heart rate
alpha
  amplitude
arousal
reaction
  time

E 2.   Stennett, R.G.: The relationship of alpha amplitude to the level of palmar conductance. *Electroencephalogr Clin Neurophysiol, 9:*131, 1957.

Thirty-one male subjects between the ages of seventeen and twenty-three were given an auditory tracking task while sitting blindfolded. EEG's and skin conductance levels were recorded for the three- to four-hour session under task conditions which were designed to create different levels of arousal. The tasks involved resting, performance under a zero reward contingency performance with a twenty-five cent reward for each correct response, and performance in a condition where two to five dollars and shock avoidance were used as reinforcement. The overall relationship established between alpha amplitude and skin conductance was an inverted U which the author used to account for the failure of some investigators to obtain consistant correlations between alpha and skin conductance measures.

ANS
GSR
alpha
  amplitude
arousal
auditory
  stimula-
  tion
motivation

E 3.   Sulg, I.A., and Ingvar, D.A.: Correlation between regional
        cerebral blood flow (rCBF) and EEG frequency spectrum.
        *Electroencephalogr Clin Neurophysiol, 27:*617, 1969.

        One hundred and sixteen neurological patients were used in   *ANS*
        an analysis of the relationship between the frequency spectra *cerebral*
        of the EEG and cerebral blood flow rate. Positive correlations   *blood flow*
        were found between mean EEG frequency and rate of blood   *alpha*
        flow to both the gray and white matter of the brain with the   *frequency*
        flow to the gray matter having the highest correlation with
        frequency.

E 4.   Faber, J., Tuhacek, M., and Mestan, J.: Synchronization of
        EEG activity with respiration. *CS Neurol, 33:*296, 1970.

        A comparison of EEG recordings with respiration rhythms   *ANS*
        was made on thirty-five patients (20 normal and 15 neu-   *respiration*
        rotics). Using graphic summation techniques for analysis the   *EEG*
        neurotics showed an irregularity and lack of synchronization   *synchrony*
        between EEG and respiration.   *neuroses*

E 5.   Surwillo, W.W.: Relation of latency of galvanic skin reflex
        to frequency of the electroencephalogram. *Psychon Sci, 1:*
        303, 1967.

        Forty-two male subjects were selected on the basis of having   *ANS*
        well-developed resting alpha rhythms, over twenty-five micro- *reaction*
        volts peak-to-peak, greater than 75 percent of the time. Sub-   *time*
        jects were required to press a key in response to a 250 Hz   *GSR*
        tone for twenty trials. GSR latency and EEG alpha period   *alpha*
        were found to be positively correlated while reaction time   *frequency*
        was found to be unrelated to these measures.

E 6.   Darrow, C.W.: Problems in the use of the galvanic skin re-
        sponse (GSR) as an index of cerebral function: implications
        of the latent period. *Psychophysiology, 3:*389, 1967.

        The author reviewed the findings on relationships between   *ANS*
        EEG activity and the occurrence of the GSR. Not all GSR's   *alpha*
        were found to be centrally mediated. Alpha blocking, which   *blocking*
        occurs to any attention-centering stimulus, precedes the GSR   *phase*
        during the latent period and acts as an indicator of central   *GSR*

nervous system involvement. The author noted that EEG phase relationships, particularly diphasic activity in the latent period, may prove to be more important as an indicator of central involvement in the GSR.

E 7. Darrow, C.W., Pathman, J., and Kronenberg, G.: Level of autonomic activity and electroencephalogram. *J Exp Psychol, 36:*355, 1946.

One hundred and twenty subjects having a resting systolic blood pressure greater than 110 mm Hg were used for an analysis of the relationships between EEG, skin resistance, systolic blood pressure, relative blood pressure, heart rate and respiration rate in a resting condition. There were negative correlations between EEG frequency and resting skin conductance levels and between EEG frequency and heart rate. There were positive correlations between EEG amplitude and resting skin conductance and EEG amplitude and heart rate. These correlations were in the opposite direction of findings when a person is responding to stimuli indicating a nonlinear relationship between EEG parameters and autonomic arousal.

ANS arousal EEG patterns

ENDOCRINE

E 8. Gupta, S.P., Gupta, P.C., Kumar, V. and Ahuja, M.M.S.: Electroencephalographic changes in hypothyroidism. *Indian J Med Res, 60:*1101, 1972.

Nine thyroid patients were studied by serial EEGs prior to and during thyroid replacement treatment. Eight patients showed increased alpha frequency from 8 cps to 9 cps. Significant correlations between frequency of alpha activity and (1) protein bound iodine (PBI) values and (2) half relaxation time measured by photomotogram were observed. Epileptiform activity was seen in three cases with no clinical correlate. Thus, EEG activity is of value in monitoring thyroid replacement therapy as well as in evaluating the effect of thyroid hormone deficiency on the central nervous system.

endocrine thyroid levels

E 9. Siersbaek-Nielsen, K., Hansen, J., Molholm, S.M., Kristensen, M., Stoier, M., and Olsen, P.Z.: Electroencephalographic changes during and after treatment of hyperthyroidism. *Acta Endocrinol (Kbh), 70:*308, 1972.

Thirty-two hyperthyroid patients with EEG abnormalities such as increase in alpha rhythm, slow rhythms, spikes and sharp waves and fast activity were studied for EEG activity and thyroid function before, during and after antithyroid treatment. EEG abnormalities and severity of hyperthyroidism were found to be statistically correlated and a slight decrease in the abnormalities occurred after treatment. These changes included normalizing of the dominant frequency within two weeks and disappearance of the large spikes and sharp waves. Although these decreases were small, except for the slow activity they were statistically significant. Furthermore, continued EEG abnormalities long after antithyroid therapy suggest that irreversible brain damage may result from hyperthyroidism.

endocrine
thyroid
levels
alpha
abundance

E 10.   Hermann, H.T., and Quarton, G.C.: Changes in alpha frequency with change in thyroid hormone level. *Electroencephalogr Clin Neurophysiol, 16:*515, 1964.

Eleven hyperthyroid and six hypothyroid subjects were tested for EEG frequency while in a comfortable, relaxed state. The subjects were given treatments for their thyroid conditions during the recording sessions to determine the relationships between changing thyroid levels and alpha frequency. The alpha frequency was found to be highly correlated with thyroid levels and changed as a function of changes in thyroid level in treatment as measured with protein-bound iodine and basal metabolism rate.

endocrine
thyroid
levels
alpha
frequency

E 11.   Garrel, S., Gautray, J.P., and Eberhard, A.: The numerical treatment of the EEG in the course of the spontaneous menstrual cycle and that induced by clomid. *Grenoble Medico-Chirurgical, 8:*331, 1970.

In observations of the EEG's of women at various stages in their menstrual cycle, variations in alpha and theta frequencies were noted. Variations in alpha were predominant in posterior areas while those in theta were predominant in anterior areas. A high level of theta activity occurred prior

endocrine
menstrual
cycle
alpha
frequency
theta

to ovulation, dropping to a low level following ovulation. Alpha was attenuated prior to ovulation, rising to a high level following ovulation.

E 12.   Gautray, J.P.: Quantitative analysis of EEG variations during spontaneous or restored menstrual cycle. *Neuroendocrinology, 5:*368, 1969.

Results of EEG analysis during the menstrual cycle included a predominance of theta waves before ovulation and depressed alpha activity during ovulation.

endocrine
menstrual
cycle
alpha
patterns
theta

E 13.   Sugarman, A.A., De Bruin, A.T., and Roth, C.W.: Quantitative EEG changes in the human menstrual cycles. *Res Commun Chem Pathol Pharmacol, 1:*526, 1970.

Twenty-three female subjects, eight using oral contraceptives and fifteen not, were measured for EEG amplitude through their menstrual cycle. The left occipital area was used for analysis. No differences were found between the two groups. The amplitude and variability of the EEG's were reduced during the second half of the menstrual cycle or during the premenstrual period. The authors hypothesized that EEG arousal accompanies feelings of premenstrual tension.

endocrine
menstrual
cycle
alpha
patterns
arousal

E 14.   Matousek, M., Volavka, J., and Roubicek, J.: Electroencephalogram in normal population. II. Influence of physiological changes on EEG. *CS Psychiatr, 63:*73, 1967.

The influence of age, drowsiness, anxiety, satiation, general conditions during examination and, in females, the interval from the last menstruation was studied using 109 normal subjects. A decrease in both slow and fast activity causes the ratio between them to be relatively constant. This ratio closely approximates results of visual EEG evaluations during which normality or abnormality are estimated and is therefore very important. Age influence proves to be less evident during visual evaluation of EEG's because of this constant ratio. Menstruation seemed to be associated with a

endocrine
menstrual
cycle
EEG
amplitude
theta

decrease of EEG amplitude and a relative increase in theta activity.

E 15. Roubicek, J., Tachezy, R., and Matousek, M.: Electrical activity of the brain in the course of the menstrual cycle. *CS Psychiatr, 64*:90, 1968.

Thirty-three females were used as subjects in a comparison of EEG characteristics and estrogen levels. Automatic frequency analysis of the EEG's revealed a shift occurring during the menstrual cycle. Decreased amplitude of all frequencies was observed as well as an increase in the incidence of alpha and theta in frontal areas of the brain during menstruation. The attenuation of alpha and theta activity was less than for other frequencies.

endocrine
menstrual
  cycle
EEG
  patterns
alpha
  abundance
theta

E 16. Gautray, J.P., Garrel, S., and Fau, R.: Electroencephalographic correlates of the human menstrual cycle. II. Results and discussion. *Acta Eur Fertil, 2*:15, 1970.

A correlation of presumed ovulation data with quantitative analysis of EEG variations during the menstrual cycle (spontaneous or restored by clomid therapy) showed theta activity (4 to 8 cps) to predominate prior to ovulation while alpha activity (8 to 12 cps) is lowest during this period. After ovulation theta waves decrease and alpha waves increase. A discussion of significance and new perspectives in clinical neuroendocrinology is included.

endocrine
menstrual
  cycle
theta

E 17. Vogel, W., Broverman, D.M., and Klaiber, E.L.: EEG responses in regularly menstruating women and in amenorrheic women treated with ovarian hormones. *Science, 172:* 388, April 1971.

Photic driving stimuli were presented to subjects at various points during the menstrual cycle or with varying levels of estrogen and progesterone administered. Estrogen alone was found to reduce the driving response while a combination of estrogen and progesterone enhanced the driving response to photic flicker.

endocrine
menstrual
  cycle
photic
  flicker

E 18. Fenton, G.W., Tennent, T.G., Comish, K.A., and Rattray, N.: The EEG and sex chromosome abnormalities. *Br J Psychiatr, 119:*185, 1971.

Twenty-two subjects with XXY, XYY, or XXYY chromosome abnormalities and twenty-two matched control subjects were recorded for EEG to determine parameters which would differentiate the groups. The abnormal group showed a higher incidence of EEG abnormalities including dominant rhythm below 8 Hz, marked asymmetries in background activity, spike and sharp wave patterns, theta activity and delta activity. The records associated with chromosome abnormalities were characterized by slow alpha, slow dominant frequencies, and an excess of theta activity. XXY and XYY patterns had equal incidence of abnormal EEG recordings.

endocrine
chromo-
somes
EEG abnor-
malities
alpha
frequency
theta
delta

STRESS

E 19. Kamp, A., Troost, J., and Van Rijn, A.J.: Influence of mental and physical stress on the alpha rhythm in normal subjects and patients (provisional communication). *TNO Nieuws, 25:*368, 1970.

A sixteen-channel EEG telemetering device was used to record EEG's from patients and normal subjects engaged in physical and mental tasks. EEG changes are provoked by alerting the subjects' behavioral conditions. Other recordings such as ECG, respiration and eye movement were made and a frequency analyzer quantified the data. Results showed shifts in the peak alpha activity related to the behavioral situation.

stress
motor per-
formance
mental tasks
telemetry

E 20. Turovskaya, Z.G.: Electroencephalographic changes during stress and its after effects. *Vopr Psikhologii, 16:*53, 1970.

Twenty subjects were studied during problem solving under frustrating conditions. It was found that: (1) beta activity changed very little; (2) alpha activity decreased under stress; and (3) theta waves increased, decreased, or did not change during stress and after stress depending upon the individual. The hypothesis that EEG changes under stress are a function of the type (Pavlovian) of nervous system was presented.

stress
mental tasks
alpha
abundance
beta
theta

E 21.   Gofman, S.S., and Freidin, Y.V.: Results of multichannel radioelectroencephalographic investigation of persons with nervous and emotional stress. *Bull Exp Biol, 70:*1242, 1970.

Changes in the electrical activity of the human brain during intensive mental activity when subjects are in a stress state were investigated in this experiment. Multichannel radio-electroencephalographic recordings were taken from ten subjects during examinations in physiology, history and mathematics. Results showed that a slow, high amplitude (60 to 90 μv, 11 to 13 cps) in the occipital region of one or both hemispheres dominated the EEG while the subjects with eyes open thought over their answer in preparation for a formal answer. Periodically, this was replaced by a lower amplitude and frequency rhythm or was totally extinguished and replaced by a low-amplitude activity. This desynchronized activity occurred most frequently in the middle or end of the preparation period, during tranquility. The interpretation of these findings is that, even though slow activity has been found to decrease during mental activity, unfavorable environmental factors contribute to the high-amplitude slow waves seen in this investigation. This slow rhythm is not felt to be a predominance of inhibitory processes but a sign of increased cortical and subcortical activity.

stress
mental tasks
EEG
  responses
alpha
  amplitude
data
  collection
telemetry

E 22.   Sawhney, B.B., and Singh, B.: Effects of mannitol on EEG rhythms in increased intracranial tension with specific reference to the alpha rhythm. *Neurol India, 16:*151, 1968.

Fifty-three patients with intracranial hypertension due to a variety of lesions were given treatments of 20 percent mannitol. In thirty-seven cases improved slow-wave activity was seen. Thirty-nine of forty-four cases studied for quantitative alpha activity using percent time and mean voltage showed improvement. It was postulated that the earliest EEG change in intercranial hypertension is deterioration of the alpha rhythm.

stress
physical
  illness
drugs
alpha
  frequency

VISUAL SYSTEM

E 23.   Shimazono, Y., Ando, K., Sakamoto, S., Tanaka, T., Eguchi, T., and Nakamura, H.: Eye movements of waking subjects with closed eyes. *Arch Gen Psychiatry, 13:*537, 1965.

Data from fifty normal subjects and fifty chronic schizophrenics at rest and following various types of stimulation
may be summarized as follows. From these observations it
may be concluded that schizophrenics seldom show slow
lateral movements, but frequently show rapid movements.
There was no significant correlation between the mean rate
of rapid, low amplitude (r-type) movement and the rating
scale of the clinical picture in schizophrenics. There was no
remarkable correlation between the mean rates of r-type eye
movements and the values of percentage time alpha of the
EEG for schizophrenics and normals. On the other hand,
we found a significant difference in the mean r rates distribution between both groups, but no remarkable difference in
percentage time alpha. Changes due to stimulation were less
demonstrable in schizophrenics than in normals, and were
sometimes paradoxical. However, this might be related to
the differences in the EOG pattern which existed between
these groups before stimulation. It was noted that findings
suggestive of tension and anxiety states were often obtained
in chronic schizophrenics who apparently seemed to be in a
nonanxious, deteriorated and indifferent state during this
study.

*visual
system
eye
movements
alpha
abundance
schizo-
phrenia*

E 24. Gaarder, K., Koresko, R., and Kropfl, W.: The phasic relation of a component of alpha rhythm to fixation saccadic eye
movements. *Electroencephalogr Clin Neurophysiol*, 21:544,
1966.

The two experimental variables—fixation saccadic (jump-
ing) eye movements and occipital alpha rhythm—have been
studied by simultaneous recording. Noting the quadrant of
alpha cycle during which a saccade occurs establishes a reliable concrete relationship between the occurrence of a saccade and a particular quadrant in some subjects. Use of
saccades to trigger a Mnemotron Computer of Averaged
Transients establishes that alpha-like activity in the evoked
response is phase-locked to saccades both before and after
the saccade. This was found in all twelve subjects studied
when alpha activity was present. Since the alpha-like component is phase-locked before as well as after a saccade, this
argues against the saccade as stimulus linearly causing the
locking, and points to the component pacing saccades or to

*visual
system
eye
movements
alpha phase*

both saccades and the component being paced by something else. The results are interpreted in the light of a model of visual information processing in which saccades generate discontinuous packets of edge information which are cycled as short-term templates at a rate reflected by the alpha component frequency.

E 25.   Gaarder, K., Alterman, A., and Kropfl, W.: The relation of the phase-locked fixation saccade-linked component of alpha rhythm to change of stimulus illuminance. *Psychon Sci, 5:* 445, 1966.

Systematic variation of the stimulus illuminance of a fixation target was carried out while recording fixation eye movements and EEG. The summated EEG activity following fixation saccadic eye movements was collected and it was found that the latencies of the alpha-like component of the summated activity did not vary significantly with stimulus change. The amplitude of the alpha-like activity did, however, follow the expected pattern of decreasing with increased stimulus illuminance.

visual system
eye movements
alpha patterns

E 26.   Kris, C.: EOG and EEG measurement while learning to position the eyes when the lids are open and closed. *Electroencephalogr Clin Neurophysiol, 24:*189, 1968 (abstr).

EEG and EOG recordings were made from (1) neonates and during the first four months; (2) four normally sighted adults while learning precision eye calibrations; (3) four recently blinded diabetics; and (4) three subjects before and after brain surgery. Results among group 1 showed a few binocularly coordinated eye movements, frequent divergent, noncoordinated, uni-ocular deviations and those who were premature had a higher incidence of spontaneous mystagmoid eye motions. Rotation-induced mystagmus was found in both full-term and premature subjects. The alpha wave EEG patterns were not associated with blinking and Bell's phenomenon in this group. Improved binocular coordination in older infants is thought to be due to visual feedback and practice in "looking." Both groups 2 and 3 were able to learn to position their eyes, (group 2 with eyes closed and

visual system
proprioception
eye movements
eye opening
biofeedback

with visual or verbal cues), and this suggests proprioceptive elements are involved in eye positioning. Alpha EEG activity was associated with upward motions of the eyes during slow blinks and with lids closed and also with eye positioning during eyes-open conditions in some subjects. Alpha-like activity disappeared after surgery in group 4 and prefrontal lobotomy also disorganized eye positioning capabilities.

E 27. Mulholland, T.B., and Peper, E.: Occipital alpha and accommodative vergence, pursuit tracking, and fast eye movements. *Psychophysiology, 8:*556, 1971.

The parieto-occipital EEG was recorded while subjects performed various fixation, accommodation and tracking maneuvers with stationary and moving targets. For some experiments the target was continuously in view and independent of the EEG; in others, a feedback path connected the occurrence of parieto-occipital alpha with the visibility of the target. The results show that alpha attenuation or blocking is not due to visual attention but to processes of fixation, lens accommodation and pursuit tracking. Saccadic movements were not reliably linked to alpha or alpha blocking. The utility of feedback methods for testing the hypotheses that visual control processes are linked to the parieto-occipital alpha rhythms was demonstrated.

visual system eye movements alpha blocking biofeedback

E 28. Berger, R.J., Olley, P., and Oswald, I.: The EEG, eye movements and dreams of the blind. *Q J Exp Psychol, 14:*183, 1962.

In a significant number of cases, a characteristic frontal EEG wave was found to precede rapid eye movements (REM) of dreaming. Three subjects who were blind for life or for extended periods of time did not have REM, but three others who were blinded for less than 15 years did exhibit such REM activity.

visual system eye movements dreams

E 29. Fenwick, P.B.C., and Walker, S.: The effect of eye position on the alpha rhythm. In Evans, C.R., and Mulholland, T.B. (Eds.). *Attention in Neurophysiology.* London, Butterworths, 1969, p. 128.

The authors investigated results of past work by Mulholland and Evans in which marked increases in alpha during eye movements in the upward direction were reported in a few subjects. In addition an explanatory model is discussed and a warning is issued against indiscriminant use of alpha activity as a measure of physiological state.

visual system
eye position
alpha abundance

E 30.   Mulholland, T., and Evans, C.R.: An unexpected artifact in the human electroencephalogram concerning the alpha rhythm and the orientation of the eyes. *Nature, 207:36, 1965.*

There is more alpha when open-eye position is up. Also, when the eyes are closed, normally the eyes relax upward. Thus the classic eyes-open and eyes-closed test for alpha may not in fact reflect reduced visual input as has been almost universally supposed, but rather some such rather prosaic variable as the tendency for eyes to turn upward under such conditions. Whether this is sufficient to account for all such differences seems unlikely, but it is now evident that (a) there is a need to re-evaluate previous experiments, and (b) no alpha work will be meaningful unless eye position is monitored.

visual system
eye position
alpha abundance

E 31.   Peacock, S.M., Jr.: Averaged "after-activity" and the alpha regeneration cycle. *Electroencephalogr Clin Neurophysiol, 28:287, 1970.*

EEG electrodes were placed on thirty subjects (adults and children) as for routine occipital placements to study relations between so-called after-activity and the alpha rhythm. Photic stimulation was used to induce the after-activity and the visual evoked response was averaged. Neither a buildup of averaged response and after-discharge in relation to the number of stimuli nor lateralization of this buildup was observed. After-activity was seen during a long flash, and, therefore, it cannot be an off response. Then, suggests the author, this after-activity seen readily in animals is not seen in the human occipital cortex, but instead, the alpha regeneration cycle is of sufficient stability to result in averaging of its stimulus-blocked regeneration.

visual system
visual stimulation
after-discharge
theory

E 32. Kooi, K.A., and Bagchi, B.K.: Observations on early components of the visual evoked response and occipital rhythms. *Electroencephalogr Clin Neurophysiol, 17*:638, 1964.

Twenty-nine males and six females who were free of any opthalmological or neurological problems were studied to see whether characteristics of the resting occipital EEG pattern could be used to anticipate variations in the form of visual evoked response. Results showed that the initial (35 to 60 msec) occipital surface negative wave had longer peak latency in subjects with (1) low voltage resting records and (2) low alpha persistence during response stimulation. Variation in amplitude of the occipital (80 to 110 msec) and occipital (100 to 140 msec) waves surface negative and positive respectively, seemed to parallel latency and was inversely related to the resting alpha frequency. Although the vertex sharp wave did not vary with respect to the resting alpha amplitude, incidence or frequency, it and the occipital waves surface negative (35 to 60 msec), positive (55 to 90 msec), negative (80 to 110 msec), and the positive (100 to 140 msec) were found to have longer latencies corresponding to higher amplitudes. Low orders of relationship were found but were expected by the authors for reasons detailed in the article. It is suggested that further studies would make clear the precise meaning of these results.

visual system visual evoked response alpha patterns

E 33. Aleksandrova, N.I.: On the relationship of indices of background alpha-activity in the human EEG to characteristics of the components of evoked potentials. *Probl Differentsial Psikhofiziol, 6*:84, 1969.

Characteristics of the components (amplitudes and latencies) of occipitally recorded evoked responses to photo stimulation (1 cps) and background alpha-rhythm indices (alpha-index, amplitude and frequency of alpha-rhythm) were studied in fifty subjects. Shorter latent periods for the II and IV evoked response components tended to correlate with low magnitude of alpha index and amplitude of alpha rhythm. Amplitudes of I to IV components were directly related to alpha rhythm amplitude, while a higher alpha rhythm frequency resulted in a shorter latent period of the I to IV components.

visual system visual evoked response photic flicker alpha patterns

E 34. Tulmay, K.U., and Nichols, D.J.: Fluctuations in target visibility as related to the occurrence of the alpha component of the electroencephalogram. *Vision Res, 7*:859, 1967.

visual system retinal images alpha abundance

Two subjects were given the task of reporting the presence or absence of visual images of a target stimulus under three experimental conditions. In the stabilized image condition, the target stimulus was presented through a device attached to a contact lens. Subjects reported spontaneous fading and reappearance of the image. In the second condition the target image was not consistent, with the eye free to move independently. The target was either blurred or dimmed until the subject reported fading. In the third condition the target was presented at threshold level so that it was reported present 50 percent of the time. A monopolar EEG recording was obtained from the right occipital electrode placement to determine the relationship between the alpha rhythm and the visibility of the target. In the stabilized viewing condition the disappearance of the image was preceded by the appearance of an alpha burst and the reappearance of the image was preceded by the termination of an alpha burst. In the second condition dimming the image to the disappearance point resulted in sharp bursts of alpha and the amount of alpha was inversely related to the brightness of the target image. In the third condition there was no relationship between the occurrence of alpha and target visibility. Not all alpha bursts resulted in target disappearances and not all alpha terminations resulted in target reappearance in the stabilized viewing condition.

E 35. Childers, D.G., and Perry, N.W.: Alpha-like activity in vision. *Brain Res, 25*:1, 1971.

visual system · after-discharge alpha patterns theory

Attempts were made to relate and integrate the diverse findings from experiments covering the spectrum of psychophysiological, EEG, visual evoked response, electroretinogram, ganglion cell response, and lateral geniculate body response, focusing upon responses evoked by visual stimuli. The relationship of the resonance and after-discharge phenomena to classical alpha rhythm and alpha-like activity is discussed. Various models and theoretical considerations advanced in the literature to explain these findings are considered.

E 36. Mulholland, T., and Evans, C.R.: Oculomotor function and the alpha activation cycle. *Nature, 211:*1278, 1966.

A biofeedback system which presented a light or tone when EEG alpha waves were present was utilized to study oculomotor functioning. Findings in five subjects showed more abundant alpha activity with eyes elevated in both eyes-open and eyes-closed conditions. Therefore, it is concluded that oculomotor function and the cortical or subcortical processes connected with the EEG alpha-activation cycle may be related. In particular, the alpha-activation cycle may in some way indicate eye movements, accommodation and position.

visual system biofeedback eye position alpha abundance

MISCELLANEOUS INFLUENCES

E 37. Elul, R.: Gaussian behavior of the electroencephalogram; changes during performance of mental task. *Science, 164:*328, April 1969. (Copyright 1969 by the American Association for the Advancement of Science) .

The probability distribution of the amplitude of scalp electroencephalogram has been investigated in an adult subject in the idle state, and during performance of a mental arithmetic task. Based on a large sample, the electroencephalogram in this subject in the idle state follows a Gaussian (normal) probability function 66 percent of the time. During performance of the arithmetic task, the portion of Gaussian electroencephalogram decreases to 32 percent. The probability function characterizing gross electroencephalographic activity is determined by the degree of mutual interaction of individual cellular generators of wave activity in the tissue underneath the recording electrode. The data imply an increase in the cooperative activity of cortical neuronal elements during performance of a mental task.

miscellaneous influences brain physiology EEG amplitude theory neuronal activity

E 38. Sulg, I., and Ingvar, D.H.: Regional cerebral blood flow and EEG frequency content. *Electroencephalogr Clin Neurophysiol, 23:*395, 1967 (abstr) .

Attempts to correlate in man regional determinations of the cerebral blood flow with the frequency content of the EEG generated from the same areas have resulted in high correlations for the slow band of 3 to 5 cps (r = .85) and 9 to 11 cps (r = +.73). Regional blood flow has been successfully predicted from the correlation diagrams in some cases. In general, slow-wave activity runs parallel with decreases in regional blood flow. Several problems do exist: for example, severe tissue anoxia may void this relationship. The author also admits that some EEG patterns cannot be explained by cerebral blood flow changes.

miscellane-
ous
influences
cerebral
blood flow
EEG
frequency
theta

E 39.   Harter, M.R.: Effects of carbon dioxide on the alpha frequency and reaction time in humans. *Electroencephalogr Clin Neurophysiol, 23:*561, 1967.

The effects of acute exposure (5 min) to carbon dioxide (0% to 7.9%) on the EEG's and reaction times of five humans were investigated. Alpha frequency and amplitude were recorded from the central and from the occipitoparietal areas of the scalp while subjects reacted with their right index finger to flashes of light. Variance analyses indicated that the percentage of CO_2 inhaled significantly affected alpha frequency and reaction time. Alpha frequency and reaction time were significantly faster under the 0 to 5.5% CO_2 conditions than under the 7.9 percent CO_2 condition. A slight increase in alpha frequency and decrease in reaction time were evident under the 3.5 and 5.5 percent CO_2 conditions as compared to the 0 and 1.5 percent CO_2 conditions.

miscellane-
ous
influences
carbon
dioxide
reaction
time
alpha
frequency
alpha
amplitude

E 40.   Querol, M.: The electroencephalogram in a group of native highlanders at 4540 meters altitude and at sea level. *Electroencephalogr Clin Neurophysiol, 18:*401, 1965.

EEG recordings were taken on eight subjects who were born and live 4540 meters above sea level. These EEG's were normal, but after descending to sea level an increase in voltage of background activity was seen with a statistically significant decrease in the mean frequency of parieto-occipital rhythms (11 to 10.5 cps). At the same time, slow wave voltage and quantity both increased. No correlation be-

miscellane-
ous
influences
environ-
ment
alpha
patterns

tween EEG frequency and factors such as alveolar oxygen and carbon dioxide pressures and the pH values were found. The EEG changes observed were regarded as acclimatization of the highlanders to sea level.

E 41.   Cobb, W.A., Hornabrook, R.W., and Sanders, S.: The EEG of kuru. *Electroencephalogr Clin Neurophysiol, 34:*419, 1973.

This study was conducted because of the similarity between the EEG's of people suffering from kuru and those with other "viral" diseases. Normal EEG's and severe disability were found to be compatible. Abnormalities such as alpha rhythm slowing, increased slow activity including theta waves and irregular delta activity were observed but no signs of repetition could be found. Some of the difficulties of field recording are included in the discussion.

miscellaneous influences
physical illness
alpha frequency
theta
delta

ALPHA RESPONSES

AUDITORY STIMULATION

F 1. Lille, F., Provaznik, K., and Pottier, M.: Effects of auditory and visual stimuli on electroencephalograms during psychosensory tasks. *Travail Humain, 33:*77, 1970.

Subjects were presented with auditory, visual, and alternating auditory and visual stimulus trains to determine the differential effects on the alpha rhythm. The presentation of auditory stimuli was associated with a mean increase in alpha incidence of 10 percent. Visual stimuli were associated with a mean reduction in alpha incidence of 35 percent. The alternation of the two types of stimuli resulted in greater reduction of alpha incidence than the presentation of visual stimuli. The integrated EEG and the incidence of alpha were positively correlated while alpha incidence was negatively correlated with heart rate.

auditory stimulation
alpha abundance
EEG integration
heart rate

F 2. Mimura, K., et al.: On the physiological significance of the EEG changes by sonic stimulation. *Electroencephalogr Clin Neurophysiol, 14:*683, 1962.

In an attempt to demonstrate that depression of alpha waves with enhancement of beta activity, normally seen during sensory stimulation, may also be caused by continuous auditory stimulation with a bell and, also, to confirm the "transforming action" (Sato et al., 1957; Sato, 1959) or "average activity of EEG generators" (Sato et al., 1961) which are extensions of the "excitability" concept of physiology, the frontal, parietal, temporal and occipital EEG of normal adults was studied. The frequency spectrum average frequency pattern of the autocorrelogram or average time pattern as well as the frequency response or frequency characteristics of the EEG were used for analysis. Results showed the alpha blocking did occur under auditory stimulation, but

auditory stimulation
alpha blocking
alpha enhancement
alpha frequency
frequency analysis

habituation to such auditory stimulation may be incomplete. Slower and faster alpha waves were seen to appear and/or be augmented in some cases and were even built up by stimulus repetition. Nevertheless, the waves did return to the original frequency of the dominant alpha activity seen in resting conditions. Some theta wave enhancement was also observed.

F 3.   Doroshenko, V.A., Muraviev, V.I., and Pudovkin, A.I.: On evaluation of amplitude changes in the main human EEG rhythms in response to sensory stimulation. *Electroenceph-alogr Clin Neurophysiol, 29*:97, 1970 (abstr).

The task consisted of comparing the main human EEG rhythms' sensitivity to an auditory stimulus; i.e. the problem was, what EEG frequency component is the most informative for judgment of the presence of sensory stimulation? Seven trials were carried out on two healthy subjects. Quantitative evaluation of the EEG was done by Kozhevnikov's method: the EEG was submitted to wide-band filtering followed by integration. To reveal the response and to evaluate it, the results of all the stimuli were averaged and 95 percent reliable intervals were calculated for every value of the averaged curves. Under these conditions stimulation enhanced alpha waves (during 15 sec after stimulation was started), decreased theta waves (most distinct during the first 15 sec with return to the initial level during the next 4 min) and increased heart rate (time course similar to that for theta waves). Differences in response clarity between the averaged curves of heart rate, alpha waves, theta waves and general EEG were not statistically reliable; i.e. all these parameters proved to be equal for judgment of the presence of a signal. The authors discuss the evaluation of correlations between rhythm amplitude in the preceding background and clarity of response for alpha range, as well as confluence of responses in different EEG frequency bands.

auditory stimulation
alpha enhancement
theta
heart rate

F 4.   Rogge, K.E.: Changes in EEG after delayed acoustic speech feedback. *Z Exp Angew Psychol, 19*:641, 1972.

Delayed speech feedback was used to produce stress in 120 male subjects divided into three experimental groups and one control group. The experimental groups were rested for different time periods following the stress. With five or ten minutes of rest, EEG changes due to stress were a decrease in alpha waves, increase of beta and a repeated interruption of a particular type of waves (intermittent EEG). After fifteen minutes of rest EEG's did not differ from control records. The changes due to stress appeared to be those of an active EEG.

auditory stimulation verbal stimulation

F 5. Giannitrapani, D.: EEG changes under differing auditory stimulations. *Arch Gen Psychiatry, 23:445,* 1970.

Subjects were presented with three types of auditory stimulation while being recorded for bilateral EEG to determine frequency and phase characteristics of the changes induced by the stimulation. White noise, music and a verbally presented story were used for auditory stimulation. Noise presentations were characterized by anterior leading alpha in a comparison of the left prefrontal and occipital areas and an increase in beta activity in the left temporal area. Music presentation was associated with increased bilateral symmetry in prefrontal-occipital alpha phase, anterior leading of alpha in the left central and occipital areas, and little change in EEG amplitude from the resting EEG. Verbal stimuli were associated with posterior leading of alpha in the prefrontal and occipital areas and a bilateral increase in temporal beta activity.

auditory stimulation auditory perception alpha phase alpha symmetry verbal stimuli beta

F 6. Giannitrapani, D.: Frequency analysis of the EEG under different behavioral states. *Electroencephalogr Clin Neurophysiol, 27:694,* 1969 (abstr).

Thirty-two male subjects were given a number of tasks to determine effects on the EEG; auditory, visual and mental involvement were checked. The mental arithmetic task resulted in more fast frequency activity (21 to 33 Hz) in frontal EEG while white noise resulted in more of this frequency range in both frontal and temporal EEG. Music produced effects similar to noise with an additional increase in

auditory stimulation auditory perception mental tasks alpha blocking beta

33 Hz and a decrease in 19 Hz activity in the left occipital EEG. Verbal stimuli produced effects similar to noise with additional decreases in alpha activity in right occipital and post temporal EEG.

VISUAL STIMULATION

F 7.   Chapman, R.M., Shelburne, S.A., and Bragdon, H.R.: EEG alpha activity influenced by visual input and not by eye position. *Electroencephalogr Clin Neurophysiol, 28:*183, 1970.

Recent investigations have suggested that elevation of the eyes is associated with a marked increase in EEG alpha activity. The experiments showed that vertical eye elevation had no direct influence on alpha activity. In preliminary and main groups of thirteen and twenty-two subjects, an EEG electronic scorer was used to measure the amount of time that alpha activity was present from the left and right hemispheres in the following comparisons: (a) eye positions ahead versus up in the light, (b) eyes ahead versus up in the dark, and (c) eyes open versus closed in the light. In the main group, fixation targets for the eye-ahead and eye-up positions and electro-oculogram records of eye position were added. In the dark, where differential visual input was eliminated, the alpha index did not increase when the eyes were elevated. Differences in alpha activity related to eye position in the light condition were decreased when differential visual input was decreased by the use of fixation targets. The effects of variables confounded with eye position, (e.g. patterned visual input to the retina, accommodation, fixation, and effort required to maintain a specified eye position) are discussed. In these experiments, the main variable that determined increase in alpha activity was reduction in visual input, either by closing the eyes or extinguishing the lights.

visual stimulation alpha abundance eye position visual system eye opening

F 8.   Lehtonen, J.B., and Lehtinen, I.: Alpha rhythm and uniform visual field in man. *Electroencephalogr Clin Neurophysiol, 32:*139, 1972.

Eighteen male subjects were recorded for temporo-occipital EEG bilaterally while being presented with photic stimuli under three conditions: eyes closed, eyes open and eyes open with an unpatterned white field in front of the eyes. The uniform visual field was found to increase the incidence of alpha to levels near those produced in the eyes-closed condition, significantly higher than in the normal eyes-open condition. Alpha frequency was significantly higher in the normal eyes-open condition than in the other two conditions. Alpha was found to occur independently of the EMG levels of the laryngial muscles. Occular fixation on a spot in the uniform visual field caused a prolonged alpha desynchronization, but flash counting with a uniform field did not. Alpha blocking was found to be more related to occular fixation than to perception or attention.

visual stimulation eye opening eye position alpha patterns

F 9.   Lehmann, D., Beeler, G.W., Jr., and Fender, D.H.: Changes in patterns of the human electroencephalogram during fluctuations of perception of stabilized retinal images. *Electroencephalogr Clin Neurophysiol, 19:*336, 1965.

Three subjects were presented with constant retinal images through the use of contact lenses. Subjects were asked to report spontaneous fadings and regeneration of the perceptual image while EEG alpha was being recorded. The presence of the alpha rhythm was significantly related to image fadings while the absence of alpha was related to the occurrence of clear images. Subjects who viewed the same target in normal vision showed an EEG pattern in which alpha appeared after the experimenter had manually faded out the target by defocusing or lowering illumination level. Alpha disappeared following reintroduction of the target. Spontaneous fading appears to be related to the occurrence of the alpha rhythm.

visual stimulation retinal images alpha abundance

F 10.   Eberlin, P., and Yager, D.: Alpha blocking during visual after-images. *Electroencephalogr Clin Neurophysiol, 25:*23, 1968.

Three subjects observed visual after-images while simultaneous recordings were made of the occipital EEG. According to instructions, subjects observed the after-images attentively, ignored them or searched for traces when none were present. Alpha blocking was greatest under the condition of attentive viewing of after-images, at a medium level under conditions of searching in the absence of after-images, and least when the after-images were ignored. The effect of after-images and attention together was greater than the sum of the two factors separately, indicating a positive interaction between after-images and attention in blocking alpha rhythms.

visual stimulation after-images alpha blocking attention

F 11. Papkostopoulos, D., Cooper, R., Walter, W.G., and Kellenyi, L.: Measurement of phase relationships of the EEG and photic driving response. *Electroencephalogr Clin Neurophysiol, 30:470,* 1971.

The sine and cosine components of the Fourier analysis of multi-channel data can be displayed using a PDP 12 computer and the technique described in this experiment. Ten healthy subjects were studied for phase or time relationships of intrinsic and widespread driven EEG activity using six sagittal or parasagittal electrodes (referred to mastoid or chin) using 8, 10 and 17 cps photic flicker. Anterior recordings were found to lead the posterior ones in a midline arrangement for both intrinsic and driven activity. Driven rhythms which occurred when the same frequency was observed in similar but parasagittal arrangements showed posterior waves leading frontal ones. The fronto-occipital phase angle remained independent of the common electrode site and photic flicker frequency. In the case of harmonics, patterns similar to the above but with phase shifts of opposite direction were seen. Further discussion of significance and consequences of these results is also included.

visual stimulation photic flicker phase harmonics theory

F 12. Karp, E., Pollack, M., and Fink, M.: Critical flicker frequency and EEG alpha: A reliability study. *Electroencephalogr Clin Neurophysiol, 14:60,* 1962.

Nine staff members and thirty psychiatric patients were studied for correlations between resting percent time alpha and critical flicker frequency. Although test-retest correlations were high, intercorrelations proved insignificant. The results are interpreted as an indication of the uselessness of investigating resting EEG variables and psychological measures. Brain reactivity or change and behavior are suggested as an alternative.

visual
* stimulation*
photic
* flicker*
alpha
* abundance*
variability

F 13.   Mundy-Castle, A.C.: An analysis of central responses to photic stimulation in normal adults. *Electroencephalogr Clin Neuropsychol, 5*:1, 1953.

EEG's were recorded from 154 young normal adults and 40 mentally normal seniles during rhythmic photic stimulation. Two results were attributed to resonance effects: (1) associations between the existence of spontaneous rhythms of alpha and beta frequencies and responses elicited by stimulation at these frequencies, and (2) a similar relation between spontaneous beta activity and the occurrence of second and third harmonics of the stimulation frequency. There was no observable connection between theta and occurrence of subharmonics nor were there any significant sex differences or differences in flicker following characteristics between young and old. A smaller incidence of the second subharmonics, probably due to maturation, and a greater incidence of occurrence of third harmonics—possibly a result of a trend toward larger amplitude beta rhythms with age—were noticed in the old group. There were greater incidences of following in the beta region and in second and third harmonics in subjects with mean alpha frequency above 10.3 cps when compared with those with mean alpha frequency below this level. Subjective sensations were ascribed to interaction between spontaneous and evoked activity and/or augmentation of harmonically related rhythms, while subharmonic responses were thought to be possibly a result of instability or immaturity of cortical development.

visual
* stimulation*
photic
* flicker*
harmonics
beta
theta
aging
subjective
* states*

F 14.   Barry, B.J., and Beh, H.C.: Desynchronization of the alpha rhythm of the EEG as a function of intensity of visual stimulation. *Psychon Sci, 26*:241, 1972.

Twenty male students were recorded for EEG while being stimulated with flashes of diffuse white light of different intensities and in a resting condition to determine the relationship between flash intensity and alpha blocking. The reduction of alpha activity with increasing flash intensity was the shape of an inverted U. Recovery time, or the delay of alpha return following a light flash was linearly related to flash intensity.

visual stimulation
photic flicker
alpha blocking

F 15.   Carels, G.: Facilitation and inhibition of cortical visual response in man. *Electroencephalogr Clin Neurophysiol, 14:* 714, 1962.

An inertia characterized often by a long latency, by the slow and gradual increase in amplitude of successive responses, and by the transitory persistence of the reactive potentials after photic stimulus cessation is seen during the driving of the occipital rhythms by photic flash exceeding 5 to 6 cps. Eye opening and closing prior to the flicker causes blocking of this inertia. This facilitation is thought to be reticular in origin. It is also noted that sensory stimuli, other than visual ones, and mental work can depress occipital driving, and sometimes for extended periods of time when superimposed on photic stimulation.

visual stimulation
photic flicker
alpha responses
eye opening
mental tasks

F 16.   Lansing, R.W., and Barlow, J.S.: Rhythmic after-activity to flashes in relation to the background alpha which precedes and follows the photic stimuli. *Electroencephalogr Clin Neurophysiol, 32:*149, 1972.

Five adults subjects with visible alpha activity in their EEG and rhythmic after-activity in their evoked responses to photic stimuli were recorded for EEG from the 01, 02, Pz and Cz electrode placements during photic stimulation to determine the relationships between alpha blocking and rhythmic after-activity in the evoked response. Although the blocking response and the after-activity of the evoked response were temporally associated, no systematic relationships between duration, latency or amplitude of the two were found. The after-activity had no consistent relation to the return of alpha following the blocking response. Ampli-

visual stimulation
photic flicker
after-discharge

tude of the after-activity was correlated with the amplitude of background alpha.

F 17. Baker, G., and Franken, R.: Effects of stimulus size, brightness and complexity upon EEG desynchronization. *Psychon Sci, 7:289, 1967.*

Subjects exposed to a series of slides showed EEG desynchronization which correlated in duration to the complexity of the slide. The duration of desynchronization did not relate to size or brightness of the slide. Habituation to both the temporal and spatial aspects of complexity was observed.

visual stimulation desynchronization

F 18. Vogel, W., Broverman, D.M., Klaiber, E.L., and Kun, K.J.: EEG responses to photic stimulation as a function of cognitive style. *Electroencephalogr Clin Neurophysiol, 27:186, 1969.*

Thirty-six male students were assessed for ability to perform routine repetitive tasks or automatization prior to the presentation of public stimuli. The photic driving response to light flashes presented at frequencies ranging from ten to thirty per second was assessed. Subjects who scored low on the tests for automatization were found to produce significantly more driving responses than those who had scored high.

visual stimulation photic flicker cognitive style motor performance

F 19. Wilson, G.F., and Lindsley, D.B.: Differential effects of repetitive visual stimulation on alpha rhythm and average visual evoked potentials. *Electroencephalogr Clin Neurophysiol, 27:704, 1969 (abstr).*

The purpose of this study was to contrast the effect of visual stimulation upon a diffuse alpha generator mechanism and that of locally generated rhythmic potentials. The alpha averages and the AEP's to repetitive stimulation produced relatively simple sinusoidal wave forms whose amplitude was largest when stimuli were presented at 10 cps and decreased when the stimulus frequency was varied either above or below 10 cps. The amplitude of alpha averages was considerably greater than that of the rhythmic AEP's recorded

visual stimulation visual evoked responses alpha patterns generators

from the same electrode. Alpha amplitude was smallest at the inion and largest over more anterior occipital and parietal areas. The amplitude of AEP's was maximal at the inion and was reduced at more anterior recording sites. As frequency of photic stimulation varied, frequency of alpha remained constant while frequency of AEP's followed the rate of stimulation. Out-of-phase flashes presented to the two eyes or to the two visual fields produced amplitude reductions and wave form changes in the AEP's at all stimulus frequencies, but produced only amplitude reductions in the alpha averages when the repetitive stimulation was in the neighborhood of 10 cps. These results provide a basis for the differentiation of diffusely distributed alpha activity, presumably controlled by a nonspecific thalamic generator, and regionally confined rhythmic potentials which closely follow the frequency of the repetitive stimulation and apparently reflect the influence of local generators associated with specific thalamic control centers.

F 20. Danilova, N.M.: Electroencephalographic responses to flickering light in the alpha-rhythm frequency range. *Pavlov J Higher Nerv Activ*, 2:8, 1961.

In an investigation to study the driving response of cortical potentials in healthy adult human subjects during wakefulness, natural sleep and subsequent awakening, it was found that the stimulus caused a clear depression of the alpha rhythm along with the driving response. Observations showed that it might be better to look at the harmonic components of the driving response which depend to a degree upon the functional state of the brain and the stimulus intensity. These harmonics seem to be one of the main indicators of level of excitation of cortical neurons. The driving response contained the higher harmonics except during the transition to sleep when they disappeared in favor of the first harmonic. An auditory stimulus before or during the flickering light will intensify the higher harmonics while diminishing the lower ones. In accordance with past observations of Mundy-Castle, it was noted that persons with a predominance of either beta or high-frequency alpha activity, apparently indicating that the central nervous system is ex-

visual stimulation
alpha blocking
harmonics
EEG activation
sleep

cited, better display these higher harmonics. The flickering light caused greater excitation and evoked the higher harmonics. The harmonic components of the driving response diminished with increased stimulus intensity during sleep; the overall effect, when viewed along with the intensified harmonics under similar conditions during wakefulness, was a relatively constant harmonic composition of the driving response. A parodoxical stage in the development of sleep inhibition is suggested as a possible explanation for these changes.

F 21. Gale, A., Dunkin, N., and Coles, M.: Variation in visual input and the occipital EEG. *Psychon Sci, 14:262*, 1969.

Ten subjects with a mean age of twenty-one were measured for EEG changes in three conditions of visual stimulation: eyes closed, eyes open with a black viewing surface, and eyes open with geometrical patterns on the viewing surface. EEG frequencies from 2 to 20 Hz were analyzed. EEG amplitudes at all frequencies were greater in the eyes-closed condition than in either of the eyes-open conditions. Beta activity (14 to 20 Hz) was the same for both eyes-open conditions while all other frequencies were higher for the black viewing surface than for the patterned surface. There was an overall decrease in eyes-closed alpha and an increase in 2 to 6.5 Hz activity between the start and finish of the sessions.

visual stimulation
visual perception
alpha amplitude
EEG frequency
eye opening

F 22. Gale, A., Christie, B., and Penfold, V.: Stimulus complexity and the occipital EEG. *Br J Psychol, 62:527*, 1971.

The study demonstrates discrete variation in EEG during relatively long-term exposure to a visual stimulus of two, four, eight, sixteen or thirty-two randomly located white squares on a black background. Specifically, mid-alpha activity of 8.5 to 10.5 cps decreased linearly as $\log_{2n}$, N = number of squares in the stimulus array (P < 0.01); beta activity of 12.5 to 16.5 cps followed a quadratic trend (P < 0.02); and theta activity of 5.5 to 7.5 cps increased linearly with ascending complexity (P < 0.05). No significant trends were observed for low alpha (7.5 to 8.5 cps) or high alpha (10.5

visual stimulation
visual perception
alpha patterns
EEG patterns

to 12.5 cps) and brightness variation showed no effects parallel to above.

F 23. Berkhout, J., and Walter, D.O.: Temporal stability and individual differences in the human EEG: An analysis of variance of spectral values. *IEEE Trans Biomed Eng, 15:*165, 1968.

Eight channels of bipolar EEG were recorded from forty-seven subjects during programmed stimulus response and rest situations. The alpha band (7 to 13 cps) was used in order to reduce artifact contamination. Normalized power spectra were used for an analysis of variance to determine dispersion characteristics. Results showed statistically significant spectral differences between individuals when compared to differences within individuals and that temporal stability of the EEG was a significant discrimination factor between individuals. During the performance of a visual task, frontal-temporal spectral characteristics became less distinct, while the parieto-occipital area maintained distinctness. Other specific frequency characteristics are pointed out, and the article suggests that alpha intensity differences between individuals may reflect different quiescent state levels of consciousness, arousal or metabolic activity which are apparently overridden when the subject reacts to events external to the central nervous system.

visual stimulation
visual perception
variability
topography
consciousness
spectral analysis

F 24. Gale, A., Coles, M., and Boyd, E.: Variation in visual input and the occipital EEG: II. *Psychon Sci, 23:*99, 1971.

This investigation replicates and extends to five the number of viewing conditions of a previous study by A. Gale, N. Dunkin and M. Coles in which it was found that resting EEG varied with different viewing stimuli. Twenty-nine undergraduates were recorded for EEG during periods of eyes shut, eyes open in the dark, viewing a blank screen, viewing a simple pattern, and viewing a more complex pattern. The stimuli were presented twice randomly at 2 min/trial. For alpha and beta activity, EEG amplitude varied inversely with increasing visual complexity. Except for the last two conditions, this inverse relation also held for theta activity.

visual stimulation
visual perception
EEG patterns

F 25.   Gastaut, H.J., and Bert, J.: EEG changes during cinemato-
        graphic presentation. *Electroencephalogr Clin Neurophysiol,*
        6:433, 1954.

        Sixty-eight male and twelve female adults were presented   *visual*
        with a controlled film to determine the effects of ideational   *stimulation*
        visual stimuli on the EEG. The film was a newsreel with two   *visual*
        1-minute intervals of blank film inserted. Opening eyes dur-   *perception*
        ing an initial rest period produced a ten-second blocking of   *cognition*
        alpra and a continued lower amplitude than with eyes closed.   *alpha*
        The start of the movie and the start of each segment follow-   *blocking*
        ing a blank period was associated with a thirty-second block- *theta*
        ing period and still lower amplitude of alpha. Each blank
        was associated with a clear increase in amplitude of alpha.
        Seven subjects showed increased theta activity during the
        film presentation.

F 26.   Ali, M.R.: Pattern of EEG recovery under photic stimula-
        tion by light of different colors. *Electroencephalogr Clin*
        Neurophysiol, 33:332, 1972.

        The response habituation of the central nervous system as   *visual*
        measured by the amount of alpha recovery after stimulation   *stimulation*
        of red and blue light was investigated in ten normal adults.   *visual*
        Results showed that the cortical habituation response is de-   *perception*
        layed more under red than blue light (greater alpha recovery   *habituation*
        under red stimulation). Conclusions of a greater cortical   *EEG*
        arousal under conditions of red light stimulation are pre-   *activation*
        sented.

F 27.   Kanoh, M., and Kitajuna, S.: Some psychological determi-
        nants of alpha attenuation after patterned flashes. *J Psychol,*
        82:155, 1972.

        Alpha attenuation was found to be higher after patterned   *visual*
        flashes as opposed to diffused flashes, but after thirty trials   *stimulation*
        the difference was quite small. Pattern complexity affected   *alpha*
        the attenuation, and habituation was transferable to new   *patterns*
        patterns provided that the primary pattern remained.   *desynchroni-*
                                                                        zation

REACTION TIME

F 28.   Morrell, L.K.: EEG frequency and reaction time—a sequential analysis. *Neuropsychologia, 4:*41, 1966.

Twelve young adult subjects, with an alpha incidence greater than 85 percent with eyes closed, were given a reaction time task of pressing a key following light flashes with their eyes closed. EEG recordings were made from the occipital leads for analysis. Fastest reaction times were obtained when the EEG was dominated by the alpha rhythm as opposed to lower frequencies. Variability of reaction time was greatest when delta and theta slow wave activity was dominant.

*reaction time
alpha abundance
theta
delta*

F 29.   Surwillo, W.W.: The relation of simple response time to brain wave frequency and the effects of age. *Electroencephalogr Clin Neurophysiol, 15:*105, 1963.

One hundred male subjects ranging in age from twenty-eight to ninety-nine were given a key-press response task with a tone as the response stimulus. Frontal and occipital leads were used for recording EEG. Significant correlations were found between response speed and alpha frequency (inverse of reaction time), age and wave period (inverse of frequency), and age and reaction time. With partial correlations factoring out age and period, age was negatively correlated with reaction time and alpha frequency was positively correlated with response speed. The author concluded that the brain-wave cycle is a basic timing unit of the nervous system for behavior.

*reaction time
alpha frequency
phase of wave period
age*

F 30.   Bjerner, B.O.: Alpha depression and lowered pulse rate during delayed actions in a serial reaction test. *Acta Physiol Scand (Suppl), 65:*7, 1949.

Five subjects were tested over a twelve-hour period between 10 PM and 10 AM to determine the physiological correlates of delayed action or long pause in the reaction to a tone stimulus. Pauses lasting longer than two seconds were accompanied by a transient drop in pulse rate proportional to the duration of the delay. A drop in alpha frequency also occurred with this delay. Pauses longer than five seconds showed physiological signs for all stages between wakefulness

*reaction time
alpha frequency
heart rate
wakefulness
sleep
biorhythms*

and sleep. There was some indication of diurnal variations in alpha frequency with an overall decrease during the night.

F 31.   Surwillo, W.W.: Frequency of the "alpha" rhythm reaction time and age. *Nature, 191*:823, 1961.

Eighteen subjects were recorded for EEG activity with bi-   *reaction*
polar electrodes over the occipital and frontal areas in order   *time*
to investigate a possible relation between alpha frequency of   *alpha*
the EEG and reaction time during the time lapse between a   *frequency*
stimulus and a response. Only thirteen subjects had alpha   *age*
rhythms which could be easily measured, but it was found
that slower alpha frequency corresponded to slower responses
in these individuals. Observations also indicated that older
people with longer reaction times show lower alpha frequencies during the period between stimulus and response
than younger subjects with shorter reaction times. The
article suggests the alpha cycle, or some multiple thereof,
could act as the unit of time in nervous system programming,
but it is also noted that further verification and study is required.

F 32.   Callaway, E., and Yeager, C.L.: Relationship between reaction time and electroencephalographic alpha phase. *Science, 132*:1765, 1960.

A technique is described to verify a proposed correlation be-   *reaction*
tween phasic behavior changes and 8 to 13 cps alpha brain-   *time*
wave activity. The report is an advancement on past experi-   *alpha phase*
ments in that it identifies the part of the alpha cycle likely
associated with slow reaction times prior to statistical evaluation and requires only moderately dominant alpha, thereby
allowing use on an unselected adult population. A predetermined phase and amplitude of the alpha wave triggers a
signal which is followed in 10 to 90 msec by a flash. The subject responds to the second signal by pressing a key and the
response time is measured. Problems in measurement and
analysis, due for example to signals triggered by artifacts and
the fact that alpha waves are not perfect sine waves with
preset frequency, do exist and are taken into consideration.
The slowest reaction times resulted from stimuli presented

nearest the point of maximum occipital positivity, and statistical analysis showed a significant correlation between visual reaction time and phase of alpha at stimulation.

F 33. Boddy, J.: The relationship of action time to brain wave period. A reevaluation. *Electroencephalogr Clin Neurophysiol, 30:229*, 1971.

Two attempts were made to replicate an experiment by Surwillo in which a significant positive correlation between reaction time and alpha wave period was found. Seventeen subjects were used in each experiment. In the first experiment, EEG alpha samples were obtained in a resting period prior to training. The wave period obtained in this manner was not significantly correlated with reaction time in high motivation, visual reaction time tasks. In a second experiment, the wave period preceding each response was analyzed in relation to reaction time. No significant correlation was found. Surwillo measured wave period in the stimulus-response interval rather than prior to the stimulus presentation.

reaction time
phase of wave period

F 34. Callaway, E., III: Factors influencing the relationship between alpha activity and visual reaction time. *Electroencephalogr Clin Neurophysiol, 14:674*, 1962.

Nine subjects were given a reaction time task in which a visual reaction stimulus was triggered by different phases of the alpha wave in the EEG. Individual subjects showed enduring tendencies to respond fastest and slowest to particular phases of alpha, but there were no reliable intersubject relationships between phase of alpha and reaction time. Although reaction times were slowest with lower brightness of the reaction stimulus, brightness did not alter the relationship between slow responding and alpha phase.

reaction time
phase of wave period

F 35. Surwillo, W.W.: Relationship between EEG activation and reaction time. *Percept Mot Skills, 29:3*, 1969.

Ninety-nine adult male subjects between the ages of twenty-eight and ninety-nine, having average alpha amplitudes greater than 15 microvolts, were given an auditory reaction time task to determine the relationship between the charac-

reaction time
alpha responses

teristics of the alpha rhythm and reaction time. EEG's were recorded from bilateral frontal and occipital electrode placements. Measures of alpha were analyzed for the period between the reaction stimulus and the response. Correlations between reaction times and alpha frequency within subjects were all high and positive with most reaching significance. No relationship was found between reaction time and alpha amplitude.

F 36.   Dustman, R.E., and Beck, E.C.: Phase of alpha brain waves, reaction time and visually evoked potentials. *Electroencephalogr Clin Neurophysiol, 18:433*, 1965.

Twenty adult subjects, having a prominent alpha rhythm in their EEG, were presented with flashes of light on a uniform visual field in a button-press reaction time experiment. The flashes of light were triggered by the alpha of the subjects at particular phase points on the wave; (1) at the start of the rising portion of the wave, (2) at the zero point, (3) just prior to peak, (4) just following the peak, (5) at the zero point, and (6) just prior to the trough. Subjects had the fastest response times when the light was triggered at phase 1. Slowest response times were associated with flashes occurring at phase 2. Characteristics of the resulting evoked potentials are discussed.

reaction time
visual stimulation
phase of wave period

F 37.   Robinson, D.N.: Visual reaction time and the human alpha rhythm: The effects of stimulus luminance, area, and duration. *J Exp Psychol, 71:16*, 1966.

Subjects were given a key-press reaction time task under a variety of stimulus conditions to determine the inter-relationships between alpha blocking, reaction time and stimulus luminance, area and duration. Latency of the alpha blocking response was found to be constant with a constant luminance x time product. With stimulus areas greater than 1°, alpha blocking latency was not constant for a constant luminance x area product. The duration of the blocking response was functionally related to stimulus area rather than luminance. Reaction time was negatively correlated with both luminance and area of stimulus. The author concluded that

reaction time
visual stimulation
alpha blocking

relationships found between reaction time and the alpha rhythm are largely related to stimulus variables.

F 38.   Hayes, R.W., and Venables, P.H.: EEG measures of arousal during RFT performances in "noise." *Percept Mot Skills, 31:*594, 1970.

Twenty-one students (10 male and 11 female) were given an upright rod and frame task with acoustical noise present and absent. In the noise trials, white noise was presented to a subject whenever EEG alpha exceeded 80 percent of the resting level. No significant differences were found in performance or alpha incidence under the two conditions even though noise was present between 18 and 60 percent of the time in the noise condition.

reaction time
auditory stimulation
alpha abundance
arousal

F 39.   Surwillo, W.W.: Some observations on the relationship of response speed to frequency of photic stimulation and conditions of EEG synchronization. *Electroencephalogr Clin Neurophysiol, 17:*194, 1964.

Forty-eight male subjects ranging in age from 34 to 101 years were given photic stimulation to regulate the frequency of the alpha rhythm produced by photic driving. Reaction times for a key-press to a tone stimulus were determined under conditions of slow and fast induced alpha. Five subjects responded successfully to the driving stimulus under all conditions. Three of these subjects demonstrated significant correlations between alpha frequency and response speed.

reaction time
photic flicker
alpha frequency

F 40.   Thompson, L.W., and Botwinick, J.: Age differences in the relationship between EEG arousal and reaction time. *J Psychol, 68:*167, 1968.

Twenty-six elderly and twenty-six young adult subjects were given an auditory reaction time task involving a key-lift response. A warning tone was presented .5, 3.0, 6.0 or 15.0 seconds prior to the reaction stimulus in both random and regular sequences. Changes in alpha amplitude were measured from parietal and occipital leads during stimulus presentations. The greatest change in amplitude was found with

reaction time
preparatory interval
aging
alpha amplitude

the .5 second warning interval. EEG changes were greater for the elderly group which also had the longest reaction times. The length of preparatory interval was significantly related to both reaction time and alpha change for the regular series. Intra-subject correlations between reaction time and alpha change were all nonsignificant.

F 41. Thompson, L.W., and Botwinick, J.: The role of the preparatory interval in the relationship between EEG alpha-blocking and reaction time. *Psychophysiology, 3:*131, 1966.

reaction time preparatory interval alpha blocking

Two experiments were performed to determine the effects of variations in preparatory intervals on the alpha blocking and reaction time relationships. In the first experiment, thirty-seven young adult subjects were given a key-release response task with a 400 Hz warning tone and a 1000 Hz reaction stimulus tone. Left parieto-occipital EEG recordings were used for analysis. Preparatory intervals of .5, 3.0, 6.0 and 15.0 seconds were given in regular and irregular sequences to each subject. Reaction time increased as a function of preparatory interval for the regular sequences of presentation. Longer reaction times were found for the irregular sequences. No significant correlation was found between reaction time and either alpha amplitude or changes in alpha amplitude. In the second study, fourteen male subjects were given a key-lift task with the tone warning signal and a light flash reaction stimulus. Preparatory intervals of .5, .75, 1.0 and 1.5 seconds were presented in random sequences. Although both reaction time and alpha amplitude changes were significantly altered by preparatory interval, and the overall functions appear to show covariance, individual correlations between reaction time and alpha amplitude changes were nonsignificant.

F 42. Leavitt, F.: EEG activation and reaction time. *J Exp Psychol,* 77:194, 1968.

reaction time alpha blocking

This author investigated the covariation of reaction time and alpha desynchronization at foreperiods of 200, 500, 1500 and 4000 msec with sixty-four male students. The results demonstrate that reaction time and alpha desynchronization are significantly influenced by variations in the foreperiod condition. Reliably faster reaction time and maximal alpha desynchronization occurred 500 msec after the warning signal; however, within the context of the foreperiod, the two variables did not covary. A unitary underlying arousal process was rejected in favor of multiple neural arousal processes.

F 43.   Stamm, J.S.: On the relationship between reaction time to light and latency of blocking of the alpha rhythm. *Electroencephalogr Clin Neurophysiol, 4*:61, 1952.

Twenty young adult students having an eye-closed incidence of alpha greater than 70 percent were presented with a series of reaction time tasks. A diffuse light and a door buzzer were used as reaction stimuli. Subjects were given instructions not to respond (passive), press a key to either stimulus when it occurred (simple responding), or respond only when the light occurred (discrimination). Stimuli were introduced only when alpha was present in one condition and at 2.5 second intervals in a second condition. A significant correlation was found between latency of alpha blocking and reaction time. No significant relationships were found between reaction time and any of the other variables.

reaction time
alpha blocking

F 44.   Dustman, R.E., Boswell, R.S., and Porter, P.B.: Beta brain waves as an index of alertness. *Science, 137*:533, 1962.

Twenty young adult male and female subjects were presented with a reaction time task of pressing a button following a light flash triggered by either spontaneous alpha or spontaneous beta burst activity in the EEG. The authors were equating reaction time with levels of alertness. Forty responses were obtained for each subject under each triggering condition. Reaction times were 12 milliseconds faster when the stimulus was yoked with beta activity than when yoked to alpha activity.

reaction time
alert
alpha abundance
beta

F 45.   Lansing, R.W., Schwartz, E., and Lindsley, D.B.: Reaction time and EEG activation under alerted and nonalerted conditions. *J Exp Psychol, 58*:1, 1959.

Adult subjects were given visual reaction time tasks with and without an auditory forewarning stimulus. In the alerted condition, a buzzer preceded the visual stimulus by intervals ranging from 50 to 1000 milliseconds. With forewarning intervals of less than 250 milliseconds, alpha blocking could not occur prior to the reaction stimulus. The alerted condition resulted in faster response time than the nonalerted condition. In the nonalerted condition, no differences in reaction time were found when the reaction stimulus was presented with alpha present or absent. In the alerted condition, forewarning intervals greater than 250 milliseconds were associated with the fastest reaction times. The authors attributed part of the increase in reaction time to the combination of the alerting stimulus and the absence of alpha at the time the reaction stimulus occurred.

reaction time
alert
alpha abundance

F 46.   Surwillo, W.W.: The relation of decision time to brain wave frequency and to age. *Electroencephalogr Clin Neurophysiol, 16:*510, 1964.

Fifty-four male subjects between the ages of thirty-four and ninety-two were given an auditory reaction time task with a key press response to two different tone stimuli which each subject had adjusted to equal loudness. Three experimental conditions were used; a nonalerted practice session with stimuli three seconds long, an alerted session with three-second stimuli in which subjects were told to respond as fast as possible, a discrimination condition with three-second stimuli in which subjects were told to only respond to 1000 Hz tones, and a discrimination condition with three-second stimuli with the same instructions. Alpha frequency was calculated for the interval between the stimulus and the response. No differences were found for frequency or reaction times between the two tones in the simple reaction tasks. For both the simple reaction time and the discrimination tasks the correlations between brain wave frequency and response speed were significant with different slopes to the regression lines. Partial correlations revealed that both age and brain wave frequency were independently related to discussion time with older persons and lower frequencies being related to longer time.

reaction time
alert
perceptual tasks
alpha frequency
age

MOTOR PERFORMANCE

F 47. Scheich, H., and Simonova, O.: Parameters of alpha activity during the performance of motor tasks. *Electroencephalogr Clin Neurophysiol, 31:357,* 1971.

Twenty-five students were tested for alpha index, frequency and standard deviation while performing rhythmic arm and leg movements as well as walking. Subjects with a low alpha index under either eyes-closed or eyes-open conditions tended to show an increase in alpha activity during performance while those with a high alpha index tended to have reduced alpha incidence. The differences were greater when the data was separated on the basis of eyes-open alpha and when high reliability samples were taken from individuals rather than pooled data. Performance of motor tasks appears to remove differences between groups of subjects with alpha going to intermediate levels.

*motor per-
formance
alpha
patterns
eye opening*

F 48. Scheich, H., and Simonova, O.: The influence of motor activity on the alpha rhythm. *Electroencephalogr Clin Neurophysiol, 28:215,* 1970 (abstr).

Two groups of subjects were selected on the basis of the alpha index of the EEG under eyes-open testing. One group had a high alpha index, the other had a low alpha index. Subjects were given motor performance tasks involving the use of the dominant hand or the dominant leg. Those having a low eyes-open alpha had an increased incidence of alpha and frequency stabilization with use of the hand and an increased incidence of alpha with larger variance of alpha duration using the leg. Those having a high alpha index showed alpha blocking or reduction under both performance conditions. When separated on the basis of eyes-closed alpha, no differences between subjects in performance were found.

*motor per-
formance
alpha
patterns
eye opening*

F 49. Mundy-Castle, A.C., and Sugarman, L.: Factors influencing relations between tapping speed and alpha rhythm. *Electroencephalogr Clin Neurophysiol, 12:895,* 1960.

Sixty-seven adults were given tasks involving tapping a telegraph key and a metal stylus at normal and fast speeds under both eyes-opened and eyes-closed conditions. Alpha frequency, amplitude, range and percent time present were determined in all conditions. Two groups were given the tasks in different orders. The order of tasks significantly affected the data such that effects of alpha on performance were masked. Tapping speed was significantly slower with the telegraph key but was significantly correlated between the two conditions. Alpha amplitude was positively correlated with percent time present while alpha frequency was negatively correlated with percent time present.

motor performance
tapping speed
alpha patterns

F 50. Suenaga, K., Goto, K., and Suenaga, H.: Study of EEG of bus drivers while driving and at rest. *Kurume Med J, 14:* 43, 1967.

Bus drivers were separated on the basis of their accident-prone and nonaccident-prone groups. The alpha rhythms of these individuals were tested under resting eyes-open, resting eyes-closed, and bus driving conditions. Accident-prone individuals had lower frequency alpha with eyes closed, a higher incidence of alpha in the resting eyes-open condition, and more frequent dominant alpha while driving a bus.

motor performance
bus driving
accident proneness
alpha patterns
eye opening

F 51. Legewie, H., Simonova, O., and Creutzfeldt, O.D.: EEG changes during performance of various tasks under open- and closed-eyed conditions. *Electroencephalogr Clin Neurophysiol, 27:*470, 1969.

Eight male subjects ranging in age from twenty to twenty-seven were given a variety of motor and cognitive tasks to determine the effects on the EEG recorded from left frontocentral and temporo occipital electrode pairs. Two writing tasks, two tracking tasks, and a mental arithmetic task were involved in the experiment. The eyes-open condition resulted in about a 50 percent reduction in alpha incidence while theta and beta activity were doubled. Frontocentral alpha was found to decrease during performance while temporo-

motor performance
mental tasks
alpha abundance
theta
beta
alpha blocking
alpha enhancement

occipital alpha remained at intermediate levels. During performance, closing the eyes produced a desynchronization while eye opening synchronized alpha.

F 52. Denier Van der Gon, J.J., and Van Hinte, N.: The relation between the frequency of the alpha rhythm and the speed of writing. *Electroencephalogr Clin Neurophysiol, 11:*669, 1959.

Sixty-nine hospital patients were tested simultaneously for speed of writing and the frequency of the alpha rhythm. Persons having no abnormal motor mechanisms were found to have a significant rank-order correlation between alpha frequency and writing speed. No relationship was found between abnormal EEG and writing speed.

motor per-
formance
alpha
frequency

F 53. MacNeilage, P.F.: Changes in electroencephalogram and other physiological measures during serial mental performance. *Psychophysiology,* 2:344, 1966.

Twenty RCAF technician trainees, ranging in age from seventeen to twenty-four, were given the tasks of writing and adding numbers while being recorded for EEG, EMG, EKG, respiration rate and skin conductance. The writing task involved auditory presentation of 60 two-digit numbers as a control condition. The adding task involved 61 one-digit numbers each of which was to be added to the previous number in the sequence. Alpha and beta activity were lower in the adding condition than in the writing condition. Both frequencies were lowest just prior to making a response and highest immediately following the response. Alpha activity showed an overall increase during the session while EMG, respiration rate, skin conductance and heart rate declined.

motor per-
formance
mental tasks
alpha
patterns
beta
ANS

ALPHA BLOCKING

F 54. Milstein, V.: Phase of alpha wave, habituation and contingent blocking. *Electroencephalogr Clin Neurophysiol, 27:* 692, 1969 (abstr).

Subjects having a relatively high alpha incidence of moderate intensity were presented with light flashes and auditory clicks triggered by various points on the alpha sine wave; peak, trough and midpoints of the up-going and down-going wave. Subjects with phase-locked stimuli habituated more rapidly than those having random presentations. Flash stimuli at the midpoint of the surface negative wave resulted in more rapid habituation while clicks did not.

alpha
  blocking
phase of
  wave
  period
habituation
visual
  stimulation
auditory
  stimulation

F 55.   Pollen, D.A., and Trachtenberg, M.C.: Some problems of occipital alpha block in man. *Brain Res, 41:*303, 1972.

This study looks at the attenuation or blocking of the occipital alpha rhythm with reference to the role played by the visual system and mental tasks. Results from ten subjects including the investigators themselves showed that the degree of attentiveness to detail is the key factor in the blocking process. In the case of mental tasks the extent of alpha attenuation increases with the amount of mental effort required. The significance of the alpha blocking phenomenon is discussed.

alpha
  blocking
visual system
attention
mental tasks
eye
  movements

F 56.   Mulholland, T.: Electroencephalographic activation: Nonspecific habituation by verbal stimuli. *Science, 152:*1104, 1966.

Subjects were presented with a series of verbal stimuli including emotional, neutral and scrambled words to determine the course of habituation of alpha blocking. Neutral words consistently resulted in shorter blocking responses across habituation. This was interpreted as indicating that habituation is a general process rather than a process related to the content of specific stimuli.

alpha
  blocking
verbal
  stimuli
habituation
mental tasks

F 57.   Putney, R.T.: Conditioned alpha blocking re-examined with the measurement of individual wave amplitudes. *Electroencephalogr Clin Neurophysiol, 34:*485, 1973.

Peak amplitudes of alpha waves were measured in nine subjects in order to study conditioning of the alpha blocking phenomen. First, random lights and sounds were presented as a pseudoconditioning control session. Then, a tone conditioned stimulus and a light unconditioned stimulus were presented one second apart. Amplitude reduction across waves during conditioning was found to be constantly decreasing. The largest difference between reductions during conditioning and the smaller reductions during the control pseudoconditioning period came before the light unconditioned stimulus. It was concluded that neither pseudoconditioning nor sensitization to the orienting response greatly affect conditioned reduction of alpha activity.

*alpha blocking
conditioning
alpha amplitude
habituation
orienting*

F 58.   Torres, A.A.: Sensitization and association in alpha blocking "conditioning." *Electroencephalogr Clin Neurophysiol, 24:*297, 1968.

Subjects were presented with tone and light stimuli in contingent and noncontingent arrangements to determine conditioning, sensitization and habituation effects on the alpha blocking response. A delayed conditioning paradigm was employed for evaluation of the effects of contingent pairings. The contingent condition produced more blocking responses than other conditions.

*alpha blocking
conditioning
sensitization
habituation*

F 59.   Darrow, C.W., Vieth, R.N., and Wilson, J.: Electroencephalographic "blocking" and "adaptation." *Science, 126:*74, 1957.

The authors review the phenomena of alpha blocking and adaptation. The presentation of any new stimulus or activity which requires attention and integration results in the blocking of the alpha rhythm. After repeated occurrence of the stimulus alpha is no longer attenuated. The authors hypothesized that the common denominator in alpha blocking situations is the necessity of integrative processes involving the cortex. Once processing of a stimulus or activity becomes automatic, it can be turned over to subcortical areas. A discussion of the application of this model to various subcortical and alpha blocking phenomena is presented.

*alpha blocking
adaptation
integrative cortex
theory*

F 60.   Mulholland, T.: Variation in the response-duration curve of successive cortical activation by a feedback stimulus. *Electroencephalogr Clin Neurophysiol, 16:*394, 1964.

The purpose of this note is to present illustrative examples of a seemingly nonrandom variation in the duration and latency of successive cortical activation responses, which were obtained using a stimulus-brain feedback loop (Mulholland and Runnals, 1962). Variation in the durations and latency of successive cortical activation responses was illustrated by examples from seven normal subjects. It was concluded that some subjects exhibit a variation of successive cortical activation latencies and durations which was not exclusively random nor strictly periodic. However, the relevant variables were not identified.

alpha blocking
EEG activation
biofeedback

F 61.   Oswald, J.: The human alpha rhythm and visual alertness. *Electroencephalogr Clin Neurophysiol, 11:*601, 1959 (abstr).

Thirteen subjects listened with eyes open for a faint tone preceded by a regular recurring warning signal. Initially, the EEG showed no alpha activity, then it appeared and became more or less continuous. In five subjects during the intermediate stage, alpha appeared at times of intense auditory alertness. Alpha activity was accompanied by loss of ocular fixation and accommodation. The author proposed that alpha blocking represents an increase of specific visual alertness which may be but one component of general arousal, and that specific auditory alertness may be accompanied by reciprocal inhibition of visual function, at the periphery, during transmission, and centrally.

alpha blocking
alerting
visual system
theory

F 62.   Wilson, N.J., and Wilson, W.P.: The duration of human EEG arousal responses elicited by photic stimulation. *Electroencephalogr Clin Neurophysiol, 11:*85, 1959.

Subjects were presented with light flashes of ten-second intervals for thirty minutes to determine the effects on the duration of alpha blocking responses with greater than 50 percent reduction in amplitude. The authors found that a drop in duration of the blocking response occurred early in the

alpha blocking
arousal
visual stimulation
adaptation

stimulus train, but that little change in response duration occurred with later stimuli.

F 63.   Visser, S.L.: Correlations between the contingent alpha blocking, EEG characteristics and clinical diagnosis. *Electroencephalogr Clin Neurophysiol, 13:*438, 1961.

The alpha blocking reaction to a visual stimulus was turned into a contingent reaction in this experiment with a visual stimulus as the unconditioned stimulus and an acoustic stimulus as the conditioned stimulus. In 250 subjects it was found that the contingent reaction is established in just a few trials, but it tends to fade as the test continues. High intensity of contingent reaction and high frequency of alpha as well as low intensity of contingent reaction and high quantity of alpha were associated. It was concluded that these findings in conjunction with past literature indicate that the intensity of formation of contingent reaction may be a good criterion of consciousness and the formation of new situation-adapted patterns of reaction, and that alpha activity carries much psychological or psychiatric information concerning the condition of psychiatric patients. Delta, theta and beta brain waves and contingent reaction formation could not be correlated. Test repetition only served to decrease the intensity of the reaction.

alpha blocking psychopathology

F 64.   Davidoff, R.A., and McDonald, D.G.: Alpha blocking and autonomic responses in neurological patients. *Arch Neurol, 10:*283, 1964.

Twenty-two patients and twenty-two control subjects were conditioned for blocking of EEG alpha activity while skin resistance, heart rate and vasoconstriction in the finger were also monitored. Care was taken to avoid confusing of anticipatory conditioned responses and the orienting reflex. All parameters of the orienting reflex adapted to tone in control subjects, but vasoconstriction and heart rate failed to adapt in persons with brain damage. EEG conditioning easily differentiated patients from controls. Conditional autonomic responses could not effectively be produced by the tone-light procedures used and no clear temporal correlations between EEG's and autonomic activity were observed.

alpha blocking neurologic problems ANS

ALPHA ENHANCEMENT

F 65. Doroshenko, V.A., Muraviev, V.I., and Pudovkin, A.: On evaluation of amplitude changes in the main human EEG rhythms in response to sensory stimulation. *Electroencephalogr Clin Neurophysiol, 29:*97, 1970 (abstr) .

Two subjects were tested with repeated presentations of a tone to determine the EEG changes which would predict the presence of such a stimulus. Thirty tones of one-minute duration were presented at eight-minute intervals. Frequency analysis of the fronto-occipital EEG revealed that alpha amplitude was enhanced overall during the fifteen seconds following tone onset while theta activity was attenuated during this period with reference to levels prior to stimulation.

alpha enhancement
auditory stimulation
theta

F 66. Morrell, L.K.: Some characteristics of stimulus-provoked alpha activity. *Electroencephalogr Clin Neurophysiol, 21:* 552, 1966.

Subjects with prominent resting alpha were presented with photic stimuli in one of two conditions. One group was required to make a response (clench their fist or press a button) to each stimulus while the other group did nothing. When the stimuli were presented in the presence of alpha, blocking occurred with the response group having the greatest incidence of blocking. When stimuli were presented in the absence of alpha, elicitation of alpha was observed with the passive group having the highest incidence of elicitation. Response latency was greatest when alpha was elicited.

alpha enhancement
alpha blocking
visual stimulation
motor performance

F 67. Kreitman, N., and Shaw, J.C.: Experimental enhancement of alpha activity. *Electroencephalogr Clin Neurophysiol, 18:* 147, 1965.

Eight subjects were given a series of discrimination tasks (auditory, visual and tactile) and a mental arithmetic task to determine the effects on EEG frequency patterns. The tasks were found to produce both alpha blocking and alpha enhancement. The enhancement effect occurred on twenty-four of sixty-four trials with tactile discrimination being

alpha enhancement
mental tasks
alpha blocking

most often associated with alpha enhancement and visual discrimination being least often associated. EMG amplitude was found to be positively correlated with the amount of alpha blocking. Alpha blocking decreased over time while the enhancement effect continued to increase.

CONDITIONING

F 68. Muskina, N.A.: Dynamics of formation of conditioned reflexes present and after reflexes of depression of alpha rhythm and their differentiation. In *The Central Nervous System and Human Behavior.* Translations from the Russian Medical Literature. Bethesda, Russian Scientific Translation Program, 1959, p. 569.

Three stages (phases) in the development and establishment of a conditioned trace alpha rhythm suppression reaction are shown: a phase of generalization, a phase of gradual concentration and a phase of total concentration. These appear to indicate in the establishment of a temporary connection that the process of inhibition which takes part in effecting the concentration of the conditioned alpha rhythm suppression reaction arises in this case in the region of the visual analyzer and then later encompasses the region of the acoustic analyzer. The dynamics of the formation of differentiation between stimuli which cause the alpha rhythm suppression is demonstrated. It was established that during the development of differentiation of alpha rhythm suppression the reaction takes place in a different fashion in the cortical regions of the acoustic and visual analyzers. A study was made of the three stages in the development of differentiation which indicate that the process of inhibition leading to the extinction of the alpha rhythm reaction arises in this case in the region of the visual analyzer and only later spreads to the region of the acoustic analyzer. The experimental material cited shows that not only the extinction of the orientation reaction, but also the development of temporary connections under different experimental conditions is reflected in the alpha rhythm reaction, which may thus serve to study the dynamics of the higher nervous activity in man.

conditioning
alpha abundance

F 69. Hofer, M.A., and Hinkle, L.E., Jr.: Conditioned alpha blocking and arousal: The effects of adrenaline administration. *Electroencephalogr Clin Neurophysiol, 17:*653, 1964.

Twenty-nine adult subjects were given injections of adrenaline and saline solutions on different days to determine the effects of adrenaline-induced arousal on the alpha rhythm in a Pavlovian conditioning paradigm. Adrenaline had no significant effect on the alpha blocking response to tone presentations prior to tone-light pairings. During conditioning, adrenaline increased the number of blocking responses produced by the tone while having a lesser effect during extinction. The duration of the blocking response to light was significantly greater with adrenaline administration. Measures of subjective arousal were significantly higher on days when adrenaline was administered and were significantly correlated with number of responses to tone on days when saline was administered. Adrenaline had no measurable effects on the resting alpha rhythm.

condition-ing
adrenaline
alpha
blocking
arousal

F 70.   Albino, R., and Burnand, G.: Conditioning of alpha rhythm in man. *J Exp Psychol, 67:*539, 1964. (Copyright 1964 by the American Psychological Association and reproduced by permission.)

Conditioning of the alpha rhythm to a tone was attempted in three experiments. In two of these, inspection of the records showed no conditioning. No conditioning was observed in four subjects to a kinesthetic stimulus. In a third experiment eight subjects were given twenty conditioning (CS tone) and four extinction trials with control on attention. Significant suppression of the alpha rhythm occurred, but it was small and variable between individuals. The effect seemed to be due to conditioning to the tone; temporal conditioning of the alpha rhythm can occur, but the phenomenon is unstable and highly variable.

condition-ing
alpha
blocking

F 71.   Jasper. H., and Shagass, C.: Conditioning the occipital alpha rhythm in man. *J Exp Psychol, 28:*373, 1941.

The disappearance of the occipital alpha rhythm in man was conditioned to auditory stimuli in the classical Pavlovian manner. The following types of conditioned response were

condition-ing
alpha
blocking

established: simple, cyclic, delayed, trace differential, differential delayed and backward. In some cases extinction and spontaneous recovery were shown. After several trials with the backward conditioning technique, a sound stimulus reestablished the alpha rhythm if introduced during its depression by light (counteraction effect). With further conditioning, the sound alone produced blocking of the alpha rhythm. This suggests simultaneous facilitation and inhibition processes during conditioning. A state resembling sleep was produced during conditioning of long delay and trace intervals, that is, slow waves appeared in the electroencephalogram and the subjects failed to give the usual manual response. The relation of electroencephalographic studies to general problems of conditioning was discussed.

F 72. Shagass, C.: Conditioning the human occipital alpha rhythm to a voluntary stimulus. A quantitative study. *J Exp Psychol,* *31*:367, 1942.

conditioning
alpha blocking

The conditioning of the response of the occipital alpha rhythm of the human EEG to a voluntary stimulus (clenching of the fist) was quantitatively studied by determining the alpha amplitude and activity level (AL) indices of a specific segment of record. This segment consisted of two seconds of activity starting 0.67 seconds after the beginning of the voluntary stimulus. Neither the conditioned stimulus alone nor the unconditioned stimulus (light) alone was effective in producing the response. However, pairing of these stimuli produced significant differences in the measured response to the fist-clench. The conditioned response so produced was extinguished by lack of reinforcement and the curve of extinction was a decelerated one. In the measurement of these events, the AL index is found to be the most useful of the three measures employed. The results are discussed from the viewpoint that they represent a central neurophysiological parallel of events which have hitherto been studied at a more peripheral level.

F 73. Stern, J.A., Das, K.C., Anderson, J.M., Biddy, R.L., and Surphlis, W.: "Conditioned" alpha desynchronization. *Science, 134*:388, 1961. (Copyright 1961 by the American Association for the Advancement of Science.)

Results casting doubt on the reported findings of Wells and Wolff on conditioned alpha desynchronization are presented. The experimental findings indicate that these authors were most likely dealing with the phenomenon of adaptation to a complex stimulus. These results are compared to similar phenomena in the conditioning of the galvanic skin response.

conditioning
alpha blocking

F 74.   Gershuni, G.V.: Conditioned cutaneous galvanic reactions and reactions of depression of alpha rhythm following sub-threshold and suprathreshold sound stimulation in man. In *The Central Nervous Stystem and Human Behavior.* Translations from the Russian Medical Literature. Bethesda, Russian Scientific Translation Program, 1959, p. 587.

Responses of conditioned GSR and alpha suppression responses were studied following both subliminal and above threshold auditory perception. The latency of conditioned GSR responses to subliminal stimulation was considerably longer than to suprathreshold stimulation. The alpha suppression response to subthreshold stimulation was of shorter duration than that to suprathreshold stimulation. The effects described were interpreted as indicating reorganization of central excitation of the analyzer to a higher level. It was conjectured that the phenomena related to orientation motor reactions.

conditioning
alpha blocking
GSR

F 75.   Milstein, V.: Contingent alpha blocking: conditioning or sensitization? *Electroencephalogr Clin Neurophysiol, 18:* 272, 1965.

Subjects were presented with tone stimuli following a sensitization procedure and a respondent conditioning procedure to determine the nature of contingent alpha blocking. In the sensitization procedure tones were presented to subjects following independent flashes of light. In the conditioning procedure light-flash and tone pairs were presented to subjects in the absence of the alpha rhythm. The conditioning procedure resulted in a greater blocking effect of tone than did the sensitization procedure.

conditioning
alpha blocking
sensitization

F 76.   Shagass, C., and Johnson, E.P.: The course of acquisition of a conditioned response of the occipital alpha rhythm. *J Exp Psychol, 33*:201, 1943.

The acquisition curve for the conditioned response of the occipital alpha rhythm to voluntary clenching of the fist was determined by using a conditioning procedure in which one half of the trials were reinforced. The curve was an accelerated one, nearly the mirror-image of the extinction curve. The curves of acquisition and extinction for EEG conditioning are similar to those obtained when peripheral responses are conditioned. The effect of a conscious attitude of expectancy was investigated by telling the subjects whether or not to expect a light. It was found that, after a short reinforcement series, responses were given when a light was not expected. These trials yielded an extinction series. Responses were always given when light was expected. It was concluded that the effect of conscious expectancy in the formation of the conditioned response is limited. The results were discussed from the viewpoint of established conditioning concepts.

condition-ing
alpha
 blocking
expectancy

F 77. Birbaumer, N.: Präventive alpha-inhibition und agst. *Studia Psychologica, 12*:179, 1970.

The relationship between EEG alpha and avoidance periods was determined for subjects in a discriminated avoidance paradigm. During the pre-shock interval some subjects showed a blocking or desynchronization response. The subjects with increased alpha in the pre-shock interval showed more signs of anxiety than the subjects which had desynchronization of alpha.

condition-ing
alpha
 blocking
alpha en-
 hancement
anxiety

SECTION G

STATE OF CONSCIOUSNESS

WAKEFULNESS

G 1.   Martin, W.B., Viglione, S.S., Johnson, L.C., and Naitoh, P.:
Pattern recognition of EEG to determine level of alertness.
*Electroencephalogr Clin Neurophysiol, 30:*163, 1971 (abstr).

Pattern recognition technology has been applied to FM recordings of awake and all-night sleep EEG activity from fourteen young adult male subjects to develop a computer scoring system for awake and sleep stages. The pattern recognition processing and analysis consisted in performing a frequency analysis of the EEG and extracting the Fourier
amplitude spectrum from 0 to 26 cps at 0.2 cps frequency
resolution. These 130 coefficients, computed every fifteen
seconds, become the input to the pattern recognition. Recognition systems have been designed for a single subject and for
composite data taken from six subjects. Sleep-stage scoring
systems, designed in individual subjects and used to classify
other recordings from the same subject, achieved 81 percent
agreement with manual scoring. Those systems designed on
composite data achieved 75 percent agreement with manual
scoring. Awake and stage 4 had the highest percent of agreement and stages 1 and 3 the lowest. Detectors for known
properties of certain sleep stages such as spindles and K complexes have also been investigated as potential inputs to the
pattern recognition system. The spindles are detected by performing a Fourier transform on overlapping four-second
epochs and comparing the energy in the sigma band with
energy in the same band over a thirty-second interval. A
peak-and-valley detector to measure the major parameters of
the K complex correctly detected 76 percent of the K complexes over a four-hour period which included all stages of
sleep. The energy in selected frequency bands was computed
as an additional indicator of sleep stage. Preliminary findings

wakefulness
alerting
sleep
EEG
 patterns
data analysis

indicate that delta activity may be the most important input for sleep staging. All-night plots of delta activity revealed a cyclic pattern with a smooth buildup of intensity through stages 2, 3 and 4 with an abrupt decline as the subject entered REM sleep. The amplitude of each cycle decreased as sleep progressed. Spindle intensity was highest in stage 2, decreased during stages 3 and 4 and spindles were absent during REM sleep.

G 2.   Lehmann, D., Jacewitz, M.M., Koukkou, M., and Madey, J.M.: Multichannel EEG field analysis: sleep and wakefulness in humans. *Electroencephalogr Clin Neurophysiol, 30:* 255, 1971.

Spatial maps of EEG activity were made using forty-eight electrode placements and simultaneous recording. Relatively simple equipotential maps were found for waking alpha with maximal positive and negative values remaining in two or three limited areas of the scalp for 70 to 80 percent of the time, with values stepping from one perferred area to the next. Clockwise as well as counterclockwise sequences were observed. Average amplitude of the field reached its peak when maximum alpha activity was in perferred areas. Maximum values for sleep spindles appeared to be limited to one precentral-central area. Fluctuations in average amplitude of alpha per electrode appeared at approximately 20 Hz while fluctuations in sigma were less regular and at approximately 28 Hz. Although the slow waves showed the highest relief in the precentral-central areas, the field distributions were complex with some bilateral symmetry.

wakefulness
sleep
spatio-temporal characteristics
topography
EEG
frequency measurement techniques

G 3.   Goldie, L., and Green, J.M.: Paradoxical blocking and arousal in the drowsy state. *Nature, 187*:952, 1960.

The authors describe a situation in which the appearance of the alpha rhythm indicates increased arousal. The appearance of alpha accompanying increased arousal is known as "paradoxical blocking." This sign of arousal can be found in awakening from sleep. The authors tested the hypothesis that hypnotically suggested sleep is associated with EEG patterns of both drowsiness and waking. Suggested deep sleep

wakefulness
drowsiness
hypnosis
alpha abundance

was accompanied by short periods of EEG associated with drowsiness. The paradoxical blocking signs of arousal appeared after the suggestion to wake up, and all conditions of the suggestion were complete in an all-or-none manner rather than in a gradual manner.

G 4.   Liberson, W.T., and Liberson, C.W.: EEG records, reaction times, eye movements, respiration, and mental content. *Recent Adv Biol Psychiatry, 8:*295, 1966. (Published by Plenum Publishing Corp., Joseph Wortis, Ed.)

A subjective impression of whether one is asleep or not may not be consistent with the apparent EEG patterns. A systematic study of the observation, to the effect that no-slow-wave sleep is a behavioral reality, has been inaugurated by Aserinsky and Kleitman. It was found to be associated with rapid eye movements (REM) and high incidence of dream reports. This original observation made by Loomis et al. has been the subject of numerous studies (see Kleitman). A second observation, namely, the presence of characteristic drowsy patterns in subjects who deny being drowsy, has received less attention. Curiously, this phenomenon is often preceded by, and associated for awhile with, slow eye movements (SEM). It is this phase of sleep research that this paper is concerned with. The authors became interested in determining precise time relationships of alpha depression of drowsiness and of changes in mental content, as well as of the following objective phenomena: motor reaction times, respiration and slow eye movements.

wakefulness
drowsiness
subjective
 reports
reaction
 time
respiration
eye move-
 ments

G 5.   Daniel, R.S.: Electroencephalographic pattern quantification and the arousal continuum. *Psychophysiology, 2:*146, 1965.

Eighteen young adult subjects were presented with situations varying in emotional arousal to determine the related changes in the EEG. Electronic analysis of amplitude, frequency, power, autocorrelation and cross-correlation were used. It was found that behavioral arousal is inversely related to rhythmicity and total power at the dominant frequency. No increase in low voltage, fast activity was found in high-arousal conditions. The dominant frequency spectrum was

wakefulness
emotion
arousal
EEG
 analysis
alpha
 patterns

found to range from 6 to 15 Hz rather than the 8 to 13 Hz typically used.

G 6. Henry, C.E.: Electroencephalogram individual differences and their constancy: II During waking. *J Exp Psychol, 58:* 236, 1959.

Four subjects from a previous experiment, one from each category of waking alpha percentages, were given a number of tasks while awake. Tasks ranged from resting in a dark room with eyes closed to rotational addition in a lighted room with eyes open. The high alpha group showed a greater decrease in alpha with mental activity and individual EEG differences were reduced to nonsignificant levels. The author concluded that similar psychological activities produced similar EEG patterns and that these activities are more important than individual differences in determining the EEG pattern.

wakefulness
mental tasks
alpha
  abundance
alpha
  responses

G 7. Jones, B.N., Binnie, C.D., Fung, D., and Hamblin, J.J.: Reversible coma with an EEG pattern normally associated with wakefulness. *Electroencephalogr Clin Neurophysiol, 33:* 107, 1972.

A case report is presented of a sixty-three-year-old woman who exhibited what resembled a waking EEG while unconscious; that is, her record was dominated by rhythmic activity in the alpha range. Although the symptoms, spells of unconsciousness, tiredness, headaches, deafness, etc., and the EEG records indicated a vascular disorder of the brain stem which had been previously thought fatal, she recovered from the spells without any apparent ill effects. It is suggested that the above diagnosis was correct, but that in this case the disorder was reversible.

wakefulness
brain
  damage
alpha
  patterns
conscious-
  ness

SLEEP

G 8. Brazier, M.A.B., and Beecher, H.K.: Alpha content of the EEG in relation to movements made in sleep and effect of a sedative on this type of motility. *J Appl Physiol, 4:*819, 1952.

Nine normal subjects were recorded for EEG's on two occasions for approximately three hours per session. Quantitative measures of alpha activity, especially the mean alpha content of the EEG, showed a trend toward wakefulness in the period of twenty to zero seconds before and zero to ten seconds after movement during sleep. With delta as an additional index, this evidence of a decrease in depth of sleep prior to movement was supported. The administration of sedatives such as 90 mg sodium pentobarbital did not stop this wakefulness trend, but the incidence of movements did decrease. It was concluded that the number of movements can be used as an index of depth of sleep when comparing drugs for hypnotic power.

sleep
alpha
  abundance
drugs

G 9. Hauri, P., and Hawkins, D.R.: Alpha-delta sleep. *Electroencephalogr Clin Neurophysiol, 34:233,* 1973.

This report defines a new sleep stage called alpha-delta sleep as 5 to 20 percent delta waves mixed with large amplitude alpha waves. It is thought that this type of sleep replaces delta sleep in some patients suffering from chronic, somatic malaise and fatigue and that it involves some brain dysfunction which may be metabolic.

sleep
alpha
  amplitude

G 10. Henry, C.E.: Electroencephalogram individual differences and their constancy: I. During sleep. *J Exp Psychol, 58:*117, 1959.

Twenty male subjects ranging in age from twenty to forty-five years were selected on the basis of the amount of alpha present in their EEG's while awake. Five subjects were selected from each category: 1 to 25 percent, 26 to 50 percent, 51 to 75 percent and 76 to 100 percent time alpha present. The author found that while the groups were heterogeneous with respect to waking alpha, they were homogeneous with respect to sleep rhythms at all stages of sleep. There were no significant differences immediately following waking.

sleep
alpha
  patterns

G 11. Larsen, L.E., and Walter, D.O.: On automatic methods of sleep staging by EEG spectra. *Electroencephalogr Clin Neurophysiol, 28:*459, 1970.

An attempt was made to develop an automated analysis of the EEG which would discriminate stages of sleep on the basis of frequency patterns. The automated analysis involved multiple regression and multiple discriminant techniques. High levels of waking alpha were associated with errors in scoring REM and low waking alpha levels were associated with errors in scoring stage 1 sleep. Quadratic discriminant functions were found to improve scoring. The authors concluded that the frequency spectra provide an adequate basis for discrimination of all sleep stages with the possible exception of stage 1 versus REM sleep.

sleep measurement techniques special analysis

G 12.   Rosandi, G., and Rossi, G.F.: Spectral power analysis of the electroencephalogram during physiological sleep in man. *Activ Nerv Sup (Praha), 11*:106, 1969.

Seven adult subjects were used in a computerized Fourier transformation analysis of sleep EEG's. Frequencies ranging from .39 to 100 Hz were analyzed from two-minute recordings from each stage of sleep. The waking eyes-closed EEG showed a sharp dominant peak at 8 to 10 Hz from the centro-occipital leads and a second low peak at around 5 Hz from the fronto-central leads. Stage 1 sleep was characterized by the sharp reduction or disappearance of a smaller and more variable peak around 2 to 4 Hz. Stage 2 sleep was characterized by the appearance of a peak in the 9 to 14 Hz band predominantly in the fronto-central area and small or absent in the temporal area. A 1 to 4 Hz peak of small amplitude was present in all areas. Stage 3 sleep was characterized by the increased amplitude of the 1 to 4 Hz peak and a reduction in the 9 to 14 Hz peak below the amplitude of the delta peak. Stage 4 and REM were characterized by small amplitude delta and theta peaks with no alpha peak present.

sleep measurement techniques spectral analysis EEG frequency

G 13.   Evans, F.J., Gustafson, L.A., O'Connell, D.N., Orne, M.T., and Shor, R.E.: Verbally induced behavioral responses during sleep. *J Nerv Ment Dis, 150*:171, 1970.

Nineteen male subjects with an alpha index of greater than 40 percent in the waking EEG were given verbal suggestions for various behaviors in portions of stage 1 sleep where alpha was absent. In a second session subjects were given a cue

sleep verbal stimuli alpha enhancement

word which elicited appropriate behaviors in sixteen out of nineteen subjects. The average of appropriate responses was 18.2 percent of alpha ranging from 0 to 48 percent in various subjects. The suggestions and cues tended to elicit alpha in the EEG's with the suggestions eliciting more than the cue words.

G 14.   Jus, K., et al.: Experimental studies on memory during slow sleep stages and REM stages. *Electroencephalogr Clin Neurophysiol, 27:688,* 1969 (abstr).

Thirty subjects were presented verbal and nonverbal stimuli while in stages 2, 3, 4 and REM sleep. Subjects were awakened after each series of stimuli and tested for spontaneous recall and recognition of the stimuli. An activation pattern following stimulation of alpha activity associated with a vegetative EMG did not result in significant recall. An "arousal-awakening" autonomic pattern with EEG alpha activity was associated with partial recall.

sleep
verbal
  stimuli
memory
alpha en-
  hancement
recall
EEG
  activation

G 15.   Johnson, L., et al.: Spectral analysis of the EEG of dominant and non-dominant alpha subjects during waking and sleeping. *Electroencephalogr Clin Neurophysiol, 26:361,* 1969.

Thirteen subjects, nine with a high incidence of alpha and four with a low incidence of alpha, were used in a spectral analysis of the P3 lead of the EEG. A delta peak appeared at all stages of sleep with a frequency of approximately 1 Hz increasing in amplitude through stages 1 to 4. REM delta amplitude was approximately equal to stage 1 sleep. A 13 Hz peak was found for all subjects in stage 2 with lower amplitudes during other sleep stages and none during the waking period. The two groups showed a similar pattern during stages 2, 3 and 4. All frequencies showed greater amplitude and variability for the high alpha group than for the low alpha group. The high alpha group had a waking alpha peak at 10 Hz which changed to approximately 9 Hz in stage 1 and REM. Waking amplitudes of alpha, theta and delta were found to be positively correlated with corresponding sleep amplitudes while no correlations were found for theta and sigma.

sleep
wakefulness
alpha
  abundance
spectral
  analysis

G 16. Goldstein, L., Burdick, J.A., and Lazslo, M.: A quantitative analysis of the EEG during sleep in normal subjects. *Acta Physiol Acad Sci Hung, 37:*291, 1970.

Using electronic integrators and unfiltered accumulated amplitude measurements in successive ten-second segments, the EEG from left and right parietal leads was analyzed for time course variability. The lowest variability occurred during waking states and the highest was during S4 sleep, while REM sleep fell somewhere in between these extremes. Variability correlations between hemispheres were greatest during S4 sleep and least during REM sleep.

sleep wakefulness measurement techniques temporal stability

G 17. Barnett, T.P., Johnson, L.C., Naitoh, P., Hicks, N., and Nute, C.: Bispectrum analysis of electroencephalogram signals during waking and sleeping. *Science, 172:*401, 1971.

EEG's of eight subjects were recorded in waking and sleeping conditions to determine the degree of interaction between various frequencies of the EEG. A bispectrum analysis technique was used in which phase locking or quadratic coupling of frequencies could be determined. Significant bicoherence values were obtained in the awake state for the four subjects with high alpha activity and one of the four subjects with low alpha activity in the left central and occipital leads. The analysis revealed a phase locked 20 Hz, 7 Hz and 2 Hz. The phase locking only accounted for one half of the 20 Hz amplitude in the awake state. No clear bicoherence patterns were observed in sleep with peaks being low and diffuse.

sleep wakefulness bispectrum analysis alpha abundance alpha harmonics

G 18. Lubin, A., Johnson, L.C., and Austin, M.T.: Discrimination among states of consciousness using EEG spectra. *Psychophysiology, 6:*122, 1969.

EEG recordings were made during waking (W) and the five sleep stages (REM, 1, 2, 3 and 4) on thirteen young adult males. For each stage, one-minute sections of the parietal EEG trace were digitized and subjected to Fourier analysis. The resulting spectral intensities were divided into five frequency bands: delta, theta, alpha, sigma and beta. Linear

sleep wakefulness spectral analysis

discriminators for all six stages were calculated using stepwise multiple regression. The overall percent agreement with visual scoring was very poor, ranging from zero for stage 3 to 91 percent for stage 4. Linear discrimination between pairs of stages yielded slightly better results, but stages 1 and REM were indistinguishable. Delta is the best overall discriminator, increasing significantly through stages W, 1, 2, 3 and 4. Sigma is unique to sleep and is highest for stage 2. Theta is unimportant and beta plays no role at all. Spectral analysis of the parietal EEG lead is not sufficient to differentiate among the six states of consciousness studied here. The use of detectors for such phasic events as eye movement and K complexes might aid sleep stage discrimination considerably.

G 19.   Jovanović, U.J.: Subclinical sleep activity in the EEG. *Psychiatria Clinica, 2:*338, 1969.

The author defines features of the waking drowsy EEG as "subclinical sleep activity." Two states of subclinical sleep are defined as A and B. The A state is divided into three segments: one in which the EEG is undifferentiable from the waking pattern, a second in which continuous alpha is present without change in frequency and amplitude, and a third in which only flat EEG rhythms are present. State B is similarly divided into three segments: one in which small fast theta waves are present, a second in which medium frequency theta waves are present, and a third in which signs of clinical sleep appear. One thousand fifty nine subjects were tested and eighty-two showed the subclinical sleep activity defined here.

sleep
drowsy
EEG
    patterns
alpha
    abundance
theta
beta

G 20.   Rodin, E.A., Luby, E.D., and Gottlieb, J.S.: The electroencephalogram during prolonged experimental sleep deprivation. *Electroencephalogr Clin Neurophysiol, 14:*544, 1962.

Sixteen subjects were recorded for EEG activity while being deprived of sleep for as much as 120 hours. The EEG's remained desynchronized as long as alertness was maintained. After forty-nine hours all subjects showed drowsiness as evidenced by a progressive inability to sustain alpha activity.

sleep
sleep deprivation
alpha
    abundance

Small decreases in alpha amplitude and increases of about 1 cps in alpha frequency were also observed. Alpha activity with eyes open during sleep loss appeared to be of the same frequency as that with eyes closed in some subjects but varied to lower frequencies in others, indicating the presence of an unknown factor in addition to drowsiness which affects such eyes-open alpha activity. Five subjects had high voltage paroxysmal activity including excessive diffuse theta in the first forty-eight hours similar to that in patients with centrencepalic convulsive disorders. This paroxysmal activity was not associated with drowsiness since it disappeared as sleeplessness continued. These same subjects had low Megimide® thresholds. Therefore, prolonged sleep loss seems to be associated with increased cerebral irritability or excitability for the first forty-eight hours of sleep deprivation. Certain people may even exhibit epileptic-like characteristics under these conditions.

alpha amplitude
alpha frequency
theta
EEG patterns

G 21. Naitoh, P., Kales, A., Kollar, E.J., Smith, J.C., and Jacobson, A.: Electroencephalographic activity after prolonged sleep loss. *Electroencephalogr Clin Neurophysiol, 27:2,* 1969.

Four subjects were totally deprived of sleep over 205 hours. EEG recordings were taken before, during and after the sleep deprivation. Alpha activity was markedly reduced during sleep deprivation with an associated reduction in tracking performance, deteriorated subjective ratings for both effort and feeling states, and an increase in hypnogogic imagery. One hundred and twenty hours after the onset of sleep deprivation alpha activity, subjective ratings and temperature showed some increase while corticosteroid levels returned to normal. Pre-deprivation levels of all variables were achieved after two nights of sleep following deprivation. Alpha index and subjective rating scales provided the only reliable indicators of sleep deprivation while autonomic measures were found to be unrelated.

sleep
sleep deprivation
alpha patterns
subjective states
ANS

REM Sleep (Dreams)

G 22. Johnson, L., Naitoh, P., Nute, C., Lubin, A., Martin, B., and Viglione, S.: EEG spectral and coherence analysis during awake and sleep. *Electroencephalogr Clin Neurophysiol, 31:* 293, 1971 (abstr).

Eight subjects were tested for EEG patterns during six stages of sleep: awake, stage 1, stage 2, stage 3, stage 4 and REM. Spectral profiles of the frequencies from .49 to 20 Hz were calculated for the F3, C3 and O1 leads. Coherence values were calculated for each of the pairs. The F3-O1 pair had the lowest average coherence value of .12, while the F3-C3 pair showed a coherence value of .60 with highest coherence values for 8 to 10 Hz in the waking and REM conditions. The 12.5 to 14.5 Hz coherence values were higher during stages 2, 3 and 4 than during waking, stage 1 or REM. Delta activity did not become increasingly coherent across stages of sleep. The authors suggest that there is a single source for sigma in stages 2, 3 and 4 while there are multiple sources for delta.

sleep
dreams
wakefulness
spectral
  analysis

G 23. Itil, T.M.: Digital computer analysis of the electroencephalogram during rapid eye movement sleep state in man. *J Nerv Ment Dis, 150:*201, 1970.

The EEG's of seven subjects were analyzed for drowsy, awakening and REM sleep conditions to determine discriminant features. Analysis of variance and discriminant function analysis were applied to individual and group data revealing that REM can be discriminated from both awakening and drowsy EEG. REM is characterized by lower voltage, less alpha activity, more slow wave activity, and more fast frequency activity. The author theorized that the increased fast activity reflects increased mental activity associated with dreaming.

sleep
dreams
computer
  analysis
EEG
  patterns
beta
awake
drowsy

G 24. Stoyva, J.: Can electrophysiological studies of dreaming be used as a paradigm for other research in psychophysiological relationships? In Hartmann, E. (Ed.) : *Sleep and Dreaming.* Boston, Little, Brown, 1969.

It is suggested that the combined use of physiological indices and verbal reports as utilized in the study of dreaming can be expanded to other areas with the addition of biofeedback procedures. This approach would include measurement, amplification, feedback and shaping and would be of considerable practical value.

sleep
dreams
biofeedback
applications

G 25.   Gresham, S.C.: Alcohol and caffeine: Effect on inferred visual dreaming. *Science, 140*:1226, 1963.

A large amount of alcohol was consumed by seven subjects before retiring for the night causing a decrease in duration of stage 1-REM sleep during the first five hours of sleep. The transitional period into stage 1-REM sleep was as follows: spindles and random slow activity changed to 4 to 7 cps waves which in turn became 8 to 12 cps alpha waves. Alpha activity was then reduced in amplitude marking the beginning of low-voltage fast activity with rapid eye movements, low-voltage 3 to 6 cps waves with sharp peaks and scattered alpha waves. Moderate dosage of caffeine had no significant effect and it was concluded that this may have resulted from an insufficient dosage or a lack of sustained stimulation during the sleep period.

sleep
dreams
drugs

ATTENTION

G 26.   Evans, C.R., and Mulholland, T.B.: Attention as a concept in neurophysiology. *Science, 163*:495, January 1969. (Copyright 1969 by the American Association for the Advancement of Science.)

This article reviews findings of a conference on neurophysiological aspects of the psychological concept of attention. Issues examined include: (a) relation of visual control systems to EEG occipital alpha rhythm, (b) evoked responses, (c) the role of the reticular activating system in the acquisition of CR's, and (d) habituation of response from single cells in brain and behavioral reactions.

attention
theory
alpha
  patterns

G 27.   Shagass, C., Overton, D.A., Bartolucci, G., and Straumanis, J.J.: Effects of attention modification by television viewing on somatosensory recovery functions. *Electroencephalogr Clin Neurophysiol, 27*:662, 1969 (abstr).

Eighteen adult clinical patients were recorded for standard EEG as well as evoked responses to electrical stimulation of the median nerve while watching television and resting. Interstimulus intervals ranged between 10 and 100 msec. Differences in attention between the resting and television

attention
television
nerve
  stimulation
alpha
  blocking

viewing conditions had no measurable effect on the evoked responses. Attenuation of alpha produced by the viewing condition was found to be proportional to the resting amplitude of alpha.

G 28. Mulholland, T.: The electroencephalogram as an experimental tool in the study of internal attention gradients. *Trans NY Acad Sci, 24*:664, 1962.

A simple electronic apparatus so filtered the EEG that selected frequencies in the alpha range (recorded from parieto-occipital locations) automatically caused a stimulus to occur. When alpha was then suppressed, the stimulus was automatically removed. When alpha reoccurred, the stimulus automatically occurred again. During this feedback stimulation the following phenomena were observed: (a) alpha tended to occur in a series of short bursts separated by periods of no-alpha activity; (b) the changes of duration of the alpha component and the no-alpha component over time were not necessarily inverse. Durations of alpha increased slowly while durations of no-alpha at first decreased rapidly and then decreased more slowly. The variance of the alpha component showed a marked decrease while the variance of the no-alpha durations showed less decrease during feedback stimulation for some individuals. (c) The temporal pattern of alpha and no-alpha response durations was significantly different for conditions of viewing and silently counting feedback flashes (more attention) compared to simply viewing the feedback stimulus. In general, alpha durations were shorter, no-alpha durations longer, and the variance of alpha durations was reduced during the period of internalized, silent counting of the stimulus. (d) The hypothesis was presented that the system fractionates phasic alerting response latencies from tonic and phasic alerting response durations. (e) Some applications of the system to the study of habituation and attention and the effect of psychopharmacologic agents on these processes were suggested.

attention
alpha
blocking
biofeedback

G 29. Mulholland, T., and Runnals, S.: Increased occurrence of EEG alpha during increased attention. *J Psychol, 54*:317, 1962.

Three experiments were performed to determine the relationships between the presence of the alpha rhythm and various attention sets in the presence of two visual illusions. In the first study, six male subjects were given the tasks of simply viewing a rotating rectangle, trying to perceive the vertical motion, or trying to see the illusion. An increased incidence of alpha was bound to occur when the object was stationary as opposed to moving, and also during the attention set conditions as contrasted to simple viewing, as well as following verbal reports. In the second experiment a rotating disc illusion was used with different illuminating backgrounds and different levels of perceptual task difficulty. In this condition the incidence of alpha was lower with attentional sets. For attentional sets, the incidence of alpha increased as a function of background luminance while the opposite was true for the simple viewing condition. In a third experiment, no difference was found between alpha incidence in attention-set and simple viewing. The authors conclude that the typical phenomenon of alpha reduction with attention is a product of defining attention in terms of transient external stimulation. With extended internal stimulation, alpha has a complex relationship to attention.

attention
perceptual tasks
visual illusions
alpha patterns
subjective reports
definitions
theory

VIGILANCE

G 30. Gale, A., Haslum, M., and Lucas, B.: Arousal value of the stimulus and EEG abundance in an auditory vigilance task. *Br J Psychol, 63*:515, 1972.

Ten college students were recorded for EEG's during an auditory vigilance task in order to compare EEG subjective states, alertness, etc., across rather than within the six signal types presented. The wanted signal was three consecutive odd digits and each signal was followed by a rest period. Results included: (1) a decrease in alpha abundance with an increase in arousal value of the signal; (2) insignificant and weak effects in the theta and beta ranges; (3) a very low value for the odd-odd-even signal in the 2.0 to 4.5 Hz range; (4) alpha abundance increase during the rest periods following the three most arousing signals while the reverse was observed for rest periods associated with the least arousing signals; (5) a generally smaller abundance of theta activity

vigilance
alpha abundance
theta
subjective states

during rest periods than during signals and a much smaller
theta abundance during the rest following the wanted signal;
(6) less activity in the 2.0 to 4.5 Hz range during rest following the three least arousing signals than during the signals;
and (7) a subject self-rating indicating them to be more
keyed up as signal arousal value increased and more alert
during rest periods following signals of increased cue value.
These variations in subjective state were also seen as systematic changes in the EEG. The results of this research were
interpreted as supporting in some respects arousal models
of vigilance and Lindsley's activation theory.

G 31. Davies, D.R., and Krkovic, A.: Skin-conductance, alpha-
        activity, and vigilance. *Am J Psychol, 78*:304, 1965.

Skin conductance and alpha brain waves were recorded in   *vigilance*
order to investigate a possible relationship between perform- *alpha*
ance in vigilance tasks and electrophysiological activation.   *abundance*
Decreased alpha activity, skin conductance, level of perform- *GSR*
ance and subjective reports showed that subjects get drowsy
over the course of a ninety-minute auditory vigilance task.
Lack of varied stimulation from the task and the environment were given as probable causes of the drowsiness.

G 32. Mangan, G.L., and Adcock, C.J.: EEG correlates of per-
        ceptual vigilance and defence. *Percept Mot Skills, 14*:197,
        1962.

EEG changes were monitored in eleven subjects trained to a   *vigilance*
defense criterion and ten others trained to a vigilance cri- *EEG*
terion. Critical and neutral stimuli presented to defensive   *patterns*
subjects and critical but not neutral stimuli presented to
vigilance subjects caused a significant decrease in frontal
limits (F1) index measures. Differentiation between the
two types of subjects was possible through responses to
neutral and critical stimuli. The results from F1, a negative
measure of emotion, indicated defensive subjects to be emotional under test conditions with a less specific reaction to
critical words when compared to vigilance subjects.

G 33. Daniel, R.S.: Alpha and theta EEG in vigilance. *Percept
        Mot Skills, 25*:697, 1967.

Nineteen male subjects between the ages of eighteen and twenty-two years were presented with a series of tape-recorded digits in random order and were asked to press a key whenever a sequence of three odd digits appeared in sequence. Left and right occipital EEG's were recorded. The decline in performance across the five 12-minute time blocks was closely paralleled by increases in two measures of alpha abundance. The incidence of theta frequency activity was lowered prior to vigilance errors. The theoretical relationships between alpha, theta and performance were discussed.

vigilance
reaction
time
alpha
abundance
theta

G 34. Gulian, E.: Effects of noise on EEG latency changes in an auditory vigilance task. *Electroencephalogr Clin Neurophysiol, 27*:637, 1969 (abstr).

Subjects were given the task of reporting the occurrence of an auditory signal in the presence of background noise at either high or low intensity and either constant or intermittent. Four other auditory stimuli were presented randomly, increasing the complexity of the discrimination task. The EEG alpha blocking response latencies were measured following each stimulus. Blocking response latencies were shorter for correct responses than for false positive or false negative responses in the discrimination. The longest blocking latencies were found when low intensity, continuous noise was present.

vigilance
auditory
stimulation
alpha
blocking

G 35. Thorsheim, H.I.: EEG and vigilance behavior. *Psychon Sci, 8*:499, 1967.

Thirty subjects were presented with a vigilance monitoring task of pressing a button each time the number *30* was replaced by the number *70* on a display screen. Half of the subjects were given physical exercises during the experimental sessions while half were used as controls. The subjects having motor exercises had lower alpha amplitude prior to stimulation and higher amplitudes following stimulus presentation. The control group demonstrated the opposite effect. No differences in performance were found between the two groups.

vigilance
motor per-
formance
alpha
amplitude

G 36.   Roth, B.: The clinical and theoretical importance of EEG
rhythms corresponding to states of lowered vigilance. *Electroencephalogr Clin Neurophysiol, 13*:395, 1961.

Five hundred EEG recordings were analyzed to determine
the reactivity of the EEG to presentation of visual stimuli
during different states of lowered vigilance (drowsy states).
Four stages of pre-sleep lowered vigilance were defined:
state A in which subjects show a disintegration of the alpha
rhythm, state B1 in which a flattened EEG is found, state B2
in which 5 to 6 Hz appears at high intensity, and state B3 in
which high intensity activity of 3 to 4 Hz appears. In the
alert, awake EEG, photic stimulation was found to produce
a blocking response in 99 percent of the cases. State A was
associated with less blocking of alpha and more enhancement
of alpha with stimulation. States B1 and B3 were associated
with paradoxical blocking or enhancement of alpha. A return to a normal waking EEG pattern was found to occur
whenever external stimulation was presented, when hyperventilation occurred and whenever Metrazol® or Benze-
drine® were administered. The author stated that the states
of lowered vigilance seem to correspond to what Pavlov
identified as "hypnotic phases."

vigilance
drowsiness
visual
*   stimulation*
alpha
*   patterns*

G 37.   Adey, W.R., Kado, R.T., and Walter, D.O.: Computer analysis of EEG data from Gemini flight GT-7. *Aerosp Med, 38*:
345, 1967.

The two astronauts who flew on the GT-7 mission in space
were recorded for EEG while performing a variety of tasks
both in simulation sessions prior to the mission and during
the actual flight. In the simulation sessions a baseline EEG
was recorded for comparison to the flight data. The theta
and beta frequency ranges showed less than one-tenth the
intensity of the alpha frequency range. The amplitude of the
delta frequency range was intermediate. In visual discrimination tasks the amplitude of alpha was significantly attenuated
at all recording sites while the amplitudes of the delta and
beta frequencies were significantly increased. Auditory vigilance involving the recognition of particular three-tone patterns was associated with an increase in the amplitude of
alpha. In altitude chamber exposure the alpha peak disap-

vigilance
attention
space flight
EEG
*   patterns*
visual
*   perception*

peared and all frequencies above 5 Hz were attenuated. Theta activity was significantly enhanced in this condition. Similar tasks performed in space resulted in similar patterns of EEG change. The primary characteristic of the EEG's during the flight was a significantly enhanced amplitude of the theta frequency range. The arousal accompanying the pre-launch periods was associated with a sequence of changes in EEG frequency pattern. The pre-launch period involved a strong focus of attention. The overall density of theta activity was increased during this period. As the launch time came close, alpha and beta activity increased in intensity. At one minute prior to launch, theta, alpha and beta frequencies were all at high intensity levels (a factor of 10 increase for some frequencies). High intensity beta occurred in several periods during the first half-hour of the flight.

G 38. Becker-Carus, C.: Relationships between EEG, personality and vigilance. *Electroencephalogr Clin Neurophysiol, 30:* 519, 1971.

EEG and personality data were analyzed in relation to the performance of nineteen young adults in mental arithmetic and vigilance monitoring tasks. Increased task difficulty was found to be related to a decrease in the incidence of alpha. Vigilance performance was positively correlated with 8 to 9 Hz activity and negatively correlated with 12 to 13 Hz activity. Vigilance performance was negatively correlated with the alpha incidence in the rest periods preceding performance. Measures of personality rigidity were positively correlated with number of errors in vigilance. Neurotic tendency measures were positively correlated with 10 to 11 Hz incidence during vigilance and negatively correlated during the initial rest period. Errors in mental arithmetic were positively correlated with 8 to 9 Hz activity during vigilance performance.

vigilance
personality
alpha
  abundance

G 39. Gale, A., Haslum, M., and Penfold, V.: EEG correlates of cumulative expectancy and selective estimates of alertness in a vigilance-type task. *Q J Exp Psychol, 23:*245, 1971.

Twenty subjects were monitored for occipital EEG during a slow presentation rate vigilance task. EEG rating values (abundance, prevalence, etc.) decreased with increased cumu-

vigilance
expectancy
reaction
  time

lative expectancy and increased with decreased expectancy. *alpha*
Subjective alertness estimates taken prior to the trial paral- *abundance*
leled EEG changes. No correlation was found between reac- *alpha*
tion time to wanted signals and measures of pre-signal EEG. *frequency*
Although the above trends could be seen in most EEG bands,
the alpha frequency showed the best and most statistically
significant results. Possible shortcomings of the research are
admitted and explained along with further work which is
underway to remedy these deficiencies.

G 40.   Koukkou, M., Madey, J.M., and Yeager, C.L.: Memory and
vigilance: Spectral EEG analysis during learning in humans.
Electroencephalogr Clin Neurophysiol, 27:687, 1969.

In order to test the theory that the extent of vigilance during *vigilance*
learning affects the quality of memory storage, parieto-oc- *memory*
cipital EEG's were evaluated via spectral analysis after pre- *spectral*
sentation of memory material to sleeping subjects. A wakeful- *analysis*
ness-type EEG spectrum was seen in those with spontaneous
recall and recognition of the material while a sleep-type frequency distribution continued in the subjects with no recall.
In a further test a comparison of learning of new material
versus relearning of familiar material showed that within the
same class of recall higher vigilance was associated with the
learning of unfamiliar things than was associated with the
relearned material.

HYPNOSIS

G 41.   Ulett, G.A., Akpinar, S., and Itil, T.M.: Quantitative EEG
analysis during hypnosis. *Electroencephalogr Clin Neuro-*
psychol, 33:361, 1972.

The ten best and the ten poorest of forty-four previously *hypnosis*
hypnotized normal volunteer subjects were studied using *alpha*
EEG's, pre-recorded video-taped hypnotic induction, digital *abundance*
computer period analysis and analog frequency analysis to *alpha en-*
discover quantitative EEG correlates of the hypnotic state. *hancement*
Statistically significant EEG changes, which were quite differ- *alpha*
ent from drowsiness or sleep EEG's previously reported, were *frequency*
observed during both the hypnotic induction and hypnotic *variability*
trance. During the hypnotic induction period, the best hyp-

notic subjects exhibited decreased slow waves and increased alpha and beta activity along with increased amplitude and reduced amplitude variability. The outstanding feature during hypnotic trance, especially in the best subjects, was a significant enhancement of alpha activity. The increased alpha activity was interpreted as indicating some similarity between hypnosis and Yoga, Zen, autogenic training and alpha training since such augmented alpha is characteristic of all of these.

G 42. Barolin, G.S.: Bioelectric correlates in hypnoid states. Study of a biological explanation of hypnosis. *Fortschr Neurol Psychiatr, 36:*227, 1968.

The sometimes confusing nature of the bioelectric expressions of hypnosis can be clarified by an understanding of: (a) the basic hypnotic state and (b) the events occurring in the course of it. In the basic hypnotic state are found: increased synchronization of the EEG, indicating decrease of afferent impulses. There may be involvement of archaic structures and mechanisms. Central arcades may appear in EEG. The EEG events seen in the hypnotic state should be distinguished from sleep patterns. Both spontaneous and induced activity during hypnosis leads to arousal patterns. Alpha blocking by stimuli may be, but need not be, reduced. Artifacts induced by blinking may disappear during hypnosis. Sensory-evoked potentials show paradoxal inversion. The results obtained during hypnotic experimentation vary greatly, probably because of the following: the degree of hypnotic trance defies measurement; individual factors govern the degree of EEG changes; the present experimental setup may not have been adequate. The findings show, however, that there are fairly close relationships between psychotherapy and neurophysiology. Hypnotic states should be seen primarily as shifts towards a different neuro-autonomic status, which differs from both sleep and the waking state. No differences appear to exist between the neurophysiological expressions of hypnosis, autogenic training and meditative states, such as Yoga and Zen.

hypnosis
EEG
synchrony
theory

G 43. Darrow, C.W., Henry, C.E., Brenman, M., and Gill, M.: Inter-area electroencephalographic relationships affected by hypnosis: Preliminary report. *Electroencephalogr Clin Neurophysiol, 2*:231, 1950 (abstr).

Eleven subjects who were easily hypnotized were recorded for EEG from frontal, parietal and occipital electrodes before and during a hypnotic trance. The greatest change found was increased in-phase, peak-to-peak correspondence of the EEG between the parietal and occipital placements and between the frontal and parietal placements. The changes in EEG synchronization were significant at the .01 level of confidence.

hypnosis
alpha
  symmetry
alpha phase
alpha
  blocking

G 44.   Marenina, A.I.: The cortical potentials of man in hypnosis in relation to different forms of rapport. *Pavlov J Higher Nerv Activ, 11*:233, 1961.

Fourteen individuals were recorded for cerebral potentials in relation to both narrow and wide rapport in different phases of hypnotic sleep. The subjects were asked neutral questions such as "Are you cold?" during the waking and hypnotized stages and the EEG and EMG (jaw muscles) changes were noted. Questions during the waking state and the first stage of hypnosis produced changes in the masseter muscle and an accompanying shift in EEG frequency to more beta and gamma waves. In the second phase of hypnosis no significant changes were observed and no verbal response was heard. During the third or somnambulistic stage of hypnosis, the electrical reaction was delayed 1 to 1.5 seconds and the verbal response was delayed 2 to 3 seconds. Also, the EEG and EMG frequency increased. Beta wave acceleration and alpha rhythm depression characterized the EEG when the question was asked by a person brought into rapport by the hypnotist during this third stage. A gradual contraction of the limits of the focus of rapport was concluded.

hypnosis
EEG
  frequency
alpha
  responses

G 45.   Dynes, J.B.: Objective method for distinguishing sleep from the hypnotic trance. *Arch Neurol Psychiatr, 57*:84, 1947.

Five patients were hypnotized and trained to go into a trance instantaneously upon the command of the experimenter. They were then recorded for EEG before and after the com-

hypnosis
EEG
  patterns

mand to go into the trance to determine the related EEG changes in frontal, parietal and occipital leads. There were no observed changes in EEG patterns in the hypnotic trance and none of the typical patterns associated with sleep were found in any of the subjects.

G 46. Obonai, T., Fujisawa, K., and Yamaoka, K.: Electroencephalographic researches of hypnotic state. *Electroencephalogr Clin Neurophysiol (Suppl), 9:*50, 1957.

Five subjects (19 to 21 years old) were recorded for EEG during hypnotic age regression to determine if the EEG patterns would parallel the stages of development of which the subjects were being regressed. The changes in frequency associated with stages of development did not occur. Alpha frequency was the same as in the waking state, occipital alpha amplitude was attenuated, frontal and occipital EEG became similar, irregularities in the alpha rhythm appeared, and the incidence of large alpha bursts decreased with time. The EEG characteristics were described as similar to those in a drowsy state.

hypnosis
age regression
alpha patterns

G 47. Wilson, N.J.: Neurophysiologic alterations with hypnosis. *Dis Nerv Syst, 29:*618, 1968.

Fifteen subjects with greater than 50 percent incidence of alpha in the eyes-closed EEG and readily hypnotizable, were recorded for EEG alpha blocking to photic stimulation before and during a hypnotic trance. The suggestion was given that the light would not bother the subject when presented. No significant differences in EEG patterns or in latency of the blocking response were found between the two conditions. The duration of the blocking response, however, was found to be significantly shorter in the hypnotic trance.

hypnosis
visual stimulation
alpha blocking
EEG patterns

G 48. Yeager, C.L., and Larson, A.: A study of alpha desynchronization in the electroencephalogram, utilizing hypnotic suggestion. *Electroencephalogr Clin Neurophysiol, 10:*193, 1958 (abstr).

Subjects were recorded for EEG during a hypnotic trance *hypnosis*
with eye opening and closing, the presentation of visual *visual*
stimuli of various colors as well as suggestions to be unaware *stimulation*
of eye opening and unaware of the visual stimuli. Alpha *alpha*
blocking was found to be produced by eye opening regardless *blocking*
of the suggestion of awareness. The suggestion eliminating *eye opening*
awareness of the visual stimuli decreased the alpha blocking
response. Blue and green lights did not produce the alpha
blocking response regardless of suggestion. Verbal commands
did not produce blocking. The authors concluded that the
blocking produced by eye opening is a reflex while that produced by some visual stimuli is a product of awareness.

G 49.   Roberts, D.R.: An electrophysiological theory of hypnosis.
Int J Clin Exp Hypn, 8:43, 1960.

Presents an hypothesis on hypnosis which suggests an elec- *hypnosis*
trical blockage between the brain stem reticular formation *visual*
and neuronal channels. Mechanisms of attention (for exam- *stimulation*
ple, estimates of behavioral arousal) are evaluated through *EEG*
EEG activity. Delta activity is suggested as a possible means *activation*
of inhibition.

G 50.   Barker, W., and Burgwin, S.: Brain wave patterns during
hypnosis, hypnotic sleep and normal sleep. *Arch Neurol
Psychiatr, 62:*412, 1949.

Four subjects were recorded for EEG before and during hyp- *hypnosis*
notic induction and hypnotically suggested deep sleep. All *sleep*
subjects had near 100 percent alpha in their eyes-closed rest- *alpha*
ing EEG. In the hypnotic trance the alpha became more *patterns*
sporadic. The suggestion of sleep caused a reduction in alpha
activity to a near flat (low voltage, fast) EEG pattern. As the
suggestions for deeper sleep continued, some patterns of
normal sleep appeared including K waves and large slow
wave activity.

G 51.   Darrow, C.W., Henry, C.E., Gill, M., Brenman, M., and
Converse, M.: Frontal-motor parallelism and motor-occi-
pital in-phase activity in hypnosis, drowsiness and sleep.
*Electroencephalogr Clin Neurophysiol, 2:*355, 1950 (abstr) .

Subjects were recorded for EEG in hypnotic trance and sleep to determine the changes in synchronization of different scalp locations. Frontal-motor synchrony increased both in hypnosis and in the hypnogogic stage which subjects pass through when going to sleep. With deeper sleep, frontal-motor synchrony decreased and parieto-motor synchrony increased.

hypnosis
sleep
EEG
  synchrony

G 52. Fujisawa, K., Koga, E., and Toyoda, J.: The polygraphical study on the psychogenic changes of consciousness. (1). About Zen Yoga and hypnosis. *Electroencephalogr Clin Neurophysiol (Suppl), 18:*51 1959.

Five subjects were recorded for EEG in waking, sleeping and hypnotic trance states to determine the changes in EEG patterns. The hypnotic suggestion of sleep was found to be similar to actual sleep. Alpha amplitude was reduced with the hypnotic suggestion and low voltage theta and delta rhythms appeared in the EEG. No humps, K complexes or sleep spindles were found in the hypnotically suggested sleep. The GSR was found to de-adapt or increase to repeated auditory stimulation rather than habituate. The physiological responses were found to be similar to those observed in the hypnogogic stages of sleep.

hypnosis
sleep
EEG
  patterns

G 53. Diamant, J., Dufek, M., Hoskovec, J., Kristof, M., Pekarek, V., Roth, B., and Velek, M.: An electroencephalographic study of the waking state and hypnosis with particular reference to subclinical manifestations of sleep activity. *Int J Clin Exp Hypn, 8:*199, 1960.

Ten psychiatric patients were recorded for EEG during awake resting and hypnotic trance states to determine the relative incidence of EEG sleep criteria. Seven of the subjects showed no change in EEG pattern, two of the subjects showed increased sleep criteria and one subject showed increased wakefulness criteria in the hypnotic trance. A slight reduction in alpha blocking to external stimulation was found in the hypnotic trance. The suggestion that the stimulus was not present did not prevent alpha blocking.

hypnosis
sleep
alpha
  blocking

G 54. Schwarz, B.E., Bickford, R.G., and Rasmussen, W.C.: Hypnotic phenomena, including hypnotically activated seizures, studied with the electroencephalogram. *Int J Clin Exp Hypn, 122*:564, 1955.

Forty-six subjects were hypnotized through a method involving eye fixation and arm levitation and were recorded for EEG under several suggestions. Suggestion of a visual stimulus produced alpha blocking under hypnosis but not in the waking state. Suggested anesthesia and age regression produced no changes in the EEG of seven subjects who were given the suggestion of sleep, three developed flattened EEG's, three had spindles and V waves and one subject had high amplitude delta in the EEG. Subjects with a history of epilepsy were found to go into and out of seizures upon suggestion.

hypnosis
visual
* perception*
sleep
alpha
* blocking*
age
* regression*
EEG
* patterns*
epilepsy

G 55. Genkin, A.A., and Mordvinov, E.F.: Electroencephalographic correlates of the hypnotic states. *Zh Vyssh Nerv Deiat, 19*:471, 1969.

Eight subjects (18 to 21 years old) were selected for the experiment on the basis of having good hypnotizability. EEG was recorded during the process of going into a hypnotic trance and while performing mental activity in the hypnotic state to determine changes in EEG symmetry. Increased symmetry over the normal resting values was found during the precataleptic stage of hypnosis and the transition to sleep. The changes in symmetry were found to be discrete. Mental activity in the hypnotic state was associated with increased symmetry of EEG in half of the subjects and with decreased symmetry in the other half. The authors hypothesized CNS mechanisms governing EEG symmetry in different stages of consciousness.

hypnosis
mental tasks
EEG
* symmetry*

G 56. Ford, W.L., and Yeager, C.L.: Changes in the electroencephalogram in subjects under hypnosis. *Dis Nerv Syst, 9*:190, 1948.

Eight psychiatric patients with a variety of disorders were recorded for EEG before and during hypnosis to determine the effects of different suggestions on EEG patterns. One sub-

hypnosis
psychopath-
* ology*

ject with anxiety hysteria was found to have little alpha in the resting EEG, a large amount of alpha in the EEG with hypnotically suggested relaxation and no detectable alpha in hypnotically suggested tension. Two patients with anxiety states were found to have flat EEG's with little alpha present in the resting condition, no change with relaxation in the waking state, and well-developed alpha following hypnotically suggested relaxation. Three subjects with normal alpha in their resting EEG's showed no change with hypnotically suggested relaxation. The suggestion of blindness was given to these subjects and visual stimuli were presented. The alpha blocking response to eye opening and visual stimulation was unchanged from the resting condition. Four subjects were age regressed with no discernable changes in the EEG.

alpha patterns
anxiety
relaxation
alpha blocking
hypnotic blindness
eye opening
age regression

G 57.   Mezan, I., Petrov, I., and Alanassov, A.: The EEG in hypnosis. *Electroencephalogr Clin Neurophysiol, 17:*709, 1964 (abstr) .

Twenty-three hysteria patients were recorded for EEG with eyes open and closed before and during a hypnotic trance in which a suggestion of blindness was given to the subjects. No changes were found in the EEG patterns associated with either of the conditions. In both conditions eye opening produced the desynchronizing of the EEG. The suggestion of blindness had no effect on the EEG.

hypnosis
neuroses
hysteria
hypnotic blindness
EEG patterns
eye opening

HYPNOTIC SUSCEPTIBILITY

G 58.   Nowlis, D.P., and Rhead, J.C.: Relationship of eyes-closed resting EEG alpha activity to hypnotic susceptibility. *Percept Mot Skills, 27:*1048, 1968.

Twenty-one subjects (20 to 35 years old; 10 male and 11 female) were given the Stanford Hypnotic Susceptibility Scale (SHSS) and recorded for EEG to determine the relationship between alpha incidence and hypnotizability. A significant correlation between alpha incidence and SHSS scores was obtained in this study. The mean alpha incidence was 44 percent which was within normal limits for the population.

hypnotic susceptibility
alpha abundance

G 59.   London, P., Hart, J.T., and Leibovitz, M.P.: EEG alpha rhythms and susceptability to hypnosis. *Nature, 219:*71, 1968.

One hundred and twenty-five female subjects (16 to 61 years old) were given the Harvard Group Suggestibility Scale (HGSS) and recorded for EEG to determine the relationships between the two measures. EEG alpha incidence was determined for eyes-closed recordings while the subjects were resting and while they were producing mental images. HGSS scores were separated into four categories for analysis on the basis of percentile ranks. An analysis of variance showed a significant relationship between alpha incidence and HGSS scores in the resting and mental imagery conditions.

hypnotic susceptibility
alpha abundance
mental imagery

G 60.   Galbraith, G.C., London, P., Leibovitz, M.P., Cooper, L.M., and Hart, J.T. EEG and hypnotic susceptibility. *J Comp Physiol Psychol, 72:*125, 1970.

Fifty-nine subjects (24 male and 35 female) were given the Harvard Group Susceptibility Scale (HGSS) and recorded for resting EEG. Autospectrum and cross spectrum analyses of the Oz, Cz, Fz and T3 leads of the EEG revealed a total of twenty EEG variables which were predictive of HGSS scores. The overall amplitude of the EEG was higher in the subjects with high HGSS scores with alpha showing the greatest overall difference. Due to the variability of alpha amplitude, however, it was not among the five variables accounting for the variance in HGSS. The five most important variables were 5 Hz activity in Oz with eyes open, 5 Hz activity in the Oz-Cz pair with eyes open, 7 Hz activity in Oz with eyes closed, 6 Hz activity in Oz with eyes open, and 8 Hz activity in Oz-Cz with eyes open.

hypnotic susceptibility
EEG patterns
alpha patterns
theta
spectral analysis

G 61.   Mordvinov, E.F., and Genkin, A.A.: On the possibilities of predicting suggestibility in man through use of the data of the spontaneous electroencephalogram. *Zh Vyssh Nerv Deiat, 19:*1027, 1969.

Thirty-nine subjects (18 to 30 years old) were recorded for EEG to determine the relationships between EEG patterns and suggestibility. Asymmetry of EEG and mean frequency were determined for the readily suggestible and the resistant

hypnotic susceptibility
EEG symmetry

subjects. The EEG asymmetry measure was found to be significantly different in the two groups.

MEDITATION

Transcendental

G 62. Wallace, R.K., Benson, H., and Wilson, A.F.: A wakeful hypometabolic physiologic state. *Am J Physiol, 221:795,* 1971.

Thirty-six subjects (17 to 41 years old; 28 males and 8 females) trained in the transcendental meditation technique were recorded for EEG, blood pressure, heart rate, rectal temperature, skin resistance, respiration rate and volume, oxygen consumption, carbon dioxide emission and blood chemistry before, during and after the practice of their meditational exercises. Oxygen consumption, carbon dioxide emission, respiration rate and tidal volume decreased significantly during meditation and increased back to normal at the end of meditation. Systolic and diastolic blood pressure remained unchanged. Blood pH levels decreased during meditation, pO_2 and pCO_2 remained unchanged, and blood lactate levels decreased during meditation. Heart rate decreased and skin resistance increased significantly during meditation while rectal temperature remained unchanged. Increased 8 to 9 Hz alpha activity was found in the frontal and central electrode placements and 12 to 14 Hz activity decreased during meditation. Five of the subjects developed 5 to 7 Hz theta activity in the frontal electrodes during meditation.

mediation
transcendental
alpha
* frequency*
theta
ANS

G 63. Wallace, R.K.: Physiological effects of transcendental meditation. *Science, 167:*1751, March 1970.

Fifteen normal college students (no physical abnormalities) with six to thirty-six months experience at transcendental meditation (Maharishi Mahesh Yogi) were recorded for EEG, EKG, skin resistance and oxygen consumption before, during and after meditation to determine associated physiological changes. Transcendental meditation was differentiated from Zen and yoga on the basis of the types of exercises involved. Subjects were presented visual and auditory stimuli to determine the characteristics of the alpha blocking re-

mediation
transcendental
alpha
* patterns*
alpha
* responses*
theta
ANS
eye opening

sponse at different stages of meditation. Oxygen consumption rate decreased significantly after five minutes of meditation. The total respiratory volume decreased during meditation and the carbon dioxide/oxygen ratio remained constant. Oxygen consumption increased to normal following meditation. Skin resistance increased during meditation and decreased to normal following meditation. Heart rate followed the same pattern. Alpha amplitude and regularity increased during meditation, alpha frequency slowed in some subjects, and periods of low voltage theta activity were found to occur. Following meditation alpha was present continuously with eyes closed and irregularly with eyes open.

Yoga

G 64. Dostalek, C.: Research on Yoga in modern India. *CS Psychol 14:497, 1970.*

Physiological studies including neurological tests and EEG's were done with yogis. During meditation exercises the resting alpha rhythm was uninfluenced by stimuli which would have caused alpha blocking in normal consciousness. It is concluded that yoga has significant effects on the control of physiological mechanisms of regulation in the body and should therefore deserve closer study by psychology and physiology.

mediation
yoga
alpha
blocking

G 65. Anand, B.K., Chhina, G.S., and Singh, B.: Some aspects of electroencephalographic studies in yogis. *Electroencephalogr Clin Neurophysiol, 12:452, 1961.*

Four experienced yogi meditators were recorded for EEG before and during meditation and were presented external stimuli including visual, auditory, thermal and vibratory events to determine the related effects on the EEG patterns. Two additional yogis with increased pain threshold for cold water were recorded for EEG before and during cold water immersion of their arms. Some students of yoga were recorded for EEG to determine the characteristics associated with good aptitude for yoga. The first group had prominant resting alpha with a normal blocking response to external stimuli. The blocking response did not habituate in the rest-

mediation
yoga
*alpha en-
    hancement*
*sensory
    stimulation*
habituation

ing EEG, however. During the Samadhi (most intense meditation) phase, the amplitude of the alpha rhythm increased, the blocking response did not occur, and occasional "hump" activity was observed in the parietal leads. The second group showed no change in EEG activity during cold water immersion during meditation as though the sensory afferent pathways had been blocked. Those students showing the greatest aptitude for yoga and the greatest enthusiasm had more EEG alpha activity in their resting EEG's than other students.

G 66. Bagchi, B.K., and Wenger, M.A.: Simultaneous EEG and other recordings during some yogic practices. *Electroencephalogr Clin Neurophysiol, 10*:193, 1958 (abstr).

Thirteen subjects of the Hatha Yoga sect were recorded for EEG, skin conductance, heart rate and respiration rate during a variety of exercises aimed at achieving a stage of ecstasy, Samadhi. The exercises resulted in the development of a well-modulated alpha rhythm with little fast activity in the EEG. Heart rate, respiration and skin conductance lowered and stabilized during the meditational exercises.

meditation
yoga
alpha enhancement
ANS

G 67. Bagchi, F.K., and Wenger, M.A.: Electro-physiological correlates of some Yogi exercises. *Electroencephalogr Clin Neurophysiol (Suppl), 7*:132, 1957.

A pilot electrophysiological investigation was carried out in India on forty-five Indian yogic subjects in ninety-eight sessions using a portable eight-channel transistor, battery-operated, ac-dc polygraph of high sensitivity with accessories. Central nervous system and autonomic nervous system changes were recorded as manifested in electroencephalogram, electrocardiogram, electromyogram, skin resistance, skin temperature, blood pressure, breathing rate, finger blood volume during meditation in "immobile" posture for a long time, during four types of pranayam breathing exercises, pulse and heart-sound stopping, heart slowing, asan (postures), sweat controlling, relaxation, etc. This investigation seeks to indicate the general direction in which a particular type of scientific research on yoga should be

mediation
yoga
EEG patterns
ANS

carried out rather than present results on the basis of exhaustive studies. Many aspects of yoga were not touched upon. However, some new findings may be named: for instance, an extreme slowing of respiration rate four to six per minute or shallow respiration for seventeen to twenty-seven minutes during a few meditative sessions, with more than 70 percent increase of palmar electrical resistance but without change in basic waking EEG and EKG pattern; heart slowing (24 per minute) through particular maneuvers, etc. (For other results see the body of the article.) Mechanisms responsible for these and other results are not altogether clear. Pending further research, it can be said that physiologically yogic meditation represents deep relaxation of the autonomic nervous system without drowsiness or sleep and a type of cerebral activity without highly accelerated electrophysiological manifestation but probably with more or less insensibility to some outside stimuli for a short or long time.

G 68.	Das, N.N., and Gastaut, H.: Variations de l'activite electrique du cerveau, du coeur et des muscles squelettiques au cours de la meditation et de l'extase yogique. *Electroencephalogr Clin Neurophysiol (Suppl), 6:*211, 1955.

Seven yoga meditators were recorded for EEG, EMG and EKG during phases of meditation including fixation of attention, meditation proper and the final ecstasy or complete concentration. Muscular activity was found to be completely undetectable during the motionless meditation. Heart rate was found to be correlated with changes in the EEG: acceleration in deep meditation, especially ecstasy, followed by deceleration. The EEG showed a sequence of changes during meditation: increased alpha frequency (1 to 3 Hz) ; appearance of 15, 20 and 30 Hz activity; appearance of 18 to 20 Hz rolandic beta; diffuse 25 to 30 Hz activity, with low voltage; increase of the amplitude of the 25 to 30 Hz activity to 30 to 50 microvolts in the ecstatic period; and reappearance of the alpha rhythm at slow frequencies with wide distribution following ecstasy. During the ecstatic period the subjects were completely insensitive to stimulation.

mediation
yoga
EEG
 patterns
ANS

G 69.   Rao, S.: Yoga and autohypnotism. *Br J Med Hypn, 17:38,*
1965.

Yoga meditation and hypnotic trance are functionally and
methodologically similar and seen to involve a common
brain mechanism. Other similarities also exist, but EEG
records differ since the alpha rhythm is not blocked by sensory stimuli during yogic meditation, but under hypnosis it
is. Also, only men can meditate. Therefore, available evidence (exact neural mechanisms are not clearly understood)
seems to indicate that these are two different phenomena
with two different ultimate objectives.

mediation
yoga
sex
  differences
hypnosis
sensory
  stimulation

Zen

G 70.   Hirai, T.: Electroencephalographic study on the Zen meditation (Zazen)-EEG changes during the concentrated relaxation. *Folia Psychiatr Neurol Jap, 62:76,* 1960.

EEG, GSR, EKG and respiration were studied in fourteen
priests of the Soto sect of Buddhism while they practiced Zen
meditation. The EEG activity was recorded from the parietal
and occipital areas. Alpha waves proved to be much more
persistant with greater amplitude and independence of eye
opening. Later in the session the frequency of alpha slowed
to 8 to 9 cps and large bursts and sharp waves were observed.
Evidence was also seen to indicate that the effects of meditation on the alpha activity remained even after the meditation had ended. Other findings include: (1) analyzed records
detailing the slowing of the enhanced alpha; (2) enhanced
amplitude of theta waves and the appearance of theta in the
parietal region, both late in the session; (3) a gradual decrease in respiration rate and increase in pulse rate; and (4)
de-adaptation of the GSR as the meditation progressed causing more easily evoked responses and the appearance of
spontaneous GSR's. EEG data indicates a lowering of the
cortical excitatory level while GSR, EKG and respiration
infer the release phenomenon of the brain stem autonomic
function. A comparison of Zen and autogenic training techniques yields thoughts on the psychiatric importance of Zen
meditation.

mediation
Zen
alpha
  frequency
alpha
  amplitude
theta
ANS

G 71. Kasamatsu, A., and Hirai, T.: An electroencephalographic study of the Zen meditation (Zazen). *Folia Psychiatr Neurol Jap, 20:*315, 1966.

Forty-eight Zen meditators (24 to 72 years old), varying in experience in meditation from less than one to greater than twenty years, were recorded for EEG before, during and after meditation sessions. Twenty-two control subjects (23 to 60 years old) were recorded for EEG under identical conditions but without the meditation experience. The meditation took place with eyes open for approximately thirty minutes. The EEG changes found in the highly experienced Zen masters followed this sequence: low voltage, fast activity prior to meditation, appearance of alpha bursts of 40 to 50 microvolts at the start of meditation, increase in alpha amplitude and incidence to 100 percent as meditation progressed, appearance of high amplitude theta bursts toward the end of the session, and a persistance of alpha after meditation ceased. Using auditory click stimuli, the alpha blocking response was found to occur without any evidence of habituation. No similar changes were found in the EEG's of control subjects and the alpha blocking response was found to habituate in a normal manner. The degree to which the EEG changes of other meditators matched the changes observed in the masters was found to be a function of experience. No similar phenomena were found to occur in induced hypnotic trances in normal subjects.

mediation
Zen
alpha
 patterns
sensory
 stimulation
habituation
hypnosis

G 72. Hirai, T., Izawa, S., and Koga, E.: EEG and Zen Buddhism. *Electroencephalogr Clin Neurophysiol (Suppl), 18:*52, 1959 (abstr).

Twelve Zen Buddhist priests were recorded for EEG, GSR, EKG and respiration rate during the practice of their meditational exercises. EEG was recorded from parietal and occipital electrode placements. A sequence of EEG changes was found: persistant alpha developing one minute after the start of meditation with eyes either open or closed; increased amplitude and decreased alpha frequency a few minutes later; the appearance of large, sharp alpha waves and increased amplitude of theta later in meditation; a return to

mediation
Zen
alpha
 patterns
theta
ANS

persistant alpha following meditation. Respiration rate and pulse rate both slowed with the slowing of the EEG from fast alpha to slow alpha to theta development. The GSR showed the de-adaptation characteristic of hypnogogic sleep.

3 73. Kasamatsu, A., Hirai, T., and Ando, N.: EEG responses to click stimulation in Zen meditation. *Proc Jap EEG Soc,* 1962, p. 77.

Findings of this experiment that the habituation of auditory stimulation is barely seen in experts during Zazen are taken to indicate that the mental state in Zen meditation cannot be affected by either external or internal stimulus beyond more response to it. Possible electrophysiological significance of the de-habituation on EEG responses during Zazen is also included.

mediation
Zen
EEG
 patterns
auditory
 stimulation
habituation

3 74. Kasamatsu, A., and Hirai, T.: An electroencephalographic study on the Zen meditation (Zazen). *Psychologia Int J Psychol Orient, 12:*205, December 1969.

The EEG has become a reliable way to assess the state of wakefulness or sleep. Studies on EEG changes during anoxia, epileptic seizures and exogenous brain disorders were carried out. Zazen is a sitting meditation which is a kind of religious exercise in Zen Buddhism. Subjects were forty-eight priests and disciples in two sects, ranging in age from twenty-four to seventy-two years. Twenty-two other persons served as controls. Training in Zen meditation produces changes in both mind and body. In such meditation, the EEG pattern is slowed and the alpha block is de-habituated.

mediation
Zen
EEG
 frequency
alpha
 blocking

3 75. Kasamatsu, A., Okuma, T., Takenaka, S., Koga, E., Ikeda, K., and Sugiyama, H.: The EEG of "Zen" and "Yoga" practitioners. *Electroencephalogr Clin Neurophysiol (Suppl), 9:* 51, 1957 (abstr).

Experienced Zen and yoga practitioners and two control subjects were recorded for EEG during the practice of meditational exercises. Both of the experienced meditators were found to produce increasing amounts of alpha activity as meditation proceeded while the control subjects continued

mediation
Zen
yoga
alpha en-
 hancement

with poorly developed alpha during the recording sessions.   *adaptation*
Auditory stimuli (claps and bells) had little effect on the   *sensory*
EEG's of the meditators while performing their separate   *stimulation*
meditational exercises.

G 76.   Shiomi, K.: Respiratory and EEG changes by cotention of
        Trigant Burrow. *Psychologia Int J Psychol Orient, 12*:24,
        1969.

Using Zen students and masters and "ordinary, no-trained   *mediation*
men" as controls, two experiments were run measuring   *Zen*
respiration (Takei psychogalvanic reflex pneumograph) and   *respiration*
EEG's (Toshiba St-1664). It was concluded that the state of   *EEG*
contention is different physiologically from that of ditention.   *patterns*

G 77.   Watanabe, T., Shapiro, D., and Schwartz, G.E.: Meditation
        as an anoxic state: A critical review and theory. *Psycho-*
        physiology, 9:279, 1972 (abstr).

The critical role of anoxia in achieving a meditative state is   *mediation*
discussed in the article based on a critical review of the   *physiologic*
literature. The sequence and localization of EEG changes   *influences*
during early stages of anoxia are similar to those during
meditation. Reduced blood pH in meditation and delay of
normal EEG after meditation point to a biochemical cause
due to lack of oxygen. After exposure to moderate oxygen
deficiency in CO_2 therapy and in high altitude studies emotional relaxation is seen. A vision impairment is seen in both
meditation and anoxia. The article continues with a discussion of other possible mechanisms underlying meditation
in reference to the anoxic state.

G 78.   Gelhorn, E., and Kiely, W.F.: Mystical states of conscious-
        ness: Neurophysiologic and clinical aspects. *J Nerv Ment*
        Dis, 154:399, 1972.

This article reviews the trophotropic (increased parasym-   *mediation*
pathetic discharges, relaxation of skeletal muscles, and less *EEG*
cortical excitation or synchrony as in sleep) and ergotropic   *patterns*
(increase in sympathetic discharges and skeletal muscle tone   *subjective*
and a diffuse cortical excitation or desynchronization of the   *states*
                                                                habituation

EEG as in awakening) systems of autonomic-somatic integration and their relevance to emotional states and levels of
consciousness. As the subject approaches the meditative state
the EEG shows four stages: (1) alpha activity regardless of
whether eyes are open or closed; (2) an increase in amplitude of these alpha potentials; (3) a decline in frequency of
the alpha activity; and (4) the appearance of theta activity.
Decreased heart and respiration rate, reduced oxygen consumption and muscle relaxation complete the transition of
the trophotropic-ergotropic balance to trophotropic dominance with increased skin resistance indicating the decline of
the ergotropic system. The fact that sleep does not occur during the meditative state may indicate that some ergotropic
excitation still exists to counteract the trophotropic discharges. Also, the arousal reaction, blocking of the alpha
rhythm by acoustic stimulus, does not habituate during
meditation. Clinically, there is evidence that transcendental
meditation results in heightened inner-directed self-control
and improved clarity in cognitive functions and in emotion-
al-behavioral integration. Reports of this sort have come
from former drug users who have tried meditation. Evidence also points to the use of transcendental meditation for
the treatment of psychosomatic disorders such as tension
states, anxiety, essential hypertension, bronchial asthma, etc.

BIOFEEDBACK

G 79.   Adrian, E.D., and Matthews, B.H.C.: The Berger rhythm:
Potential changes from the occipital lobes in man. *Brain, 57:*
355, 1934.

In addition to its historical value, this article contains an
interesting note on a subject of current interest: biofeedback. "Adrian reported listening to the alpha rhythm recorded from himself and presented through a loud speaker.
He then tried to correlate the subjective impression of looking or not with the absence or presence of the alpha rhythm."

*biofeedback
history*

G 80.   Stoyva, J., and Kamiya, J.: Electrophysiological studies of
dreaming as the prototype of a new strategy in the study of
consciousness. *Psychol Rev, 75:*192, 1968. (Copyright 1968,
by the American Psychological Association and reproduced
by permission.)

The authors argue that the combined use of physiological   *biofeedback*
measures and verbal report, as in the rapid eye movement   *theory*
(REM) studies of dreaming, represents a new strategy in the
study of private events. Electrophysiological studies of dreaming are seen as an instance of converging operations serving
to validate a hypothetical mental state. The authors further
argue for a redefinition of dreaming. The latter is not fully
indexed by either the REM measure or by verbal report;
rather it may be best thought of as a hypothetical construct.
The possible ways of relating verbal reports of dreaming, the
REM measure, and the hypothetical dream experience are
placed within a systematic framework. That the new strategy
—combined use of verbal report and physiological measures
—need not be confined to dreaming is suggested by the experiments on learned control of the EEG alpha rhythm.
Here, the use of information feedback procedures teaches
subjects to control the physiological response and apparently,
the associated mental state as well.

G 81.   Gaarder, K.: Control of states of consciousness II. Attain-
        ment through external feedback augmenting control. *Arch
        Gen Psychiatr, 25*:436, 1971.

        This paper reviews the theory and history of biofeedback   *biofeedback*
        with specific reference to its use in psychiatric treatment.   *review*
        Special consideration is given to biofeedback as a means of   *theory*
        treating psychosomatic disease and states of anxiety. Possible   *history*
        limiting factors of feedback techniques are also discussed.

G 82.   Mulholland, T.B.: Feedback electroencephalography. *Activ
        Nerv Sup (Praha), 10*:410, 1968.

        Contents: (1) Special usefulness of feedback methods; null-   *biofeedback*
        ing a closed internal loop; environmental clasping of a bio-   *theory*
        logical control system; testing hypotheses of causality; testing   *visual*
        hypotheses of difference between causes. (2) Standardization   *system*
        of feedback EEG; the external path; stimulus functions. (3)   *applications*
        The effects of feedback stimulation; bilateral differences;
        feedback as an increase or decrease of stimulation; delayed
        feedback. (4) Visual control systems and occipital alpha;
        control of the EEG by the subject; accommodation, fixation

and target clearness. (5) The occipital alpha activation cycle as a controlled process. (6) The activation of the occipital EEG. (7) The alpha process. (8) Prospects for feedback methods in psychophysiology; voluntary control of physiological processes.

G 83.   Hart, J.T.: Autocontrol of EEG alpha. *Psychophysiology, 5:* 506, 1968 (abstr).

Subjects were trained to increase their alpha indices by placing them in a feedback loop so that every time an alpha wave of 8 to 13 cps was produced, a tone occurred. The feedback loop included the following: the subject, a polygraph, a bandpass filter, an oscilloscope, a trigger, a duration timer, an oscillator and a speaker. The results replicate those from the investigations of Kamiya in showing that subjects can learn to increase alpha. Thirteen of eighteen subjects in the experimental groups significantly increased their alpha indices within ten training sessions. The subjects in Experimental Group 1, who received both in-session feedback training and post-session information about their alpha scores, demonstrated greater alpha increases than the subjects in Experimental Group 2, who received only feedback training. However, some of the control subjects also showed alpha increments. Thus it is important to include a control group (this was not done in the earlier investigations); without a control group the influence of feedback training is likely to be overestimated.

biofeedback
alpha
abundance

G 84.   Kondo, C.Y., Travis, T.A., and Knott, J.R.: Initial abundance and amplitude of alpha as determinants of performance in an enhancement paradigm. *Electroencephalogr Clin Neurophysiol, 34:*106, 1973 (abstr).

While apparent enhancement of abundance has been seen in previous work by the authors, large individual differences in alpha amplitude and alpha abundance have also been observed. In order to investigate this phenomena, the records of thirty subjects who received five alpha training sessions of ten minutes duration with eyes open were analyzed. Initial alpha amplitude with eyes closed and initial alpha abundance

biofeedback
alpha
abundance
alpha
amplitude

with eyes open served as baselines, and data from the ten best and ten poorest performers (those with increases of alpha over trials) were compared. Large initial alpha amplitude resulted in significantly larger increases in alpha over trials than did small initial amplitude, whereas low initial alpha abundance gave way to significantly larger increases in alpha as training progressed when compared to high initial abundance.

G 85.   Kamiya, J.: Conditioned discrimination of the EEG alpha rhythm in humans. Presented at Western Psychological Association, San Francisco, Calif., 1962.

Six subjects learned to distinguish alpha from non-alpha states with nearly 100 percent accuracy in fifty to five hundred trials. It was also found that some subjects could turn on the alpha activity upon demand of the experimenter. Verbal reports of the two states generalized to visual imagination and relaxed inattention. No indication of similar results for heart and respiratory activity, eye movement and muscle activity was found.

biofeedback
alpha
  abundance
ANS

G 86.   Schwartz, G.E., Shaw, G., and Shapiro, D.: Specificity of alpha and heart rate control through feedback. *Psychophysiology, 9*:269, 1972 (abstr).

To explore the effects of repeated alpha wave training on cardiovascular functioning, twelve subjects were pre- and post-tested in the laboratory on their ability to control their alpha and heart rate after four daily one-hour sessions of feedback training to increase and decrease alpha. The pre-test data indicated that subjects were initially unable to differentially increase or decrease alpha, but they were able to produce 5 beats-per-minute differences in heart rate which were unaccompanied by alpha changes. However, after the four sessions of alpha training, subjects evidenced significant alpha control unaccompanied by heart changes, while their ability to control their heart rate was unaffected (identical to the pre-test). Analysis of the subjective report data supports the notion that the mechanisms of alpha and heart rate control are different. Implications for the direct feedback control of patterns of alpha and heart rate are discussed.

biofeedback
alpha
  abundance
heart rate

G 87. Sacks, B., Fenwick, P.B.C., Marks, I., Fenton, G.W., and Hebden, A.: An investigation of the phenomenon of auto-control of the alpha rhythm and possible associated feeling states using visual feedback. *Electroencephalogr Clin Neurophysiol, 32:*461, 1972.

The aims of this study were to investigate previous reports that voluntary control of the amplitude of the alpha rhythm could be achieved by means of a visual feedback system and to confirm whether or not there were associated feeling states. Sixteen subjects were tested. Subjects were seated with their eyes open looking at the feedback lamp and were required to control the illumination of the lamp in response to instructions presented on an illuminated panel. Each subject was given only one session. Of sixteen subjects so tested, six were able to achieve voluntary control of the alpha amplitude with their eyes open. After the recording session, subjects completed two semanic differential questionnaires which referred to their feelings and mental states when the feedback lamp was on and when it was off; they were also given an unstructured interview. No correlations were found between mental or feeling states when the subject showed small or large alpha amplitudes.

biofeedback
alpha
* amplitude*
subjective
* reports*

G 88. Hord, D., Naitoh, P., and Johnson, L.: Intensity and co-herence contours during self-regulated high alpha activity. *Electroencephalogr Clin Neurophysiol, 32:*429, 1972.

Spectral intensity and coherence analysis of EEG activity during rest and during a period of self-regulated high alpha in two subjects indicate that (1) slow frontal activity, which is due primarily to eye movements, is less intense during successful alpha regulation than during baselines; (2) there is little evidence for increased intensity in frequency ranges other than the alpha range during alpha regulation; and (3) occipital alpha tends to be more coherent with frontal than with temporal alpha during occipital alpha regulation.

biofeedback
alpha
* symmetry*
spectral
* analysis*
coherence

G 89. Brown, B.B.: Recognition of aspects of consciousness through association with EEG alpha activity represented by a light signal. *Psychophysiology, 6:*442, 1970.

Forty-seven subjects (21 to 60 years old; 16 males and 31 females) were given feedback for the presence of the alpha rhythm in their EEG's to determine whether there were particular states of consciousness associated with the alpha rhythm. The recorded EEG was filtered for alpha activity which, in turn, was used to power a display light in front of the subject. The subject received real-time information about the incidence and amplitude of the alpha rhythm in his EEG. All subjects had significant increases in alpha incidence across successive sessions and significantly decreased alpha frequency. Subjects were asked to answer a questionnaire about their experiences following each training session. The greatest alpha abundances were associated with reported feelings of losing awareness of the environment, feelings of floating, concentrating on mental imagery, and either not experiencing time or feelings that the experimental sessions were short.

biofeedback
subjective
states
alpha
patterns

G 90. Silverman, S.: Operant conditioning of the amplitude component of the EEG. *Psychophysiology, 9:*269, 1972 (abstr) .

Feedback contingent on the amplitude component of the EEG irrespective of frequency changes was presented to subjects over 4 one-hour sessions. The feedback signal (soft tone and dim light) was presented each time the subject's EEG equalled or exceeded a baseline amplitude obtained with eyes closed during the rest period of each session. There was no difference between EEG control in the fourth training session and the no-feedback session. There was a significant amplitude difference between "on" and "off" trials for sessions 4 and 5 combined. In all cases, high amplitude was associated with alpha frequencies, low amplitude with higher frequencies. It was concluded that learned control of EEG amplitude can transfer to a no-feedback condition.

biofeedback
EEG
amplitude

G 91. Smith, K.U., and Ansell, S.D. Closed-loop digital computer system for study of sensory feedback effects of brain rhythms. *Am J Phys Med, 44:*125, 1965.

A computer system with appropriate transducers for physiologic and response mechanisms was designed to record and control sensory and excitatory feedback based on delay, space

biofeedback
data
collection

displacement, kenetic modulation, etc. Experiments involving (a) the effects of brain-wave-generated stimulus feedback patterns on perception and EEG frequency patterns, (b) delay of these feedback stimuli relative to their source and the effects on perceptual or brain wave pattern and, (c) judgment of magnitude of the delay of cyclic auditory stimuli produced by the EEG showed no significant relationships. Computer-delayed auditory feedback effects of speech slowed, slurred and produced repetitive defects in reading. It is suggested that these experiments make clear problems of dynamic correlation between perception and brain wave pattern in addition to proving the value of computer-controlled feedback systems. It is also pointed out that these methods may help in developing new techniques of real-time dynamic simulation of physiologic and behavioral disorders.

theory
applications

G 92. Mulholland, T.B., and Gascon, G.: A quantitative EEG index of the orienting response in children. *Electroencephalogr Clin Neurophysiol, 33:*295, 1972.

The basic assumption that all responses of the occipital EEG relevant to the orienting response are characterized by a disturbance followed by a recovery of the series of alpha intervals alternating with no-alpha intervals was made so that a new method for analyzing the orienting response could be developed. This is described and illustrated under various conditions using alpha feedback. An index of orienting, developed from average disturbance and recovery series estimates, differentiated experimental conditions and ages. Therefore, these new quantitative methods of evaluating the alpha attenuation cycle aid in the study of EEG correlates of the human orienting response.

biofeedback
children
orienting
EEG
* activation*
alpha
* blocking*

G 93. Woodruff, D.S., and Birren, J.E.: Alpha training for the elderly. American Psychological Association Meeting, Hawaii, 1972.

Fifteen subjects between eighteen and twenty-nine years and fifteen subjects between sixty and eighty-one years were trained successfully in alpha production. It was concluded

biofeedback
aging

that these results show that alpha rhythm slowing is not an indication of irreversible deterioration in the nervous system of the aged. Hope for control of behavioral alterations associated with aging through brain wave frequency manipulation is offered.

G 94.   Green, E., Green, A.M., and Walters, E.D.: Self-regulation of internal states. Proceedings of the International Congress of Cybernetics, London, Sept. 1-6, 1969.

Techniques and tools for investigating states of internal awareness, psychological and physiological, are developed in this paper. Physiological feedback in voluntary control of normally unconscious physiological functions of the craniospinal, autonomic and central regions is used. Successful subjects have reduced muscle tension to zero levels, increased hand temperature as much as 5°C in two minutes, up to 100 percent alpha over ten-second epochs, while speaking with eyes open. The purpose of this training is to enhance and make possible the study of those psychological states which appear as functional concomitants of a passive peripheral nervous system and an "alpha-activated" central nervous system. Psychology, psychosomatic medicine, psychiatry, education and creativity research are all areas in which this ongoing project may be valuable.

biofeedback
muscle
system
alpha
abundance
subjective
states
data analysis
applications

G 95.   Machac, M., and Moravek, M.: Frekvencnizmey alfa rytmu pri psychologickych manipulacich s aktivacni urovni. *Cesk Psychol, 11:*421, 1967.

Fourteen subjects were trained to relax with an autoregulation method. Changes in the EEG occurring through stages of increasing relaxation were observed. A 0.9 Hz increase in frequency of the alpha rhythm accompanied the relaxation produced by this method.

biofeedback
relaxation
alpha
frequency

G 96.   Green, E., Green A., and Walters, D.: Voluntary control of internal states: psychological and physiological. *J Transpersonal Psychol, 11:*1, 1970.

A need to shorten the learning time of autogenic training techniques and to adapt the system to states of consciousness research have spawned the methodology used in this report. That is, a combination of the conscious self-regulation aspects of yoga, the psychological method of autogenic training and the instrumental technique of physiological feedback is used. Preliminary experiments showed that seven of twenty-one subjects could reduce muscle activity to zero levels through muscle feedback in twenty minutes with associated body image changes such as the arm feeling like a bag of cement. A larger project used triple feedback to train simultaneous reduction of muscle tension in the right forearm, increase in temperature in the right hand (autogenic relaxation), and increase in percentage of alpha activity. Projected research into imagery, etc., includes percentage-of-alpha, frequency-of-alpha and percentage-of-theta training, using visual and auditory feedback. Home training is described along with an arm balancing technique (subliminal dredging) to prevent drowsiness and aid in recognition and recall of imagery. In conclusion the possible significance of the voluntary control of internal states research is presented. Areas of important application would include education, creativity, psychology, psychotherapy and psychosomatic medicine (i.e. chronic headache, etc.). A dramatic application involves starvation and absorption of cancerous growths through blood flow control.

biofeedback
autogenic training
alpha abundance
subjective states

G 97. Rohmer, F., and Israel, L.: The electroencephalogram in "autogenic training." *Electroencephalogr Clin Neurophysiol, 9*:566, 1957 (abstr).

Subjects were recorded for EEG during autogenic training exercises and under hypnotic suggestion of autogenic training to determine related EEG pattern changes. The autogenic procedures were associated with decreased amplitude and incidence of alpha, short paroxysmal bursts of alpha, and/or spikes and generalized bursts of theta activity. The same EEG changes were found in the hypnotic suggestion of autogenic stages but were less marked and of shorter duration. The EEG changes were interpreted as similar to stages preceeding sleep but not similar to deep sleep.

biofeedback
autogenic training
hypnosis
alpha patterns
theta

G 98.   Paskewitz, D.A., and Orne, M.T.: Visual effects during alpha
         feedback training. *Psychophysiology, 9:*269, 1972 (abstr).

In a study of alpha feedback training, no increases in alpha   *biofeedback*
density were observed across six days (60 trials) when audi-   *visual*
tory feedback was presented to nine subjects in total dark-   *system*
ness. For theoretical reasons, it was predicted that the mere   *theory*
addition of low level ambient light would establish lawful
increases in alpha densities. A second sample of seven subjects, given ten trials a day for two days, confirmed the prediction. The original group of subjects, who failed to show
increases in total darkness, also increased densities in the
presence of light. Furthermore, with light, both groups
showed significantly higher densities during feedback than
during intervening rest periods. These findings may help
reconcile some of the conflicting results in the literature.
The results support the view that increases in alpha densities
can take place only if inhibitory mechanisms are initially
present to depress density. Increases in alpha activity may
reflect an increasing ability of the subject to ignore otherwise
distracting influences, and this process may account for some
of the reported subjective concomitants of alpha feedback
training.

G 99.   Mulholland, T.B.: Feedback method: a new look at func-
         tional EEG. *Electroencephalogr Clin Neurophysiol, 27:*688,
         1969 (abstr).

Application of feedback EEG is developed from basic re-   *biofeedback*
search which has shown the following: (1) Feedback from   *visual*
EEG to the display constrains the EEG alpha activation   *system*
cycle, reducing unpredictable or uninformative variation.   *EEG*
(2) The constrained system can be disturbed showing an   *activation*
initial response followed by a recovery to near baseline con-   *applications*
ditions. (3) The disturbance and recovery of the feedback
system is an index of stimulus parameters and complex variables of visual control. (4) EEG processes which are not
consciously known can be brought into awareness by information feedback and combined with training, voluntary
control of these processes can be learned. (5) By means of
the feedback path, information displays and appliances can
be automatically regulated by the EEG processes to which

they are connected and, combined with training, voluntary control of the display or appliance can be learned. (6) By controlling the parameters of the feedback path, the EEG response can be controlled. If these determine a behavioral response, then it can be controlled.

G 100. Peper, E.: Feedback regulation of the alpha electroencephalogram activity through control of the internal and external parameters. *Kybernetik, 6:*107, 1970.

Experiments with feedback stimulation triggered from the subject's electroencephalogram result in changing the sequential time series of intervals of occipital alpha and intervals of little or no alpha EEG activity. The rate of recurrence of alpha and no-alpha EEG can be changed by regulating the external feedback stimuli or by asking the subject to change his internal state. Four different paradigms were investigated and the results interpreted in terms of the hypothesis that oculomotor functions regulate the occurrence and nonoccurrence of alpha.

biofeedback
visual
system
subjective
states

G 101. Keesey, U.T., and Nichols, D.J.: Changes induced in stabilized image visibility by experimental alteration of the ongoing EEG. *Electroencephalogr Clin Neurophysiol, 27:*248, 1969.

The authors took continuous EEG recordings while judgments of stablized image disappearance and reappearance were made by two adult subjects. On-line use of a computer executing a closed-loop program made it possible to detect the alpha rhythm while it was occurring and to present a burst of white noise shortly after each onset of alpha activity. The stimulus could also be presented in random order. It was found that alpha-dependent presentation of the stimulus both lengthened the time the stabilized image stayed visible and changed the temporal patterns of alpha occurrence and image disappearance and reappearance in comparison to the condition where the stabilized image was viewed without any white noise presentation.

biofeedback
retinal
images
alpha
blocking

G 102. Dewan, E.M.: Communication by voluntary control of the electroencephalogram. *Phys Sci Res Papers, 284:*349, 1966.

Past suggestions that the alpha rhythm and eye position   *biofeedback*
could be used to send Morse code are followed up in this   *eye position*
project. Working with a computer and a teletypewriter, one
can perform this function, but over half a minute is required
per character. Messages were also sent using muscle activity
from the forehead. The possibility of practical usefulness of
these techniques is suggested but not dealt with in this
communication.

G 103. Beatty, J., and Kornfeld, C.: Relative independence of conditioned EEG changes from cardiac and respiratory activity.
*Phys Behav, 9:*733, 1972.

EEG, heart rate and respiration were recorded from fourteen   *biofeedback*
subjects who were being trained to produce occipital alpha   *heart rate*
and beta waves in order to investigate the possibility that   *respiration*
heart rate and respiration mediate the changes in the central *generators*
nervous system which are observed during learned changes
in EEG activity. No significant changes in heart or respiratory activity were seen during discriminant control of the
alpha and beta activity, suggesting relative independence of
the EEG generating system from those systems controlling
the functions of heart rate and respiration.

G 104. Bundzen, P.V.: Autoregulation of functional state of the
brain: an investigation using photostimulation with feedback. *Fed Proc Trans Suppl, 25:*551, 1966.

Ten healthy subjects and ten psychasthenic patients were   *biofeedback*
recorded for EEG from bipolar parieto-occipital and parieto- *visual*
temporal electrodes in both hemispheres. The apparatus in-   *stimulation*
cluded the usual feedback components (amplifier, filter and *EEG*
integrator), but in this case suppression of alpha by a flash   *activation*
caused stimulus (flash) cutoff. An inertia filter was used   *alpha*
which allowed alteration of the autostimulation according   *blocking*
to mean level of electrical activity. Automatic EEG analysis *theory*
gave filtered and integrated material for four ranges (1 to 3,
8 to 14, 16 to 32 and 35 to 50 cps) which was used to make
spectrochronograms showing changes in integrated values
of these frequencies over time. It was concluded that (1)
cyclical recurring changes in cortical neuron electrical activ-

ity was an important factor in stabilization of the functional state of the brain under autostimulation conditions; (2) functional state of the cortex autostabilization is done through the direct agency of nonspecific effects from subcortical structures and is separately connected with control of the afferent flow; and (3) disturbance of cerebral autoregulation by, for example, pathologic states is due to weakened corticofugal control of the activity of activating structures in the brain stem.

G 105. Bundzen, P.V.: Autoregulatory mechanisms of the central nervous system in the presence of photostimulation in the rhythm of the biopotentials. *Fiziol Zh SSSR, 54:683, 1968.*

Ten subjects were given photostimulation and autostimulation from 2 to 20 cps in order to study that part of the EEG which reflects activity of the nonspecific or diffuse mechanisms that control autoregulation of the current functional state of the brain. Amplitude and frequency of the alpha rhythm recorded from the occipital and central areas of the cortex indicated a link between alpha and the activity of the autoregulatory brain mechanisms. Autoregulation of the tonic level of activation or excitability of higher divisions of the central nervous system was found to be related, in part, to "encountered" or "attendant" inhibition which in turn is a result of the slight lability of the brain structures controlling nonspecific mechanisms. A direct connection between the process of autoregulation of the current functional state of the brain and optimization of the changing strength of afferent current was also found.

biofeedback
photic
flicker
alpha
*   amplitude*
alpha
*   frequency*

G 106. Bundzen, P.V., et al.: Method of automatic photostimulation in the rhythm of cerebral biopotentials with a selectively controlled feedback system. *Fiziol Zh SSSR, 54:1239, 1968.*

Technical details, drawings, etc., of equipment for automatic photostimulation with a direct connection between the stimulus and amplitude, frequency, form, etc., of the cerebral biopotentials which have been proven in the analysis of autoregulatory processes of the brain are given. A direct expression of the principle of "optimal interaction" between

biofeedback
photic
flicker
theory

the nervous centers in the regulation of the "general tonic functional state of the brain" has been demonstrated using this apparatus.

G 107. Spilker, B., Kamiya, J., Callaway, E., and Yeager, C.L.: Visual evoked responses in subjects trained to control alpha rhythms. *Psychophysiology, 5:*683, 1969.

Averaged visual evoked responses (AER) to sine wave light and to light flashes were recorded in seven subjects trained to control alpha rhythms. All seven subjects demonstrated a greater AER amplitude to sine wave light when there was high or abundant alpha in the EEG than when the alpha was low or almost entirely absent. Two of the early waves of the flash AER were usually greater in amplitude during periods of high alpha. A cycloplegic agent was shown to have no effect upon this finding, nor did varying the frequency of sine wave light stimulation. Period analysis of the EEG showed more activity at both low and high frequency bands during periods of low alpha. Auditory evoked response amplitudes were not significantly different between the high and low background alpha conditions. These results were discussed in relation to current views correlating AER's with attentive states.

biofeedback
visual
evoked
response

G 108. Travis, T.A., Kondo, C.Y., and Knott, J.R.: A controlled study of alpha enhancement. *Psychophysiology, 9:*268, 1972 (abstr).

The effects of no-noncontiguous and contiguous reinforcement on alpha enhancement were investigated. Three groups were employed: (1) experimental, n = 8 (contiguous reinforcement); (2) yoked control, n = 8 (noncontiguous reinforcement); (3) naive control, n = 8 (no reinforcement). All subjects experienced 6 ten-minute sessions on each of two days. The feedback stimulus was a blue light and the dependent variable was percent alpha-on time. Experimental subjects produced significantly more alpha on day 1 than subjects in either of the control groups. On day 2, both experimental and yoked control groups (who had been switched to relevant feedback) produced significantly more alpha than

biofeedback
alpha en-
hancement

the naive control group. Significant increases over trials were noted for experimental subjects on day 1 and for both experimental and yoked control subjects on day 2. Naive controls evidenced no changes on either day. Increases in alpha output in our situation appeared to be related to a crucial contiguity between alpha production and the delivery of the feedback stimulus.

G 109. Travis, T.A., Kondo, C.Y., and Knott, J.R.: A comparison of instructed and non-instructed non-reinforcement sessions following alpha enhancement training. *Electroencephalogr Clin Neurophysiol, 34*:105, 1973.

This experiment questions whether true operant control resulted from past alpha abundance enhancement experiments. The effects of removal of reinforcement following training were studied under two conditions: (1) no warning, and (2) instructions to subjects that this was a test session and that they should do whatever proved most successful during feedback sessions. Eight of sixteen subjects who received five to ten-minute enhancement training sessions with eyes open also received a nonreinforcement trial under one of the conditions mentioned. Results tended to support the assumption that operant control is not a consequence of such learned control of alpha. Subjects under condition 2 (instructions given) showed increased production of alpha during the nonreinforcement trial while the others showed no significant changes. No signs of classical extinction were seen in the nonreinforcement period.

biofeedback conditioning

G 110. Korein, J., Maccario, M., Carmona, A., Randt, C.T., and Miller, N.: Operant conditioning techniques in normal and abnormal EEG states. *Neurology, 21*:395, 1971 (abstr).

A pilot study to condition EEG's involved thirteen normal subjects, eight subjects with psychogenic and systemic disorders, and fifteen patients with seizure disorders in whom potentially induced or spontaneous spikes and bursts existed. Conditioning of the first two groups used filtered and amplified fronto-occipital 8 to 13 cps EEG activity which caused a click or photic stimulus feedback. The last group was given an auditory feedback signal when paroxysmal activity was

biofeedback conditioning psychopathology epilepsy subjective states applications

present. Of those receiving alpha conditioning 70 percent
could attain control within two weeks and they reported
alpha to be a relatively tranquil state as opposed to the non-
alpha or concentration state. Evoked response, frequency
changes, eye movements, etc., also appeared significant. Only
20 percent of the fifteen patients could control their paroxysmal spikes and this occurred during the first trials and occasionally as one trial learning. The authors conclude that
such techniques of maintaining a steady state (alpha) may
be useful in quantifying drug activity, evoked response, etc.,
and may also be associated with meditation. Lastly they say
that therapeutic aspects of operant conditioning should be
considered further.

G 111. Mulholland, T., and Runnals, S.: Evaluation of attention
and alertness with a stimulus-brain feedback loop. *Electroencephalogr Clin Neurophysiol, 14:*847, 1962.

A simple electronic apparatus was so arranged that selected
EEG frequencies in the alpha range caused a stimulus to
occur. When alpha was suppressed the stimulus was automatically removed. When alpha recurred the stimulus was
automatically presented again. During feedback stimulation
the following phenomena were observed: (1) Alpha tended
to occur in a series of short bursts separated by periods of
faster no-alpha activity. (2) The changes in the durations
of alpha and no-alpha components over time were not simple
inversions, not complements of each other. (3) The temporal
pattern of alpha and no-alpha durations were significantly
different for conditions of viewing and attempting to remain at an alert, attentive level, compared to simple viewing when no such attempt was made and, in general, alpha
durations were shorter, no-alpha durations longer and the
variance of alpha duration reduced during the condition requiring greater attention. (4) The distribution of alpha and
no-alpha response durations was not Gaussian, but resembled
a Poisson distribution. The hypothesis was advanced that the
feedback system fractionates "phasic" response latencies from
predominantly "tonic" response durations (Sharpless and
Jasper, 1956). Application of the system to the study of internal attention states was described and other applications
suggested.

biofeedback
EEG
  activation
attention
theory

G 112. Peper, E., and Mulholland, T.: Methodological and theoretical problems in the voluntary control of electroencephalographic occipital alpha by the subject. *Kybernetik, 7:*10, 1970.

Twenty-one normal humans attempted to control the facilitation and inhibition of their EEG occipital alpha rhythm. They received auditory feedback which informed them whether or not alpha occurred. Most subjects learned to inhibit alpha, only four learned to facilitate it. Further training did not bring improved control of alpha. The results are presented to illustrate problems of method and interpretation which include the following: the diversity of subjective attempts at control; day-to-day variability of the response; the control for alpha increase caused by habituation; and the feedback technique as an operant conditioning method.

biofeedback
habituation

G 113. Bremner, F.J., Moritz, F., and Benignus, V.: EEG correlates of attention in humans. *Neuropsychologia, 10:*307, 1972.

In an attempt to extend the Bremner attention model to humans, the expectancy subset, as well as a new one—internal focus—was used with twenty male college students. Ten subjects received the Silva Mind Control course while the others received a classical conditioning paradigm procedure which was similar to that used to obtain animal data for the Bermner model except that alpha activity was used instead of theta. In both groups a frequency shift was seen. When biogenic feedback was introduced, another shift or narrowing of the spectra occurred. It is therefore concluded that expectancy as defined by the model correlates with the shape of the spectra and a frequency shift. The authors also suggest that the internal focus subset is demonstrated by the Silva group since they used no external stimuli but only what could be called mental imagery to generate their data. It is recognized that further study is required to validate the subset internal focus.

biofeedback
attention
expectancy
alpha
  frequency
theory

G 114. Kaszniak, A.W.: Dichotic auditory vigilance during feedback-enhanced EEG alpha. *Psychophysiology, 10:*203, 1973 (abstr).

Two different groups of nonsense syllables were presented simultaneously in the right and left ears. Target syllables were specified and those given in the right ear were made task central through instructions to pay particular attention to them. Findings indicated decreased accuracy for target syllable detection in the left ear during alpha enhancement as opposed to alpha suppression trials, but no difference was found in right ear accuracy for the two conditions. Therefore, this supports the hypothesis of decreased peripheral perceptual awareness during alpha production, but does not suggest any accompanying increase in central perceptual awareness. A consideration of the results in the light of both trained and spontaneous alpha is also offered.

biofeedback
vigilance

G 115. Engstrom, D.R., London, P., and Hart, J.T.: Hypnotic susceptability increased by EEG alpha training. *Nature, 227:* 1261, 1970.

Thirty subjects (17 to 62 years old; 10 males and 20 females) with low scores on the Harvard Group Susceptibility Scale (HGSS) and less than 50 percent incidence of alpha were used in the experiment. Subjects were given form A of the Stanford Hypnotic Susceptability Scale (SHSS) before and after a training procedure of alpha brain wave feedback was given. Twenty subjects received binary alpha feedback (a light came on whenever the alpha rhythm was present in the EEG) and ten subjects received yoked feedback or were presented with the light which represented the alpha activity of another subject. Alpha incidence was found to have a significant positive correlation with scores on the SHSS. Alpha incidence increased significantly for both the feedback and the yoked control groups during the sessions, with the feedback group having a significantly greater increase. The scores on the HGSS were found to have increased in the same manner as alpha; the same significant relationships were found. The subjective feelings reported to be associated with the production of the alpha rhythm were described as similar to those in a hypnotic trance.

biofeedback
hypnotic
suggesti-
bility
alpha
abundance
subjective
states

G 116. Kamiya, J.: Conscious control of brain waves. *Psychology To-day, 1:*56, 1968. (Reprinted from *Psychology Today Maga-*

zine, April 1968. Copyright © Communications/Research/
Machines, Inc.)

Indicates the possibility of teaching "man to perceive and
control some of his brain functions." After subjects had
learned to distinguish between alpha and nonalpha states,
they were able to consciously produce the alpha state. Control of alpha rhythms was monitored by EEG's. Experienced
Zen meditators "learned control of their alpha waves far
more rapidly than did the average person. . . . The possible
value in studies of alpha wave control during the LSD experience" is indicated. The lack of connection between alpha
waves and extrasensory perception is stressed. "No evidence
of electromagnetic radiation to the outside world by brain
activity. . . ." was found. Studies with groups other than
college-educated subjects are suggested.

biofeedback
meditation
conscious-
ness

G 117. Regestein, Q.R.: Prolonged continuous production of EEG
alpha rhythm and desynchrony. *Psychosom Med, 34:*471,
1972.

Thirty-one subjects were trained to produce alpha waves during a four-hour session, with twenty-two being paid for success. Results included no difference between paid and unpaid
groups and greater mean amounts of alpha in thirteen men
versus eighteen women. Seven subjects who did the best in
this experiment participated in two additional twelve-hour
paid feedback conditions which took place on two days, two
weeks apart. One of the sessions involved alpha production
and the other nonalpha production with the result that the
former became easier while the latter grew more difficult. In-
nate alpha production was attributed more to relevancy of
performance than to any effects of learning.

biofeedback
motivation
alpha
abundance
EEG
activation

G 118. Beatty, J.: Similar effects of feedback signals and instructional information on EEG activity. *Physiol Behav, 9:*151, 1972.

In order to evaluate the effects of prior information about
psychological correlates of EEG activity and of EEG-based
information feedback on biofeedback of the occipital EEG,
forty-five college students participated in EEG biofeedback
training sessions under a variety of instructional and in-

biofeedback
cognition
alpha
abundance
beta

formation conditions. Those given both ideas of how to produce alpha and beta activity and online feedback did no
better than subjects who received only one form of information. Subjects provided with either no information or, in
some cases, inappropriate feedback information showed no
systematic changes. The author warns that ascribing learned
changes to effects of feedback where subjects are told the
nature of the task is dangerous in light of the similar results
from the groups that learned in this study.

G 119. Honorton, C., Davidson, R., and Bindler, P.: Shifts in subjective state associated with feedback-augmented EEG alpha.
Psychophysiology, 9:269, 1972 (abstr).

Twenty-three subjects completed one session with auditory *biofeedback*
feedback to EEG alpha activity using a closed feedback loop. *subjective*
Subjects alternated two-minute trials of alpha generation, *states*
rest periods (no feedback) and suppression. Ten trials of
each type were given with order counterbalanced by subject.
In addition to monopolar EEG (occiput-ear lobe), EOG
(supraorbital-canthus) and EMG (frontalis) were recorded.
Two verbal report measures were used to assess changes in
subjective activity: an on-line state report scale in which subjects called numbers between 0 and 4 to indicate degree of
relaxation and attention to external stimuli (elicited during
alternate feedback trials), and a postexperimental interview.
Successive trials of generation, suppression and resting alpha
were compared: generated mean alpha = 40 percent, suppression = 16 percent, rest = 36 percent. The three conditions differed significantly (p. < .01) for the group and each
subject individually had significant generation/suppression
differences (p. < .01). Alpha generation was associated with
mean state report = 2.01, suppression mean = 0.63 (p. =
.005). Subjects with strong shifts in state reports between
conditions had significantly larger alpha shifts than subjects
with little shift in state reports (p = .05). High state reports were associated with significantly less REM activity and
EMG activation than low state reports (p < .005). Blind-
coded interview responses related significantly to state reports (p. = .05). These converging measures support the
hypothesis that relatively high alpha is associated with nar-

rowing of perceptual awareness, relaxation and with some subjects' altered states of consciousness.

G 120. Nowlis, D.P., and Kamiya, J.: The control of electroencephalographic alpha rhythms through auditory feedback and the associated mental activity. *Psychophysiology, 6:476, 1970.*

Twenty-six subjects were given baseline tests for electroencephalographic (EEG) alpha rhythm presence and then a period of fifteen minutes to gain insight into mental activity associated with alpha presence and absence while provided with an auditory feedback loop keyed to the presence of alpha. Sixteen of the subjects worked with eyes closed, and ten, with very high initial alpha baseline scores, worked with open eyes. After the fifteen-minute practice period permitting control of alpha through feedback, the subjects were given a trial during which they attempted to produce as much alpha as possible and a trial in which they tried to produce as little as possible. The results indicated significant appropriate change for both the generation and suppression trials. Those who were able to control alpha spontaneously reported mental states reflecting relaxation, "letting go" and pleasant affect associated with maintaining alpha.

biofeedback
subjective
states

G 121. Brown, B.B.: Awareness of EEG-subjective activity relationships detected within a closed feedback system. *Psychophysiology, 7:451, 1970.*

The present report summarizes results from feedback experiments using the three EEG frequency ranges of theta, alpha and beta to operate lights of three different colors. The subjects were requested to try to isolate and identify feeling (and/or thought) activity which they felt caused successful operation of the lights. Written descriptions of this experience from one subject group (26 subjects) were compared to evaluations of subjective activity obtained in a second group of subjects (45 subjects) determined using a color Q-sort technique. Results from the latter technique were controlled for effects of color and for effects of the feedback experience using a control subject group (45 subjects). Results established two sets of relationships with subjective activity: color

biofeedback
subjective
states
theta
beta

and EEG frequency. Each set could exist independently or in relationship to the other. Several characteristics were postulated to account for development of the subjective-biological relationships in this feedback system, e.g. that generation of stimulus and response were both internal events; that both reinforcement of the process and the behavior reinforced were selected by subjective activity of the subject; and that positive reinforcement did not occur without effort by the subject to define it.

G 122. Peper, E.: Localized EEG alpha feedback training: A possible technique for mapping subjective, conscious, and behavioral experiences. *Kybernetik, 11*:166, 1972.

A subject was trained in localized control of alpha activity successfully. These preliminary results are suggestive of possible localized control to establish relationships between subjective, conscious and behavioral experiences with certain EEG patterns, thereby developing a new subjective physiological language. Particular medical and altered-states-of-consciousness-type applications are considered. *biofeedback subjective states consciousness*

G 123. Schmeidler, G., and Lewis, L.: Mood changes after alpha feedback training. *Percept Mot Skills, 32*:709, 1971.

Thirteen young adults completed a mood checklist and Breskin Rigidity Test (measuring preference for perceptual closure) before alpha training. After two training sessions, significant increases in production of alpha EEG activity, scores for moods associated with alpha by prior research, and preference for closure were observed from retest results. *biofeedback subjective states perceptual tasks*

G 124. Hefferman, M.S.: The effects of self-initiated control of brain waves on digit recall. *Dissertation Abstracts International, 31*:6404, 1971.

In order to test whether cortical desynchronization is necessary for the recall of digit series, thirty-three subjects were conditioned to elicit synchronized and desynchronized brain rhythms during phases in learning digit sequences. At digit presentation and digit rehearsal, recall performance during *biofeedback memory* synchronized rhythms was significantly better than that during desynchronized activity; but, during the digit repeat phase of learning, no significant difference in recall between the two brain rhythms was found.

G 125. Sterman, M.B., and Friar, L.: Suppression of seizures in an epileptic following sensorimotor EEG feedback training. *Electroencephalogr Clin Neurophysiol, 33*:89, 1972.

Studies of 12 to 14 cps activity in the sensorimotor cortex of cats showed it to be related to thalamocortical inhibitory discharge, suppression of phasic motor behavior and drug-induced convulsions. Similar activity of the rolandic cortex in a twenty-three-year-old female with epilepsy was fed back to the subject using biofeedback techniques. Results included enhancement of abundance of the sensorimotor rhythm, differentiation of the sensorimotor rhythm from alpha activity, changes in sleep patterns and personality and seizure suppression.

biofeedback
psychopath-ology
epilepsy
alpha
frequency

G 126. O'Malley, J.E., and Comers, C.K.: The effect of unilateral alpha training on visual evoked response in a dyslexic adolescent. *Psychophysiology, 9*:467, 1972.

This project was undertaken with a dyslexic adolescent to further elucidate the possible relationship between alpha activity and averaged visual evoked response. Baseline alpha and visual evoked response (VER) were recorded and bilateral alpha training carried out. Analysis of variance showed that alpha training significantly increased VER amplitude (p. < .001). Baseline VER and percent alpha were not correlated although baseline VER did fluctuate. Unilateral alpha training when 0.5 second of alpha appeared in the left hemisphere and 0.5 second of beta or theta in the right hemisphere caused a significant increase over five days (4 trials per day) of alpha activity on the left side and beta and theta activity on the right side. Left minus right VER amplitude difference increased and was correlated (p < .05) with percent time alpha (L) and beta and theta (R) increases.

biofeedback
dyslexia
visual
evoked
response
beta
theta

G 127. Lynch, J.J., and Paskewitz, D.A.: On the mechanisms of the feedback control of human brain wave activity. *J Nerv Ment Dis, 153:*205, 1971.

Factors influencing density of alpha rhythms are reviewed. *biofeedback* Results include three areas of influence: constitutional, *learning* physiological and cognitive-attentional. A discussion of these *review* factors as mediators of alpha activity leads to the idea that *theory* increased alpha density during feedback is due to a lessening of the factors which block alpha. Continued discussion evolves around the question of generalizability of this theory to the whole field of operant control of autonomic activity.

G 128. Kamiya, J.: Operant control of the EEG alpha rhythm and some of its reported effects on consciousness. In Tart, C.T. (Ed) : *Altered States of Consciousness.* New York, Wiley, 1969, p. 507.

Early developments by Kamiya on EEG alpha brain wave bio- *biofeedback* feedback using auditory displays including subjective reports *review* concerning mental activities during alpha are discussed. *measure-* More recent experiments involving control of alpha fre- *ment* quency through auditory feedback techniques are also pre- *techniques* sented. *subjective states*

ESP

G 129. Stanford, R.G., and Lovin, C.: EEG alpha activity and ESP performance. *J Am Soc Psychical Res, 64:*375, October 1970.

Thirty male, college-age students were each given two *ESP* recognition runs using the standard ESP symbols. For several *alpha* minutes prior to the ESP testing, and throughout the ESP *frequency* testing, monopolar right occipital EEG (referenced to the right ear lobe) was recorded. The frequency (Hz) of the alpha rhythms recorded during the pretest (relaxation) period correlated $-.41$ with the total ESP score (p $<$ .04, 2-tailed) . The frequency of alpha recorded during ESP testing did not correlate significantly with ESP scoring. Change in alpha frequency from pretest (relaxation) period to the ESP testing correlated $+$ .51 with the total ESP score (p $<$ .01, 2-tailed) . Such findings suggest that there may be an optimal level of arousal for ESP performance in a discrete-calling task. Thus subjects who relax during the pretest period but who are somewhat aroused by the actual testing seem to do best. Additionally, correlations are reported between the percentage of time alpha is present in the record and ESP performance. These latter correlations are, however, regarded by the authors as inconclusive in view of difficulties which arise in using the measure of alpha percentage employed in this and certain earlier work.

G 130. Honorton, C., and Carbone, M.: A preliminary study of feedback-augmented EEG alpha activity and ESP card-guessing performance. *J Am Soc Psychical Res, 65*:66, January 1971.

This study was performed to assess the effects of feedback-augmented EEG alpha activity on ESP card-guessing performance. It was hypothesized that increments in alpha activity following a series of operant training sessions would be associated with concomitant increments in ESP scoring level. Each of ten volunteer subjects participated in ten sessions of EEG feedback training. The subject, a digital frequency discriminator, and an audio oscillator made a closed feedback loop. Subject's alpha activity activated a 250 Hz tone. Alpha abundance was automatically registered on digital counters. Only two of the subjects showed significant increments in alpha. A significant negative correlation ($r = -0.636$, $p < .05$) was observed between percent of alpha and ESP scores in the nonfeedback condition. Results for the feedback condition were not significant ($r = -0.042$). A statistically significant decline effect was observed *post hoc* for the nonfeedback condition ($p \leqslant .006$).

ESP
biofeedback
alpha
patterns

SECTION H

EMOTIONAL INFLUENCES

PERSONALITY

H 1.   Travis, L.E., and Bennett, C.L.: The relationship between
        electroencephalogram and scores in certain Rorschach cate-
        gories. *Electroencephalogr Clin Neurophysiol, 5:*474, 1953
        (abstr).

Sixty-six adult subjects were separated into two groups on
the basis of the pattern of frequencies in their EEG's. One
group (A) was characterized by having greater than 50 percent alpha incidence in their resting EEG's (32 subjects) and
the other (B) by having a high incidence of beta activity and
a low incidence of alpha. The subjects were given the
Rorschach to determine the relationships between EEG pattern and personality. Group A had a significantly greater percentage of whole responses to the Rorschach. Group B had
a larger total number of whole responses, more total responses, more unusual detail, more space responses, more
color responses and more total time. The authors concluded
that the A group may have a more passive-receptive manner
of organizing stimuli.

personality
alpha
  abundance
EEG
  patterns
EEG
  responses

H 2.   Schmettau, A.: Two electroencephalographic clusters of
        signs and their physiologic correlates. Results of a correlative
        study by means of automatic interval analysis. *EEG-EMG
        (Stuttg), 1:*169, 1970.

EEG and personality traits were studied using 118 male
students (19 to 32 years old). One hundred and seventeen
personality variables and twenty-one EEG variables were
chosen by questionnaire and automatic frequency analyzer
respectively. Two clusters resulted: (1) voltage- and abund-
ance-related parameters—alpha index, alpha amplitude, theta
index, theta amplitude and alpha variance—and (2) speed-
or frequency-related parameters—mean alpha frequency and
beta index. In group 1 high alpha index, alpha amplitude,

personality
alpha
  patterns
EEG
  patterns
data analysis
beta
theta
neurotic
  tendency

204

theta index, and theta amplitude and low alpha frequency variation correlated with active, energetic, tense, experimental, self-sufficient, critical self-opinionated, sober, pessimistic, emotionally easily upset, achieving people with low tolerance to frustration. The group 2 traits of rapid alpha frequencies and relatively high incidence of beta waves corresponded to hypertensive, tender-minded, anxious, cautious, submissive and defensive people with neurotic tendencies. Also, there was no simple quantitative relationship between personality traits and index for theta and beta activity.

H 3.   Gastaut, H.: Conclusions d'ensemble. *Electroencephalogr Clin Neurophysiol (Suppl), 6:*321, 1957.

The author summarized the results of a number of reports on EEG methods and the relationships between EEG parameters and personality variables. Three groups of subjects were tested for EEG and personality: a normal group consisting of 113 soldiers, an affective immaturity group consisting of 309 cadet pilots, and a neurotic group consisting of 100 patients. Affective immaturity was associated with the presence of theta and slow posterior rhythms associated with hyperventilation and with deviations in alpha frequency in either direction from the normal range of 9 to 10 Hz. Rolandic beta activity was a characteristic of the neurotic group. None of the subjects in the normal group showed rolandic beta while 16 percent of the pilots and 41 percent of the neurotics showed this pattern of activity. Theta appeared in 50 percent of the records for the affectively immature group, less than 20 percent of the records in the normal group and in 36 percent of the records for the neurotic group. Mean alpha frequency was 10.04 Hz for the normal group, 9.57 Hz for the affectively immature group, and 9.79 Hz for the neurotic group.

personality
neurotic
  tendency
alpha
  patterns
beta
theta

H 4.   Costa, L.D., Cox, M., and Katzman, R.: Relationship between MMPI variables and percentage and amplitude of EEG alpha activity. *J Consult Psychol, 29:*90, 1965.

Seventy-two first-year medical students were given the MMPI and recorded for EEG to determine the relationships between personality and alpha parameters. None of the

personality
alpha
  patterns
anxiety

major personality dimensions were significantly related to alpha parameters. A significant negative correlation was found between alpha amplitude and Welsh's "A" (anxiety).

H 5.   Gale, A., Coles, M., and Blaydon, J.: Extroversion-introversion and the EEG. *Br J Psychol, 60:*209, 1969.

A review of EEG activity and extroversion-introversion is presented with criteria for their evaluation including a new measure of mean dominant frequency. In an eyes-closed condition, the EEG of the extrovert was found to be higher in integrated output over a large frequency range with greatest difference in the lower alpha frequencies. These differences in alpha activity were quite difficult to see with the large bandpass filter as above, but when the eyes were opened and monotonous visual stimulation was given the changes were large enough for this gross filter to discriminate. Theta, alpha and beta ranges were also monitored and more clearly showed such information as the increase in low frequency alpha waves mentioned above. Also, prolonged recording indicated differences in theta and beta activity which were even stronger with the eyes closed.

personality
EEG
* frequency*
alpha
* frequency*
eye opening
theta
beta

H 6.   Saunders, D.R.: Further implications of Mundy-Castle's correlations between EEG and Wechsler-Bellevue variables. *J Natl Inst Personnel Res, 8:*91, 1960.

The reapplication of factor analysis to Mundy-Castle's correlation matrix using thirty-four subjects showed alpha frequency and digit span performance comparable, and considerations with respect to the hypotheses of excitability, primary versus secondary function, and externalization-internalization are also given. Alpha Index was found to be an indicator of "Conditioned Attentiveness."

personality
EEG
* patterns*
alpha
* patterns*

H 7.   Moses, L.: Psychodynamic and electroencephalographic factors in duodenal ulcer. *Psychosom Med, 8:*405, 1946.

Twenty-five Navy servicemen who were duodenal ulcer patients were recorded for EEG to determine the relative incidence of EEG alpha. Nineteen of the patients were found to have 75 to 100 percent incidence of alpha, one was found to

personality
psychoso-
* matic*
* illness*

have 50 to 75 percent alpha, and five were found to have 0 to 25 percent alpha. The high incidence of alpha in the EEG's of patients with ulcers was considered abnormal. Personality traits of those subjects with high alpha incidence clustered around insecure feelings, "passive-dependent" traits, and a "facade of independence and aggressiveness." The author hypothesized that the ulcers may have been the product of conflict between the requirements of service life and the personality variables associated with dominant alpha.

H 8.   Rubin, S., and Moses, L.: Electroencephalographic studies in asthma with some personality correlates. *Psychosom Med, 6:* 31, 1944.

Forty-five male subjects with asthma were recorded for EEG and were given a clinical interview to determine the relationships between EEG, personality and asthma. The subjects were found to have a significantly higher incidence of alpha than normal (27 subjects with greater than 75% incidence of alpha). The subjects were also found to have a significantly greated incidence of low frequency alpha. The clinical interviews revealed tendencies for these subjects to be reserved, withdrawn, outwardly calm, desiring a dominant mate, and to not show signs of ambition or aggressive striving.

personality psychosomatic illness alpha patterns

H 9.   Rubin, S., and Bowman, K.M.: Electroencephalographic and personality correlates in peptic ulcer. *Psychosom Med, 4:*309, 1942.

One hundred male subjects with peptic ulcer were recorded for EEG and were evaluated for personality variables to isolate the relationships between these measures. The subjects were found to have a significantly higher incidence of resting alpha than normal (71 subjects with greater than 75% alpha incidence). Those subjects with high alpha incidence were found to have held jobs for a longer time, had less difficulty at work, came from smaller families, were more passive toward their mates and were more passive toward friends. Those with low alpha incidence were found to be more aggressive, outgoing and independent.

personality psychosomatic illness alpha patterns

H 10. Remond, A., and Lesevre, N.: Remarques sur l'activite cere-
       brale des sujets normaux. *Electroencephalogr Clin Neuro-*
       *physiol (Suppl), 6:*235, 1957.

Forty-six air force recruits and thirty-eight truck drivers were *personality*
tested for personality traits and recorded for EEG under a *sensory*
number of experimental conditions. The conditions in- *stimulation*
cluded hyperventilation, presentation of constant and inter- *mental tasks*
mittent light, auditory stimulation, mental arithmetic, word *intelligence*
association and the presentation of TAT images. Subjects *EEG*
were also given a battery of personality tests. One group was *patterns*
classified as hyperexcitable with hypermotionality and either
an impulsive or inhibited nature. These subjects had an EEG
pattern which was complex and polyrhythmic and had a
tendency to desynchronize to sensory-affective stimuli. A
second group with stable psychomotor performance was
characterized by an EEG pattern involving slow, mono-
rhythmic, widely distributed alpha which did not readily
block to the presentations of sensory-affective stimuli. The
third group was classified as having good emotional adaptiv-
ity and had the best performance on the tests. This group
had a higher alpha frequency with well-organized parieto-
occipital bursts and a normal blocking response to sensory-
affective stimuli.

H 11. Walters, C.: Clinical and experimental relationships of EEG
       to psychomotor and personality measures. *J Clin Psychol,*
       *20:*81, 1964.

The author summarized some of the findings concerning the *personality*
relationships between EEG and personality. Consistent rela- *intelligence*
tionships were noted as follows: (1) anxiety and alpha block- *motor per-*
ing time, (2) nonverbal intelligence and the absence of slow *formance*
waves, (3) excitability and reduced alpha activity, (4) alpha *alpha*
frequency and speed of performance, (5) slow alpha and *patterns*
stable performance, (6) complex alpha and poor performance. The data for other relationships were considered inconclusive for a number of reasons. The author proposed a
number of controls and studies which should be done to determine further relationships between personality and EEG
variables.

H 12. Henry, C.E., and Knott, J.R.: A note on the relationship between "personality" and the alpha rhythm of the electro-encephalogram. *J Exp Psychol, 28:*362, 1941.

Eighty subjects were separated into introvert and extravert groups on the basis of performance on the Nebraska Personality Inventory. Introverts were those scoring above Q2 on the scale of introversion and the extraverts were those scoring below Q2. Alpha incidence in the eyes-closed condition was classified as high if greater than 50 percent and low if less than 50 percent. No significant relationship was found between extraversion and alpha incidence under these conditions.

personality
neurotic
 tendency
alpha
 abundance
eye opening

H 13. Savage, R.D.: Electro-cerebral activity, extraversion and neuroticism. *Br J Psychiatry, 110:*98, 1964.

Twenty female students were given the Maudsley Personality Inventory and were separated into four groups on the basis of having high or low extraversion scores and high or low neuroticism scores. Parieto-occipital EEG was recorded to determine alpha amplitude for correlation with the two personality variables. In an analysis of variance, the extraversion dimension and the extraversion neuroticism interaction were significant. High extraversion was associated with higher alpha amplitudes and high extraversion combined with low neuroticism was associated with high alpha amplitudes.

personality
neurotic
 tendency
alpha
 amplitude

H 14. Broadhurst, A., and Glass, A.: Relationship of personality measures to the alpha rhythm of the electroencephalogram. *Br J Psychiatry, 115:*199, 1969.

Fifty-one students (43 male and 8 female) were recorded for EEG to determine the relationship between frequency patterns and personality traits. Extraversion and neuroticism were of primary interest. EEG parameters included alpha incidence, alpha amplitude, alpha frequency and rate of change in amplitude during blocking. An analysis of variance showed several significant relationships. Extraversion was significantly related to both alpha incidence and amplitude while neuroticism was related to alpha incidence. High

personality
neurotic
 tendency
alpha
 patterns

extraversion was associated with low incidence and amplitude of alpha. High neuroticism was associated with low
incidence of alpha.

H 15.   McAdam, W., and Orme, J.E.: Personality traits and the
         normal electroencephalogram. *J Ment Sci, 100:*913, 1954.

Forty-eight chronic alcoholics were recorded for EEG to de-   *personality*
termine the relationships between personality variables and   *alcoholism*
EEG patterns. Personality was assessed through clinical   *neurotic*
evaluation and performance on the Eysenck Ranking Ror-   *tendency*
schach. Alpha frequency and alpha incidence were nega-   *alpha*
tively correlated. Alpha incidence and performance on the   *patterns*
Rorschach were positively correlated. The subjects were   *beta*
found to fit into two basic categories. The first category included those subjects having predominantly beta activity in
the EEG. This group was characterized as extravert, nervous,
strong-willed and determined. The second group included
those with predominant alpha activity in the EEG and a
higher incidence of theta activity. This group was characterized as introvert, emphasizing external activities, and variable willpower. The definition of the personality variables
and the criteria for assessment were not clearly specified in
this study.

H 16.   Gray, J.A.: Strength of the nervous system, introversion-
         extraversion, conditionability and arousal. *Behav Res Ther,*
         *5:*151, 1967.

The author reviewed the literature on the Teplov concept of   *personality*
strength of the nervous system and compared it to the data   *neurotic*
for introversion, conditionability and arousal to see where   *tendency*
the concepts corresponded. The concept of strength of the   *alpha*
nervous system was seen to overlap with the western concept   *patterns*
of arousal. The Nebylitsyn concept of equilibrium in dynam-   *alpha*
ism or conditionability was also seen to correspond to the   *responses*
strength concept and the data differentiating personality
types on the basis of characteristics of the alpha rhythm
corresponded well with similar data on introversion. His
contention was that introverts correspond to Nebylitsyn's
excitable type and extroverts to the inhibitory type. The

Russian data on this dimension of personality show that the excitable type has longer alpha blocking duration, longer conditioned alpha blocking duration, slower speed of habituation, slower extinction, greater amplitude of blocking, lower alpha incidence, lower alpha amplitude, higher alpha frequency, lower beta incidence and frequency, lower theta frequency, and a smaller photic driving response. Similar data for introversion were discussed.

H 17. Young, J.P.R., Lader, M.H., and Fenton, G.W.: The relationship of extraversion and neuroticism to the EEG. *Br J Psychiatry, 119*:667, 1971.

Sixty-four young adult male subjects were recorded for EEG's and scored for extraversion and neuroticism. Alpha index, mean alpha amplitude, alpha attenuation response, its rate of habituation during photic stimulation and two average evoked auditory potentials under different states of attention were also measured. Four parallel broad wave-band filters were used for analysis, but no significant correlation between these variables and the extraversion and neuroticism scores could be found.

personality
neurotic
tendency
alpha
patterns
alpha
responses
visual
evoked
response
auditory
evoked
responses
attention

H 18. Saul, J.J., Davis, H., and Davis, P.A.: Psychologic correlations with the electroencephalogram. *Psychosom Med, 11:* 361, 1949.

One hundred and thirty-six psychiatric patients were recorded for EEG over a five-year period to determine the relationships between EEG variables and personality. Five general types of EEG pattern were defined and three types of relationships with personality were identified. The EEG types were (A) regular, prominent alpha with a high incidence in the EEG, (B) low alpha amplitude and incidence with beta prominent, (M) irregular alpha with both higher and lower frequencies dominant, (MS) alpha mixed with dominant slow wave activity, and (ME) alpha mixed with dominant

personality
neurotic
tendency
alpha
patterns
sex
differences

beta activity. Extreme passivity was found to be associated with A type EEG's. Masculinity in women was associated with the B type EEG. Frustrated, aggressive, impatient, demanding and hostile qualities in women were associated with M, MS and ME types of EEG. Overt hostility and aggression were associated with ME type EEG's. Repressed hostility and aggression were associated with the MS type EEG. More men were found to have A type EEG's, while more women were found to have mixed frequency types of EEG's.

H 19.   Rabinovitch, M.S., Kennard, M.A., and Fister, W.P.: Personality correlates of electroencephalographic patterns: Rorschach findings. *Can J Psychol, 9:*29, 1955.

Electronic frequency analysis of EEG's were used to determine differences in the EEG patterns among psychiatric patients, prison inmates and normal control subjects. Correlations between personality characteristics as reflected in the Rorschach test and EEG frequency patterns are presented. Hypotheses for further research into relationships between EEG patterns are discussed.

personality
EEG
*   frequency*
psychologic
*   testing*
psychoses

H 20.   Fenton, G.W., and Scotton, L.: Personality and the alpha rhythm. *Br J Psychiatry, 113:*1283, 1967.

Fifty-four medical students (21 to 30 years old) having a 50 percent or better alpha incidence in the eyes-closed EEG were tested for extraversion and neuroticism and were recorded for EEG during light flash pair presentations. Alpha blocking durations were recorded for analysis. With sixty light flash presentations, the duration of blocking responses decreased over the first twenty-five and stabilized over the last thirty-five. No significant differences were found between high and low extraversion or high and low neuroticism in the characteristics of alpha or the blocking response. Those subjects with low extraversion scores showed less stability of alpha blocking duration in the last thirty-five presentations, but no significance level was calculated.

personality
neurotic
*   tendency*
visual
*   stimulation*
alpha
*   blocking*

H 21.   Gale, A., Coles, M., Kline, P., and Penfold, V.: Extraversion-introversion, neuroticism and the EEG: Basal and response measures during habituation of the orienting response. *Br J Psychol, 62:533,* 1971.

Subjects selected by a factorial design which varied extraversion-introversion and neuroticism independently were monitored for occipital EEG during habituation trials to a regularly presented auditory stimulus. A double-blind recording, scoring and statistical analysis procedure was used. Analysis showed no differentiation between extraverts and introverts, greater EEG abundance in high neurotic groups, and no readily explicable interactions between personality variables. EEG attenuation (trials 1 to 3) and EEG augmentation (trials 4 to 20), both subject to the law of initial values, were seen in all subjects; there were no differences in response amplitudes and speed of habituation for the personality groups.

personality
neurotic
* tendency*
alpha
* patterns*
habituation
orienting

EMOTION

H 22. Becker, D.: EEG changes while listening to affective stories. *Electroencephalogr Clin Neurophysiol, 31:*411, 1971 (abstr).

In order to check the classical, conceptual and explanatory models of the relations between affective excitement and EEG, affectively toned changes have been induced in fifty-two subjects by short stories of different stimulatory content. The EEG's were stored on magnetic tape and then evaluated descriptively as well as by automatic methods of interval and partial area analysis. The results are, in part, surprising. For their explanation a model is proposed which may explain the complex alterations in the EEG while listening to the stories as a result of the joint operation of two known EEG mechanisms. The results of the analyses of the changes let one recognize that a characteristic combination of affective and activating components of the total experience corresponds to a balance of both EEG mechanisms.

emotion
EEG
* patterns*

H 23. Remond, S., and Lesevre, N.: EEG and emotion. *Electroencephalogr Clin Neurophysiol (Suppl), 6:*235, 1957.

Two populations of subjects, Air Force recruits and truck drivers, were tested for characteristic EEG patterns and re-

emotion
EEG
* patterns*

actions to affective stimuli. Three patterns emerged from the *alpha* *frequency* analysis representing different EEG relationships to psycho-physiological responsiveness. EEG patterns which were poly-rhythmic, tending to desynchronize to all affective stimuli and metabolic fluctuations were associated with hyperemo-tional or emotionally reactive subjects. The emotionality tended to interfere with performance in motor tasks. EEG patterns with a dominant slow-alpha rhythm with little tend-ency to desynchronize with affective stimuli were associated with stable motor performance. EEG patterns characterized by a fast alpha frequency partially desynchronizing to affec-tive stimuli were associated with the quickest motor perform-ance and indications of high emotional adaptation.

alpha frequency
alpha blocking
motor per-formance

H 24.   Berkhout, J., Walter, D.O., and Adey, W.R.: Alterations of the human electroencephalogram induced by stressful verbal activity. *Electroencephalogr Clin Neurophysiol, 27:457, 1969.*

Fourteen male subjects between the ages of eighteen and twenty-two were presented with a series of emotionally charged questions to determine the relationship between emotional responses and EEG patterns. The amount of emo-tional stress induced by a question and the "yes" or "no" answer was determined by analysis of heart rate and pulse volume. Perception of questions was accompanied by attenu-ation of alpha, decision was accompanied by increased co-herence in theta and beta, and anticipation was accompanied by low coherence and high amplitude alpha. High stress was associated with narrowing of theta and alpha frequency bands and a 70 percent increase in frontal beta amplitude. Phase lead and lag between frontal and occipital electrodes dis-criminated between the semantic content of the questions used.

emotion
stress
verbal stimuli
alpha patterns
phase

H 25.   Small, J.G., Stevens, J.R., and Milstein, V.: Electroclinical correlates of emotional activation of the electroencephalo-gram. *J Nerv Ment Dis, 138:146, 1964.*

Forty-four epileptic patients were presented with words hav-ing various levels of emotional content to determine the effects on the EEG. GSR, EKG and respiration rate changes

emotion
epilepsy
verbal stimuli

were observed in thirty-seven of the forty-four subjects. Increases in EEG abnormalities including epileptic discharges were observed in twelve subjects following emotionally charged words; no change in EEG was found for ten subjects; alpha blocking and increased low voltage, fast activity were observed for seven subjects; intermittent and diffuse theta was observed for six subjects; and two subjects showed a normalization of the EEG following emotionally charged words.

alpha blocking theta ANS

H 26. Emrich, H., and Heinemann, L.G.: EEG and perception. *Psychol Forsch, 29:*285, 1966.

EEG's and electrocardiograms (EKG's) were continuously recorded for subjects viewing emotional and neutral words under varied brightness conditions on a transluscent screen. Difference in EEG and EKG were observed between emotional and neutral words presented in the subliminal range: namely, under the latter conditions there was a greater predominance of alpha waves, and the former differences disappeared when the stimuli were brought above threshold.

emotion verbal stimuli alpha abundance heart rate

H 27. Heinemann, L.G., and Emrich, H.: Alpha activity during inhibitory brain processes. *Psychophysiology, 7:*442, 1970.

Three studies were made to determine the relationship between the alpha rhythm and inhibitory cortical responses. In the first study sixteen subjects were presented a series of words on a frosted glass screen, half with neutral content and half with emotional content, at increasing brightness levels from sensory threshold to recognition threshold. The second study employed ten subjects in a procedure involving the hypnotic suggestion of blindness and the presentation of diffuse photic stimulation. In the third study thirty-two schizophrenic patients were given dosages of a phentothiazine derivative to determine the cortical inhibitory effects on the alpha rhythm. The perception of emotionally significant words was associated with significantly more alpha incidence than with neutral words beginning prior to reported sensory threshold. Suggestion of blindness resulted in the increased amplitude of alpha during stimulation while in two control

emotion verbal stimuli alpha blocking hypnosis drugs

conditions the amplitude of alpha was decreased during stimulation. The phentothiazine derivative resulted in significant
increases in alpha spacial distribution and occurrence in synchronous bursts over a placebo condition. The authors concluded that alpha activity is connected with inhibitory processes of the brain. They also conclude that the awareness of
the emotional content of a word precedes the awareness of
the presence of a word and that the inhibition resulting
from emotional words is associated with the alpha rhythm.

H 28.   Dixon, N.F., and Lear, T.E.: Electroencephalograph corre-
         lates of threshold regulation. *Nature, 195*:870, 1963.

Seven subjects were tested for recognition thresholds for emo-   *emotion*
tionally charged and emotionally neutral words while their   *verbal*
EEG's were being recorded. The words were presented in   *stimuli*
random order and increased in light intensity until the sub-   *emotional*
ject had signaled both an awareness of the presence of the   *thresholds*
word on a translucent screen and recognition of the word.   *alpha*
Subjects were separated for analysis on the basis of having   *abundance*
higher or lower thresholds for emotionally charged words.
Subjects with a higher threshold for emotionally charged
words had a relative increase in alpha abundance during
awareness and recognition with reference to emotionally
neutral words, while the relationship was reversed for subjects with a lower threshold.

H 29.   Darrow, C.W., and Hicks, R.G.: Interarea electroencepha-
         lographic phase relationships following sensory and idea-
         tional stimuli. *Psychophysiology, 1*:337, 1965.

Young adult subjects were presented with stimuli varying   *emotion*
in emotional content from simple sensory stimuli to emo-   *verbal*
tional words. The phase relationships between parietal and   *stimuli*
occipital EEG leads were analyzed for the different types of   *alpha phase*
stimuli. Simple stimuli, which produced a GSR, increased
anterior leading. Disturbing verbal stimuli created rapid
diphasic reversals between leads, and neutral verbal stimuli
reduced diphasic reversals.

H 30.   Gale, A., Lucas, B., Nissim, R., and Harpham, B.: Some

EEG correlates of face-to-face contact. *Br J Soc Clin Psychol,* 2:326, 1972.

During the recording of transoccipital EEG from twelve male undergraduates, the experimenter smiled at the subject, looked at the subject or averted his gaze away from the subject in order to study the relationship between emotion (and indirectly arousal) and EEG activity. The amount or abundance of EEG activity decreased as arousal increased except in the case of theta activity (4.5 to 6.5 Hz). This finding proved to be statistically significant for low and middle alpha frequencies (8.5 to 11.5 Hz) and for activity in the 2.0 to 4.5 Hz range. It is concluded that this research supports the proposal that social interaction influences arousal as measured by the EEG. Investigations into the influence of sex and personality as well as clinical comparisons are proposed.

emotion
social
interaction
eye contact
EEG
patterns
alpha
abundance

H 31. Ulett, G.A.: The relationship of the EEG to emotions. *Psychiatr-Res Rep, 12:*176, 1960.

The status of work correlating EEG and emotions is discussed in the light of previous studies and applications by a variety of investigators. Also included are descriptions of work by the author on EEG's and emotions and on photic stimulation to determine convulsive thresholds in schizophrenics.

emotion
EEG
patterns
photic
stimulation
schizo-
phrenia

H 32. Mundy-Castle, A.C.: The electroencephalogram and mental activity. *Electroencephalogr Clin Neurophysiol, 9:*643, 1957.

Seventy-two European adults, 66 African adults and 304 clinical patients with emotional instability were recorded for EEG changes during eye-opening, eye-closing, mental arithmetic and imagery in different sensory modalities. The various tasks were given both with and without photic flicker induction of alpha. The European group showed an increase in beta activity which was greatest in visual imagery and mental arithmetic, and less in eye-opening. The following conditions are listed according to increasing intensity of the blocking response produced: kinesthetic imagery, auditory imagery, mental arithmetic, visual imagery, and eye-opening.

emotion
emotional
instability
mental tasks
imagery
eye opening
alpha
blocking
theta
ethnic
differences

African subjects produced more alpha blocking at the lowest intensity and had augmented theta activity in the eyes-opening condition. Emotional reactivity was found to be related to the incidence of theta in the EEG's of clinical patients. Theta was also found to decrease in incidence as a function of age. The author proposes a four-category classification of the theta rhythm and a two-category classification of beta activity.

H 33.   Mundy-Castle, A.C.: Electrical responses of the brain in relation to behavior. *Br J Psychol, 44:*318, 1953.

The psychologic significance of brain electrical rhythms was explored by determining the effects of rhythmic photic flicker from 1 to 30 Hz on emotional, sensory and intellectual activities. A variety of normal and of nonepileptic abnormal responses are documented. High frequencies appeared to evoke anxiety, anger or confusion, and theta frequencies tended to enhance unpleasurable emotional expression. Changes in visual perception and in body movement were also elicited and could be accompanied or enhanced by the emotional changes. High alpha frequencies were associated with quick, impulsive, variable primary function individuals and interpreted as attributable to high level cortical excitability. There were marked individual differences in frequency harmonics.

emotion
sensory
* perception*
cognition
alpha
* frequency*
harmonics

H 34.   Nencini, R., and Pasquali, E.: Amplitude variations in alpha rhythm during the controlled presentation of images. *Arch Psicol Neurol Psichiatr, 30:*337, 1969.

Positive and negative visual images were presented to subjects during the measurement of their EEG's. Presentation of stimuli produced attenuation of alpha. Removal of positive stimuli resulted in a further attenuation of alpha while removal of negative stimuli increased the amplitude of alpha.

emotion
visual
* imagery*
alpha
* blocking*
alpha en-
* hancement*

H 35.   Simonov, P.V., and Mikhailova, N.G.: Quantitative approach to studying positive emotions. *Psychophysiology, 8:*82, 1971.

Mean changes in total tension of alpha, theta and delta rhythms in twelve actors with increasing negative stress or fear and positive stress or joy/pleasure measured via heart rate are presented. Three EEG stages were observed: slight exaltation, depression and repeated increased slow rhythms associated with heart rates of 130 to 140 bpm. Under the positive stress condition, the slow waves start repeating sooner and with less stress at 120 to 130 bpm. Generating mechanisms for these emotional reactions as well as other work being done in this area are also discussed.

emotion
fear
pleasure
EEG
  patterns
heart rate

H 36.   Scherzer, E.: Low voltage EEG's as the bio-electrical measure of tense expectancy (psychogenic alpha reduction). *Psychiatr Neurol, 152*:207, 1966.

Hospital patients were tested for EEG differences under normal clinical and insurance claim examination conditions. The EEG's taken during insurance examinations showed a lower amplitude and incidence of the alpha rhythm than prior to the examination. The author related the change to the expectancy and anxiety accompanying the insurance examination.

emotion
expectancy
anxiety
alpha
  patterns

SECTION I

PERCEPTUAL INFLUENCES

SENSORY PERCEPTION

I 1.   McKee, G., Humphrey, B. and McAdam, D.: Scaled lateral-ization of alpha activity during linguistic and musical tasks. *Psychophysiology, 10:*441, 1973.

Bilateral alpha activity from temporal-parietal areas was studied in 4 students during auditory tasks. Left/right alpha activity ratios were largest during muscial tasks and decreased as linguistic tasks became more difficult.

*sensory
  perception
auditory
  perception
hemispheric
  dominance*

I 2.   Cohen, S.I., Silverman, A.J., and Shmavonian, B.M.: Neuro-physiological, humoral and personality factors in the re-sponse to sensory deprivation. *Third World Congress of Psychiatry, Montreal, 2:*1004, 1961.

This experiment sought to study the interaction of environ-mental and psychological characteristics by causing a state of uncertainty through lack of environmental information in thirty-five subjects. EEG measures such as alpha activity were used to assess cortical alerting while GSR served a similar function for autonomic arousal. Endocrinologic measures were also utilized. Results from the total group were not significant but individual subgroups based on perceptual mode (body- or field-orientated) and personality traits proved more interesting in that they did not show a random distribution of responses. It is hoped that this data will be of practical value in identifying the appropriate treatment to which different types of patients will respond.

*sensory
  perception
spatial
  orientation
alpha
  abundance*

I 3.   Gale, A., Bramley, P., Lucas, B., and Christie, B.: Differ-ential effect of visual and auditory complexity on the EEG: Negative hedonic value as a crucial variable? *Psychon Sci, 27:* 21, 1972.

As reported in past experiments, part 1 of this four-part investigation showed EEG abundance and visual stimuli complexity to be inversely related. That is, EEG abundance decreases with increased stimulus complexity. Part 2 showed the opposite to be true for auditory stimuli. In part 3 subjects rated complexity of auditory stimuli and hedonic value; results indicated the simpler stimuli to be most irritating. Part 4 expands part 3 to include both auditory and visual stimuli with findings similar to those of part 3. It was concluded that auditory and visual stimuli can be differentiated by some sort of irritation-relaxation scale.

sensory perception
EEG abundance variability

I 4. Pillsbury, J.A., Meyerowitz, S., Saltzman, L., and Satran, R.: Electroencephalographic correlates of perceptual style: Field orientation. *Psychosom Med, 29:*441, 1967.

Seventy-four medical students were separated into field-independent and field-dependent groups on the basis of their performance in a rod-and-frame task. Auditory (telephone bell) and visual (light flash) stimuli were presented to the subjects to determine the effects on the EEG alpha. Field-independent subjects had little habituation of the alpha blocking response to the auditory stimulus while they habituated rapidly to the visual stimulus. The reverse was found for the field-dependent subjects with rapid habituation to the auditory stimulus and slow habituation to the visual stimulus.

sensory perception
sensory stimulation
spatial orientation
alpha blocking habituation

I 5. Marshall, C., and Harden, C.: Use of rhythmically varying patterns for photic stimulation. *Electroencephalogr Clin Neurophysiol, 4:*283, 1952.

A pattern consisting of an expanding circle which begins as a dot and enlarges to a maximum diameter at a constant speed and then returns to a dot instantly was used to study the effect of low intensity visual rhythmic pattern stimulation on the normal human EEG. The rate of pattern repetition was varied from one to one hundred per second. For each condition, five- to ten-second epochs of alternated experimental and control recording were averaged and graphed. Results showed odd color changes and patterns like those

sensory perception
photic flicker
alpha frequency

seen with high intensity stimulation at particular frequencies and with three- to four-inch maximum diameter circles. It was also observed that a peak occurred at the pattern frequency during experimentation with no peak at the alpha frequency. The alpha peak returned during controls except when acute attention was required of the subject. It was concluded that this pattern driving effect probably affects the occipital rhythm activity. The possibility of intensity stimulation as the image moves from macular to peripheral areas caused by the gradient of stimulation threshold between these regions was ruled out because the pattern driving effect remained even at low illumination levels.

I 6. Evans, C.R., and Smith, G.K.: Alpha frequency of electro-encephalogram and a stabilized retinal image. *Nature, 204:* 303, 1964.

A study was performed to see if alpha wave suppression is actually associated with pattern perception as has been thought. Since it is known that alpha is suppressed during viewing of patterns, it was of interest to see what happens when a stabilized pattern disappears as it does when viewed as a stabilized retinal image. Experimental sessions using a simple patterned target as well as two controls for resting alpha activity and possible after-effects of the flash on the retina were conducted. The later control investigated the possibility that the flash rather than the perception of the patterned target may be the cause of alpha wave suppression. Analysis of the records indicated that the suppression is indeed related to the pattern perception, but the role of attention was not clear. The authors suggest that signals that define contours, boundaries, and maybe shape have been shown to be of independent importance by this work.

sensory perception retinal images alpha frequency

I 7. Shaw, J.C., and McLaughlan, K.R.: The association between alpha rhythm propagation time and level of arousal. *Psychophysiology, 4:*307, 1968.

Eight subjects between the ages of eighteen and twenty-four were presented with a series of tasks alternating with rest periods. The tasks involved visual, auditory and tactile discriminations as well as mental arithmetic. Skin conductance

sensory perception mental tasks alpha phase GSR

and the time delay between frontal and occipital alpha were compared. Significant positive correlations were found between mean log conductance and delay time for five of the eight subjects. A negative correlation was found in one subject while no correlations were found for the other two.

I 8.   Giannitrapani, D.: Scanning mechanisms and the EEG. *Electroencephalogr Clin Neurophysiol, 30*:139, 1971.

Thirty-two right-handed, male children (11 to 13 years old) were given a series of eight perceptual tasks while their EEG's were being recorded from sixteen scalp electrode placements. The tasks included the presentation of such stimuli as diffused pictures, white noise, an audible story and mental arithmetic. The presentation of a stimulus was associated with a reduction in alpha activity and an increase in beta activity. Perception or structuring of a stimulus was associated with a reduction in beta activity. Temporal areas showed the largest effects of the stimulus-perception process, although the same changes occurred in the occipital areas with diffused visual stimuli and in the frontal areas with white noise presentations. The author proposed that different frequencies of the EEG represent different perceptual scanning mechanisms, with higher frequencies being associated with faster and more focused scanning.

sensory
  perception
mental tasks
children
EEG
  frequency
scanning
  mechanisms

I 9.   Ciofu, I., and Floru, R.: Electroencephalographic investigations of set. *Rev Roum Sci Soc Serie Psychol, 9*:195, 1965.

Twenty-four subjects were given response sets for tasks involving motor, perceptual or intellectual activities. The presence of a response set resulted in a decreased incidence of alpha in the resting EEG. After performing the appropriate tasks, the attenuation of alpha in the presence of a set to repeat the task was of shorter duration. Amount of alpha blocking was found to be directly related to level of task difficulty.

sensory
  perception
mental tasks
motor per-
  formance
alpha
  blocking
cognition

I 10.   Beyn, E.S., Zhirmunskaya, E.A., and Volkov, V.N.: Electro-encephalographic investigations in the process of recognizing images of objects during their tachistoscopic presentation-I.

Investigations carried out on normal subjects. *Neuropsy-chologia, 5:203, 1967.*

Thirteen normal subjects were given an object recognition task in which ten to twenty images of objects were presented tachistoscopically on a translucent screen and subjects were asked to respond by pressing a button when they were aware of an image occurring and when they were able to recognize the object. Mean recognition threshold was 0.62 msec image duration. There were two patterns of EEG change which were produced by image presentation. The first pattern involved a 0.35 second latent period of no effect on the EEG followed by a 0.48 second depression of all EEG activity and a burst of alpha mixed with low frequency beta activity. The second pattern involved a 0.19 second latent period followed by a 0.40 second evoked potential, a 0.48 second period of EEG suppression and a burst of alpha and beta.

sensory
  perception
recognition
alpha
  patterns
beta

I 11.   Sklar, B., Hanley, J., and Simmons, W.W.: An EEG experiment aimed toward identifying dyslexic children. *Nature, 240:414, 1972.*

The experiment was conducted to find statistically significant spectral features of the EEG for identifying dyslexic children using twelve dyslexic children and thirteen controls. Ten-second periods of EEG activity were chosen for analysis during five situations: rest, eyes closed; attentive, eyes open; during mental arithmetic; reading word lists; and reading a text. Data gathered during the rest, eyes-closed and the reading-a-text situations proved most valuable with the former being the most significant. It appears that constrained situations cause a sameness in the EEG's, while removal of the constraints elicits the most disparate features. During this rest, eyes-closed phase the parieto-occipital area allowed the best discrimination between subject groups. In particular, the dyslexic children had on the average more energy in the 3 to 7 cps activity. Also, during the mental task period there was a higher coherence between regions in the same hemisphere in dyslexic subjects.

sensory
  perception
dyslexia
perceptual
  tasks
spectral
  analysis

SENSORY DEPRIVATION

I 12.   Heron, W., Tait, G., and Smith, G.K.: Effects of prolonged perceptual isolation on the human electroencephalogram. *Brain Res, 43*:280, 1972.

Past research has shown that EEG's of humans exposed to environments with reduced pattern stimulation exhibit slower frequencies in the alpha rhythm recorded from posterior regions. This article replicates these results and describes them fully since these EEG changes may be useful in understanding the basis of the drastic behavioral effects (changes in perception, intellectual functions and hallucinations). Deprivation effects could also be seen in REM sleep in some subjects and, along with slow onset and long recovery time for the deprivation effects, they suggest that a direct link between these changes and level of arousal may not exist. Perhaps some new organization which cannot be explained by our present understanding of neurophysiology has developed. This experiment was carried further to study the theta rhythm and 12 to 15 cps spindles of stage II sleep. Frequency and amplitude of these wavelengths were not altered by isolation.

sensory deprivation
alpha patterns
dreams
arousal
spectral analysis

I 13.   Zubek, J.P., Bayer, L., and Shephard, J.M.: Relative effects of prolonged social isolation and confinement: Behavioral and EEG changes. *J Abnorm Psychol, 74*:625, 1969.

Sixty male students were given one to three treatments: complete social isolation, confinement control, or ambulatory control for a period of several weeks. In the social isolation condition twenty subjects were placed in a chamber which was visually and acoustically isolated from the outside world and only occasional human contact with the experimenter was allowed. In the confinement condition the subjects were allowed visits from relatives and friends, and they had radio and television and auditory contact with the activities of the laboratory. The ambulatory control group lived outside the laboratory and made scheduled visits for testing. Both the social isolation and the confinement groups showed a significant decrease in alpha frequency during the

sensory deprivation
alpha patterns
subjective reports

procedure while the ambulatory control group showed no change. The social isolation group showed a significantly higher incidence of reported feelings of loneliness, hostility, temporal disorientation, loss of contact with reality and novel ideas than the other two groups. The confinement group reported more loss of contact with reality and novel ideas than the ambulatory group. Both social isolation and confinement conditions resulted in a higher incidence of reported visual hallucinations, inefficient thought, restlessness and reminiscence.

I 14.   Zubek, J.P., and Welch, G.: Electroencephalographic changes after prolonged sensory and perceptual deprivation. *Science, 139:*1209, 1963.

Forty male students were placed in one of four conditions to determine the effects of isolation on the EEG. Ten subjects were placed in total sensory isolation, ten were isolated from visual patterns and noise but had stimulation present, ten were given normal stimulation but required to stay in a prone position on a bed for the duration of the experiment, and ten were allowed to lead life as usual but come into the lab for EEG measurements at regular intervals. The first two groups showed a post-isolation decrease in mean frequency of the occipital EEG. The decrease was greater for the group which had received some stimulation than for the totally isolated subjects. Neither of the control groups differed from each other, but both showed significant differences in mean EEG frequency from the isolation groups.

sensory deprivation
EEG frequency

I 15.   Marjerrison, G., and Keogh, R.P.: Field dependency and electroencephalogram (EEG) responses to perceptual deprivation. *J Nerv Ment Dis, 152:*390, 1971.

Six chronic, nonparanoid schizophrenic patients and six normal control subjects were recorded for EEG in consecutive periods of perceptual deprivation. Destruction of auditory and visual stimuli was accomplished with masking noise from an air conditioning unit and red light projected evenly over the surface of transluscent eye coverings. Two subjects from each group were scored as field-dependent and four

sensory deprivation
schizophrenia
spatial orientation
EEG patterns

from each group as field-independent on the basis of performance in a rod-and-frame task. A monopolar occipital EEG was used for analysis of integrated EEG, coefficient of variation and mean alpha frequency. Integrated EEG amplitude increased during perceptual deprivation for field-dependent schizophrenics and field-independent control subjects. Amplitude decreased for field-independent schizophrenics and field-dependent controls. Field-dependent schizophrenics showed decreased EEG variability in perceptual deprivation while field-independent schizophrenics and field-dependent controls showed increased variability. Field-dependent subjects showed a 1.1 Hz increase in alpha frequency during perceptual deprivation while field-independent subjects showed a 0.5 Hz decrease. The interaction effect of field-dependency and EEG change during perceptual deprivation was the only parameter which differentiated the groups in this experiment.

I 16. Harrison, A., Lairy, G.C., and Leger, E.M.: The EEG and visual deprivation. *Electroencephalogr Clin Neurophysiol,* *29*:20, 1970.

The findings in seventeen children who were blind or had only a perception of light confirmed these classical findings: marked changes in background rhythm, often with a rolandic or parietal distribution of an activity of alpha frequency; and occipital foci of spikes, which occurred mainly in children over five years of age. One hundred subjects between five and eighteen years of age with significant visual defects but a useful residual acuity of 2/100 to 3/10 were used. The EEG variables were studied in relation to age, the residual acuity and the IQ, and the etiology of the ocular condition was considered as well as the possibility of organic cerebral disease, independent or not of the ocular lesion. The parameters of the background rhythm showed very little relationship with age or with residual visual acuity. On the other hand, in this very mixed population from the mental point of view, there were very significant relationships with the IQ. The foci of occipital spikes, in 47 percent of the cases, showed no statistical relationship with age, the residual acuity and the IQ, or with the possibility of old organic cerebral disease. These foci were seen equally with diseases

sensory
  deprivation
children
intelligence
EEG
  patterns

of the lens, the retina or the optic tracts. The significance of topographic changes in the background rhythm and of the occipital spike foci was studied. Statistical investigation of this population, and also the longitudinal study of some cases, support the conclusion that the interpretation of the EEG in blind or partially sighted children cannot be made in relation only to the quantitative loss of vision but must also take account of the existing adaptation to the visual defect.

VISUAL IMAGERY

I 17.   Reyher, J., and Morishige, H.: Electroencephalogram and rapid eye movements during free imagery and dream recall. *J Abnorm Psychol, 74:*576, 1969.

Ten male subjects ranging in age from eighteen to twenty-nine years, having reported high visual imagery ability, were given two tasks involving creating visual images while being recorded for eye movements and occipital EEG. In a free-imagery procedure, subjects were asked to sit quietly and press a switch each time they were experiencing visual images. After each imagery sequence, the subjects were to report the content. In a dream recall task subjects were asked to recall particularly vivid dreams which they had experienced in the past. Subjects had a higher imagery rate in the dream recall condition than in the free-imagery condition with a greater amount of reported movement and longer episodes. Alpha blocking was found to occur just prior to the report of an episode of imagery, but no difference in alpha characteristics was found during the episode.

visual imagery eye movements alpha blocking dreams

I 18.   Brown, B.B.: Specificity of EEG photic flicker responses to color as related to visual imagery ability. *Psychophysiology,* 2:197, 1966.

Two groups of subjects were selected from a previously studied population sample: a group of habitual visualizers, most of whom developed eye movements during recall of motion, and a group of nonvisualizers, most of whom did not. EEG following responses to red photic flicker differed mark-

visual imagery mental tasks photic flicker

edly for the two groups, being diminished in visualizers but enhanced in nonvisualizers as compared to their EEG following responses to blue or green. Mental and visual imagery tasks induced significantly greater alpha blocking in visualizers than in nonvisualizers. The partial or complete desynchronization of ongoing rhythmic EEG activity suggests a lower threshold for EEG desynchronization for visualizers than for nonvisualizers. The augmented EEG following of nonvisualizers to red flicker appears to represent a different aspect of the same response continuum.

EEG patterns eye movements

I 19.   Costello, C.G., and McGregor, P.: The relationships between some aspects of visual imagery and the alpha rhythm. *J Ment Sci, 103*:786, 1957.

Twenty female subjects were given tasks involving the production of visual images while being recorded for EEG changes from bilateral parietal and occipital electrode placements. Subjects were presented picture cards and after their removal were asked to visualize the pictures. A questionnaire was presented to determine the vividness of the resulting imagery including clarity, shape and movement. The amount of measured alpha suppression was a function of vividness of imagery. Higher thought processes or complexity of thinking was found to be inversely related to the amount of alpha suppression.

visual imagery alpha blocking criteria

I 20.   Barratt, P.E.: Use of the EEG in the study of imagery. *Br J Psychol, 47*:101, 1956.

The hypothesis that suppression of the alpha rhythm offers a reliable and objective index of visual imagery was examined in sixty-nine subjects. Two conditions of problem solving were employed: solving a visual problem and solving a verbal problem. Results suggested that the hypothesis was not tenable since imagery appeared to be only one of many factors causing suppression of alpha activity.

visual imagery desynchronization

I 21.   Brown, B.B.: Some observations on eye movement and EEG activity during different sensory modalities of perception and recall. *Slovak Academy of Sciences,* in press.

Twelve subjects ranging in age from twenty-one to fifty were tested for visual, auditory and tactile perception and memory using a system of random bits. Subjects were separated into visualizers and nonvisualizers on the basis of tests previously developed by the author. Subjects were required to recall the perceptions of the random bit stimuli as well as the motion of a metronome pointer, auditory rhythms presented from a tape recorder, and a variety of textured materials. Visualizers showed little difference in EEG patterns with eyes opened and eyes closed. Nonvisualizers exhibited increased amplitude rather than abundance of alpha under eyes-closed conditions. Visual perception was associated with alpha blocking for all subjects. Visual recall was associated with attenuation of alpha for all visualizers and two nonvisualizers while three nonvisualizers showed enhanced alpha activity. Auditory perception was associated with normal alpha for both groups while recall resulted in attenuation of alpha for less than half of the subjects. During tactile perception alpha was enhanced while during recall two visualizers changed to dominant theta, two nonvisualizers showed alpha attenuation and one showed enhanced alpha.

visual imagery
sensory perception
recall
alpha patterns

I 22.   Slatter, K.H.: Alpha rhythms and mental imagery. *Electroencephalogr Clin Neurophysiol, 12*:851, 1960.

Subjects were presented with a series of tasks involving the use of visual and auditory images to separate visualizer and nonvisualizer subjects and to determine the effects of imagery tasks on EEG alpha. The memory of familiar visual images (a friend or an apple) resulted in a reduction in alpha while familiar verbal images (national anthem, the Lord's Prayer) had no effect on alpha. Active vision resulted in greater alpha reduction than visual recall. The largest reductions in alpha were associated with the largest amplitude of alpha. Low amplitude resting alpha was characteristic for high visualizers while high amplitude alpha was characteristic for verbalizers. Visualizers had less rhythmic alpha, more frequent complete blocking of alpha and more often had a dominant alpha frequency of 12 Hz.

visual imagery
visual perception
alpha abundance
alpha rhythmicity
alpha frequency

I 23.   Walter, R.D., and Yeager, C.L.: Visual imagery and electroencephalographic changes. *Electroencephalogr Clin Neurophysiol,* 8:193, 1956.

EEG changes related to acute vision, visual imagery, recall and visual-motor performance were studied in 195 subjects (180 psychiatric patients and 15 blind adolescent students). Accurate diagram reproduction during nonstimulated states was found to be associated with a low potential, nonrhythmic activity in the occipital region while inaccurate reproduction during rest was associated with a higher potential, rhythmic occipital activity. Performance and age or sex, EEG abnormalities, the percent reduction during active vision or recall, or rate of alpha appearance on eye closure showed no significant correlations.

visual imagery
visual perception
alert
eye opening
blindness
desynchronization

I 24.   Drever, J.: Some observations on the occipital alpha rhythm. *Q J Exp Psychol,* 7:91, 1955.

Seventy-four subjects (half blind and half sighted) were recorded for EEG before, during and after various mental, visual and physical tasks to investigate the relationships between alpha activity and visual imagery. The groups were matched for age, sex and intelligence, and the blind group was subdivided into those who lost their sight before and after age four. The sighted wore eye pads and much effort was expended to reduce alpha reduction due to anxiety in all subjects. An overall comparison showed close agreement of alpha frequency between the groups. This was interpreted as indicating similar phenomenon occurring in both groups during this time. However, the blind group did show a smaller amount of alpha activity. Average amplitude was insignificant, but the mean of the maximum amplitude had a significance level of 1 percent. Using a normal threshold classification of alpha types (M,R,P), it was found that some blind subjects had records which were characteristic of visualizers (type M). This, concludes the author, proves the association of the alpha rhythm with visual imagery to be too simple. Further analysis of test performance indicated the alpha rhythm to be more sensitive to figure recognition than orientation and that while figure recognition test performance discriminates between sighted and unsighted, orienta-

visual imagery
blindness
mental tasks
perceptual tasks
motor performance
alpha patterns

tion performs a similar function between early- and late-blinded subjects.

I 25.   Gale, A., Morris, P.E., Lucas, B., and Richardson, A.: Types of imagery and imagery types: An EEG study. *Br J Psychol, 63*:523, 1972.

This study attempts to look at the EEG effects of passive, spontaneous, voluntary or nonimaging conditions in vivid, intermediate or weak imagers and to examine a possible inter-relation between individual differences in imagery ability and type of instruction. Alpha abundance and mean dominant alpha frequency were the main parameters extracted from trans-occipital, bipolar EEG's from thirty undergraduates chosen for their responses on the Betts Vividness of Imagery Scale. Findings included a distinction between vivid and weak imagers in that mean dominant alpha frequency was higher in vivid imagers. This difference held only under an eyes-open minimal imaging condition and there was no such finding for the more commonly used alpha abundance measure. More suppression exhibited by decreased abundance occurred during passive elicited imagery after the presentation of high imagery words than occurred after low imagery words, while the reverse was seen during voluntary elicited and autonomous imaging. It was noted that criterion groups (vivid, medium and weak imagers) were differentiable by strength of imagery elicited by high and low imagery words, and also that these groups all were able to differentiate between the high and low imagery words. Also, high imagery words elicited more imagery than low imagery words for both vivid and weak imagers, and vivid imagers reported more elicited imagery. No significant causal relation between the results and extraversion and neuroticism was found using the Eysenck Personality Inventory. On the basis of alpha suppression seen during imagery, it is felt that imaging does influence the EEG and that this may not be merely a byproduct of arousal during such imaging tasks. However, this is not directly proven. Other variables such as difficulty of imaging by variation of instruction also have an effect on the EEG as shown in this study, and it is suggested that this may explain equivocal results of earlier

visual imagery
mental tasks
alpha frequency
alpha abundance

research. It is admitted that these results do not form a systematic pattern; findings for individual differences are significant only in terms of mean dominant frequency and differences for tasks only in abundance measures. Also, the comparison of tasks lacks a design which would allow direct quantitative comparison. Nevertheless, the authors feel that the results are valuable enough to merit further investigation.

I 26. Oswald, I.: The EEG, visual imagery and attention. *Q J Exp Psychol, 9*:113, 1957.

Thirty-three subjects who reported a high incidence of visual imagery were tested for the characteristics of alpha in their EEG's while performing tasks involving the use of visual images. The presence and persistence of alpha in the EEG had no significant relationship to imagery ability with twenty-seven of the subjects having normally reactive alpha. The process of visualization was associated with momentary blocking of the alpha rhythm with an immediate return to full amplitude while visualization was continuing. With visual arithmetic, simple problems did not change the amplitude of alpha while difficult problems were associated with alpha blocking until a solution was obtained. The author concluded that alpha blocking is associated with the occurrence of new and difficult mental tasks rather than the process of thinking or visualizing alone.

visual imagery mental tasks alpha patterns attention

I 27. Simpson, H.M., Paivio, A., and Rogers, T.B.: Occipital alpha activity of high and low visual imagers during problem solving. *Psychon Sci, 8*:49, 1967.

Sixty-three male students were given a battery of tests for imagery ability to select nine subjects with high imagery ability and nine with low imagery ability. The occipital EEG of each subject was recorded during the performance of a series of tasks including eyes-closed, eyes-opened, verbal stimulation, verbal memory, visual stimulation and visual memory. Subjects which had scored high on the tests of imagery ability had a greater incidence of alpha in the rest periods than those who had scored low. The stimulation and

visual imagery mental tasks perceptual stimulation alpha patterns memory eye opening memory conditions were associated with decreased amplitude alpha with the greatest decrease occurring in the verbal conditions. Low visualizers showed some increase in alpha in the visual conditions.

I 28.   Brown, B.B.: Subjective and EEG responses to LSD in visualizer and non-visualizer subjects. *Electroencephalogr Clin Neurophysiol, 25:372,* 1968.

Subjects who reported possessing vivid visual imagery ability responded to LSD by enhanced visual perceptual and visual imagery activity, whereas subjects completely lacking this ability experienced little or no change in visual perception or imagery but responded by increased conceptual activity. Nonvisualizers, however, reported vivid visual imagery during dreaming. EEG responses of visualizers and nonvisualizers to spectral flickering light were reversed for the two groups and were affected differently by LSD. EEG responses indicated activation effects of LSD in visualizers and decreased EEG activation in nonvisualizers.

visual imagery hallucinogens photic flicker

TIME PERCEPTION

I 29.   Werboff, J.: Time judgment as a function of electroencephalographic activity. *Exp Neurol, 6:152,* 1962.

This study investigates a possible correlation between alpha activity and time judgment along lines similar to those of Hoagland who demonstrated that increased body temperature results in underestimation of time. Alpha index (or percentage-time-alpha) and wave-count per second scores (or frequency) were calculated. Of course, time judgments were made by the subjects during the experiment. Results showed that subjects with 50 percent or more alpha during eyes-closed resting EEG over-estimated time in the eyes-open condition when compared to those with less than 50 percent alpha. This supports Hoagland's cerebral metabolic clock idea to account for estimation of short temporal intervals. An inherent organic or constitutional mechanism of cerebral activity mediated by the EEG may intervene in or be correlated with cerebral metabolism and control of temporal experience.

time perception alpha patterns eye opening

I 30. Anliker, J.: Variations in alpha voltage of the electroencephalogram and time perception. *Science, 140:*1307, 1963.

Subjects were given the task of making regular key taps at subjective estimates of three-second intervals while their EEG's were being recorded. A narrow band filter tuned to the peak frequency of each subject's alpha activated a cumulative recorder. Inter-response times were recorded along with slopes of the cumulative record to determine the relationships between time estimation and alpha voltage. The relationship appears as a power function, fitting a straight line when plotted with log-log coordinates. The occurrence of higher and lower frequencies than the peak alert alpha were not accounted for in this study.

time perception
alpha amplitude

I 31. Legg, C.F.: Alpha rhythm and time judgments. *J Exp Psychol, 78:*46, 1968. (Copyright 1968 by the Amer Psychol Assoc and reproduced by permission.)

Previous studies have indicated correlations between time judgments and certain characteristics of the EEG. Here, using intervals betwen 0.5 and 8 seconds, no significant correlations were found between judgment lengths and mean alpha rate or alpha index. Reliable, if weak, associations between judgments and aspects of concurrent EEG may yet be established.

time perception
alpha patterns

I 32. Cahoon, R.L.: Physiological arousal and time estimation. *Percept Mot Skills, 28:*259, 1969.

Forty college students separated into high and low chronic arousal groups on the basis of scores on the Taylor Manifest Anxiety Scale were given a task of estimating the time interval between two tones under high induced arousal (HIA, threat of shock) and low induced arousal (LIA) conditions. Heart rate, respiration rate, alpha frequency and integrated EEG were used as measures of arousal. Values for heart rate, respiration rate and integrated EEG amplitude were greater under the HIA condition than in LIA. Using tap rates and verbal reports as time estimates, fast tap rates were associated with high respiration and low verbal time estimates were

time perception
arousal
alpha frequency
EEG integration
heart rate

associated with fast heart rates. Alpha frequency was correlated with tapping rates in the HIA condition and with verbal estimates in the LIA condition.

I 33.   Jasper, H., and Shagass, C.: Conscious time judgments related to conditioned time intervals and voluntary control of the alpha rhythm. *J Exp Psychol, 28:*503, 1941.

Eleven adult male subjects were given delayed, trace and cyclic Pavlovian conditioning of light flashes and time intervals with the alpha blocking response in one part of the experiment. In another, called voluntary conditioning, light flashes were paired with the verbalization of the word "block" at ten-second time intervals. In the photic conditioning part, time estimations were longer than the conditioned interval while conditioned alpha blocking was anticipatory or shorter than the conditioned interval. The voluntary conditioning to the word "block" was successful but no data were presented concerning time estimation under this latter condition.

time
* perception*
condition-
* ing*
alpha
* blocking*
expectancy

COGNITIVE INFLUENCES

INTELLIGENCE

J 1.   Vogel, W., and Broverman, D.M.: Relationship between EEG and test intelligence: A critical review. *Psychol Bull, 62:*132, 1964.

The authors reviewed the literature on the relationships between EEG parameters and intelligence as measured by a variety of tests. They found a relatively large number of studies which showed positive relationships and some which showed no relationships. The negative results were attributed to the use of different tests of intelligence, conditions in which EEG recordings were made, lack of control for age, and lack of control for sex. In studies of mental defectives, mongolian idiots were found to show a positive correlation between mental age (MA) and alpha incidence, and familial defectives were found to show a correlation between alpha frequency and MA with slower alpha frequency than normals. With age held constant, MA in children was found to be significantly correlated with alpha frequency. Equal numbers of studies showed negative results but the conditions of the experiments were described as different and generally lacked the controls of the studies with positive results according to the authors.

intelligence
age
alpha
 frequency
criteria

J 2.   Vogel, W., and Broverman, D.M.: A reply to "Relationship between EEG and intelligence: A commentary." *Psychol Bull, 2:*99, 1966.

In an earlier article the authors reviewed the literature on the relationship between EEG and intelligence, concluding that the data support the existence of a reliable set of relationships. Ellingson criticized the article on a number of grounds. The authors defended their earlier position in this article.

intelligence
EEG
 patterns
critique

J 3. Giannitrapani, D.: WAIS IQ. as related to EEG frequency scores. *Electroencephalogr Clin Neurophysiol, 28*:102, 1970 (abstr) .

In an attempt to investigate the relationships between in- *intelligence* telligence and a broad frequency range, this experiment *EEG* studied the average frequency of the EEG, a variable which *frequency* had received very little attention, even though the increase of *alpha* fast activity during mental work is a phenomenon observed *symmetry* by the earliest investigators. While the early expectation of a correlation between thinking-resting differences was not supported with any degree of strength, both the traditional alpha index and homologous area asymmetry scores showed varying degrees of correlation with IQ.

J 4. Wien, E.W.: Das elektroenzephalogramm bei intellektuell unterschiedlich bagabten 9-14 jahrigen kindern. *Helv Paediatr Acta, 27*:109, 1972.

Thirty-nine children (9 to 14 years old) were given tests for *intelligence* intelligence and recorded for EEG to determine the rela- *children* tionships between EEG and intelligence. The Hamburg *personality* Wechsler Intelligenztest fur Kinder and the Coloured Pro- *EEG* gressive Matrices tests were used to estimate intelligence. *patterns* Children with a dominant, high amplitude, reactive alpha rhythm and little theta and beta activity scored higher on the intelligence tests. Children with less alpha and more beta in the EEG had lower scores on the tests. The latter group was found to have personality characteristics of increased irritability, decreased ability to concentrate, and difficulty in overcoming stress. The personality factors were suggested as having interfered with test performance with the effect of creating an artifactual relationship between EEG and in- telligence.

J 5. Genkin, A.A.: Differentiation of EEG signals in various types of intellectual activity. *Byull Eksper Biol Med, 67*:120, 1969.

The EEG is discriminated statistically according to various *intelligence* kinds of intellectual activity. No reference to background *EEG* activity or background changes during the changes in intel- *patterns* lectual function are utilized in the analysis.

J 6.   Liberson, W.T.: EEG and intelligence. In *Psychopathology of Mental Development*. New York, Grune and Stratton, 1967, p. 514.

It is shown that a much stronger correlation exists between EEG abnormalities and active intelligence scores than between the former and passive intelligence scores such as those of vocabulary tests. Analysis showed that intellectual efficacy may deteriorate physiologically. Examples include conceptual efficiency and alpha blocking which are influenced similarly by age and alpha frequency and respiration rhythm and heart rate which are related to the alerting function in the deep brain structures. The significance of these and other such correlations remains for future research.

intelligence
EEG
  patterns

J 7.   Ellingson, R.J.: Relationship between EEG and test intelligence: A commentary. *Psychol Bull*, 2:91, 1966.

This article is a critique of the article by Vogel and Broverman in which they indicated that there is evidence to support a set of reliable relationships between EEG parameters and intelligence. Ellingson criticized the earlier literature review on the basis that much of the data was taken from subjects with various degrees of brain damage as indicated by EEG abnormalities and subject diagnoses. He indicated that an equal number of studies had found negative results as had found positive relationships between EEG and intelligence. His conclusion was that the data do not warrant the conclusion that there are reliable relationships between EEG and intelligence other than in neurological problems.

intelligence
EEG
  patterns
brain
  damage
critique

J 8.   Sugerman, L.: Alpha rhythm, perception and intelligence. *J Natl Inst Personnel Res, 8*:170, 1961.

Fifty subjects were given the Wechsler Vocabulary Test, the New South African Group Intelligence Test, a perception rate and were recorded for EEG to isolate the relationships between alpha characteristics and intelligence. The vocabulary test was found to be significantly correlated with age but not with alpha frequency or perception rate. Alpha frequency had a significant negative correlation with perception

intelligence
perception
alpha
  frequency
age

rate and the group intelligence test scores. The group intelligence test scores had significant positive correlations with perception rate and vocabulary but the latter two were not significantly correlated with each other.

J 9.   Beckman, F.H., and Stein, M.I.: A note on the relationship between percent alpha time and efficiency in problem solving. *J Psychol, 51:*169, 1961.

Thirty-three subjects were recorded for resting EEG and were given a test of problem-solving ability in an apparatus designed to present problems of deductive logic. Logic efficiency scores were calculated on the basis of unnecessary questions and guessing errors. Alpha incidence was calculated on the basis of amount of time alpha was present without superimposed beta activity. Efficiency was found to be negatively correlated with resting alpha incidence independent of age.

intelligence
mental tasks
alpha
  abundance

J 10.   Giannitrapani, D.: Stability of EEG components relating to intelligence scores. *Electroencephalogr Clin Neurophysiol, 34:*105, 1973 (abstr).

Previous work of the same author had demonstrated significant relationships between EEG components and IQ. It was demonstrated that when using a resting EEG log amplitude scores of selected frequency bands showed correlations with intelligence test scores. Results showed a pattern of relationships which varied among WAIS subtests both in regard to EEG frequency and brain areas. To test whether the EEG components involved in these correlations fluctuated with different organismic states, correlation matrices were produced for conditions which represented a varied spectrum of activities: initial resting, eyes closed; listening to white noise; listening to music; listening to a story; performing mental arithmetic; looking at a poster; looking through diffusing goggles; final resting. The correlation matrices obtained for fifty-six 11- to 13-year-old normal subjects for EEG periods lasting only eight seconds showed a great degree of stability. For full IQ, for instance, correlations for the 13 cps band in the central areas are significant beyond the 0.001 level of

intelligence
mental tasks
attention
alpha
  frequency
stability

confidence, for all the eight conditions. The actual rho values obtained for the left central area are from +0.48 to +0.59. For the same area the rho obtained between the sum of the activity of the eight conditions (a total of 64 seconds per subject) and full IQ is +0.60.

J 11.   Giannitrapani, D.: EEG average frequency and intelligence. *Electroencephalogr Clin Neurophysiol, 27*:480, 1969.

Eighteen subjects were recorded for EEG while performing a mental arithmetic task and scored for IQ on the basis of performance on the WAIS. Alpha index, left-right frequency differences and frequency differences between cortical areas were computed for correlation with IQ. Left parietal average frequency (thinking minus resting) was significantly correlated with both performance and full IQ. A combined frontal, temporal, parietal and negative occipital frequency score was correlated with verbal performance and full IQ scores in the thinking condition. Parietal frequency (left minus right) was correlated with performance IQ in the thinking condition and both performance and full IQ in the resting condition. Occipital frequency (left minus right) was negatively correlated with performance and full IQ in the resting condition. Alpha index was correlated with verbal performance and full IQ in the thinking condition and with verbal IQ in the resting condition.

intelligence
mental tasks
alpha
  patterns
hemispheric
  dominance

J 12.   Bry, B.H., and Daniel, R.S.: The unresponsive EEG's of college underachievers. *Psychon Sci, 9*:103, 1967.

The ten most extreme underachievers in a state university sophomore class and ten control subjects, matched for ability scores on the school and college abilities test, were recorded for EEG while performing a mental arithmetic task. The grade point averages of the two groups were 1.2 and 3.1 respectively on a 4.0 scale. The arithmetic task involved adding successive integers and determining which of the numbers— 1, 2, 3 or 4—could be divided evenly into the number. Achievers were found to be more aroused by eye opening with an overall EEG amplitude change and a 0.2 Hz slowing of the alpha rhythm. The mental arithmetic task resulted in

intelligence
mental tasks
alpha
  patterns
eye opening

a return to resting alpha frequency for the achievers. Under-achievers were found to have a higher resting alpha frequency (9.79 versus 9.30 cps) which was unaffected by any of the conditions.

J 13.   Vogel, W., Broverman, D.M., and Klaiber, E.L.: EEG and mental abilities. *Electroencephalogr Clin Neurophysiol, 24:* 166, 1968.

Two studies were done to test the relationships between mental ability and EEG parameters. In the first study, thirty-six male college students with WAIS IQ scores ranging from 111 to 151 were recorded for EEG with parietal and occipital electrodes used for analysis. In the second study twenty-five high school students with Otis IQ scores of 105 to 136 were given the same treatment conditions as the first group. All subjects were given a battery of seventeen cognitive tests before the experimental treatment began. Subjects were recorded for EEG during resting, simple arithmetic and complex arithmetic conditions. Five EEG indices were isolated: slow wave index, alpha index, beta index, alpha frequency and beta frequency. An automatization score was obtained for each subject on the basis of differential performance on repetitive or conceptual cognitive tasks. In the first study, automatization was found to be directly related to performance in mental arithmetic tasks and inversely related to beta index and beta frequency. General intelligence was unrelated to EEG parameters but was directly related to task performance, and performance on simple mental arithmetic was directly related to the presence of slow alpha during performance. In the second study, automatization was again related to arithmetic performance and inversely related to beta index. In addition, automatization was found to be related to slow wave index and beta frequency and inversely related to alpha frequency. Arithmetic performance was related to slow wave index and inversely to alpha frequency. In neither group was cognitive task performance (called general intelligence) related to any of the EEG parameters.

intelligence
mental tasks
EEG
  patterns
beta

J 14.   Clusin, W.: EEG and the measurement of visual performance. *Electroencephalogr Clin Neurophysiol, 27:707,* 1969 (abstr).

The present experiment was performed to determine whether alpha activity would be related to a subject's performance on a more specifically visual task. For this purpose, we employed the scaled score of Wechsler's Coding Subtest, which measures the speed and accuracy of transcribing digits into corresponding abstract symbols. Digitized EEG signals were recorded on magnetic tape from sixteen monopolar electrodes from a sample of thirty-two 11- to 13-year-old right-handed males. The power density of the activity in each of several frequency bands was calculated by a computer. The alpha score obtained for each electrode was a combined measurement of alpha amplitude and alpha index. We found that Spearman correlations between alpha activity and Coding were positive at all electrode loci, and significant (p = 0.005, one-tailed) in twelve of the sixteen areas. Our correlations were no less significant in anterior electrodes. The highest correlation, 0.70, reached a significance of p < 0.00005. The hypothesis that these correlations reflect an association between alpha activity and visual performance is supported by the fact that the power density of activity outside the alpha range was not significantly correlated with Coding and that the alpha scores were not related to full IQ, or other such nonvisual measurements as information, comprehension and vocabulary.

intelligence
visual
* perception*
spectral
* analysis*
alpha
* patterns*

J 15. Mundy-Castle, A.C., and Nelson, G.K.: Intelligence, personality and brain rhythms in an isolated community. *Nature, 185*:484, 1960.

Ninety-six white laborers (94 male and 2 female) from an isolated South African community were administered the South African version of the WAIS and recorded for EEG to determine the relationship between alpha frequency and intelligence. The alpha frequency correlated significantly with full IQ and five of the subtests including vocabulary. The mean IQ of the group was 75, and 50 percent of the subjects showed strong EEG evidence of organic disturbances which were discussed in terms of the nutritional and genetic conditions of the isolated community.

intelligence
personality
alpha
* frequency*
social
* interaction*
genetics

J 16. Mundy-Castle, A.C.: Electrophysiological correlates of intelligence. *J Pers, 26*:184, 1958.

Thirty-four subjects were administered the WAIS (South African version) and recorded for EEG to determine the relationships between characteristics of alpha rhythm and intelligence. Alpha frequency was found to be significantly correlated with vocabulary. A number of significant correlations were found between alpha characteristics and different dimensions of personality and a factor analysis was performed to isolate the clusters of relationships. Four primary factors were labeled: visual-concrete, verbal-abstract, age-experience and excitability. The visual-concrete factor had positive loadings of practical IQ and alpha frequency and a negative loading of alpha incidence. The verbal-abstract factor was positively loaded with verbal IQ and alpha incidence. The age-experience factor was associated with a slight positive loading of alpha frequency and verbal IQ. The excitability factor had a high positive loading of alpha frequency.

intelligence
personality
alpha
patterns

J 17.   Saunders, D.R.: Digit span and alpha frequency: A cross-validation. *J Clin Psychol, 17*:165, 1961.

Seventy-one male subjects, some of whom were brain damaged, were recorded for EEG and given the WAIS to determine the relationships between intelligence and EEG parameters. A significant positive correlation was found between alpha frequency and the difference between digit span retention and the normal performance level.

intelligence
memory
alpha
frequency
brain
damage

J 18.   Surwillo, W.W.: Digit span and EEG frequency in normal children. *Electroencephalogr Clin Neurophysiol, 31*:93, 1971.

Seventy-nine boys (54 to 207 months old) were recorded for EEG from bilateral parietal and occipital placements while performing a digit span test to determine the relationship between EEG frequency and performance. The digit span lists from the WISC were used and recalled in both forward and backward sequences. Frequency was measured from the interval in which the numbers were being presented for the longest list recalled. Digit span memory ranged from 5 to 15. When converted to log scores, digit span was significantly correlated with age and negatively correlated with wave

intelligence
children
memory
EEG
frequency

period. Age was also negatively correlated with wave period. When age was factored out, the negative correlation between log digit span memory and log wave period was nonsignificant.

J 19.   Jenkins, C.D.: The relationship of EEG slowing to selected indices of intellectual impairment. *J Nerv Ment Dis, 135:* 162, 1962.

Fifty-seven hospital patients (18 to 64 years old), having only diffuse EEG abnormalities, if any, were recorded for EEG to determine the relationship between dominant frequency and intellectual performance. Tests of intellectual ability included the WAIS, the Proteus mazes, the Revised Benton Visual Retention Test, and the weight discrimination test from the Stanford-Binet test. An analysis of variance revealed significant relationships between EEG slowing and lower scores on the WAIS digit symbol block design, object assembly, performance IQ and a discrepancy between verbal and performance IQ. The quality score on the Proteus mazes, the Benton and the weight discrimination tests also showed the relationship between lower scores and EEG slowing. Verbal performance tests showed no relationship to EEG slowing.

intelligence
cognition
EEG
  frequency

J 20.   Clusin, W.T., and Giannitrapani, D.: EEG and the short-term retention of digits. *Electroencephalogr Clin Neurophysiol, 28:*423, 1970.

Pursuing the possibility that the relationship among EEG signals is more salient to the study of cortical organization than descriptions of individual wave forms, the authors repeated Giannitrapani's correlation experiment with Walter's coherence coefficient as a criterion of symmetry. The coherence coefficient is a statistical expression of synchrony that is available through the computer analysis of digitized multichannel EEG. The Wechsler Digit Span was chosen as the intellectual variable because of the specific character of the aptitude that it is supposed to reflect. By computing Spearman correlations between the digit span and the various coherence test scores, we found that for a sample of thirty-two

intelligence
memory
EEG
  symmetry

11- to 13-year-old right-handed males short-term digit learning is inversely related to the degree of similarity among EEG signals in the occipital, lateroparietal and prefrontal areas. Although strongest in the activity between 25 and 33 cycles, this relationship is present across the entire frequency range. Although the negative correlations between the digit span and hemispheric symmetry are in agreement with Giannitrapani's data, the discovery of similar correlations among ipsilateral EEG signals suggests that short-term digit retention may be associated with a general differentiation of on-going neural activity in certain cortical regions. These findings are compatible with clinical evidence on the effects of lesions in these areas and with Luria's observations that the evolution of higher cognitive functions parallels histological differentiation of the cortex.

J 21.   Lairy, G.C., Remond, A., Rieger, H., and Lesevre, N.: The alpha average. III. Clinical application in children. *Electroencephalogr Clin Neurophysiol, 26*:453, 1969.

Eight children with scholastic and extrascholastic difficulties and six normal children were tested for IQ and EEG alpha parameters to determine the factors which differentiated the groups and the differences between adult and child EEG patterns. The normal children showed homogenous scores on verbal, motor and perceptuomotor IQ scales. The children with difficulties showed normal verbal IQ but discrepant motor and/or perceptuomotor IQ. The EEG's of normal children were found to have a lower frequency alpha with a larger spread around the mean than normal adults. Disturbed children showed a greater spread of alpha frequencies, poorer spatial organization of alpha, less symmetrical alpha, and less bilateral coordination of alpha than normal children. Normal children had lower symmetry of alpha amplitude than the disturbed children.

intelligence
children
cognition
motor performance
alpha patterns

J 22.   Shipton, J., and Walter, W.G.: Alpha and intelligence, personality, cultural differences, and social activity. *Electroencephalogr Clin Neurophysiol (Suppl), 6*:185, 1957.

When the methods of analysis and display described in a previous paper are used in the course of a psychophysiologi-

intelligence
personality

cal experiment, the personal features of a record are empha-
sized and it is possible to follow the changes in distribution
of the several alpha components which occur either spontaneously or during the performance of diverse tasks. Information collected in this way permits a classification of normal
subjects based on the responsiveness or persistence of the
various alpha components. This classification seems to correspond with psychological estimates of mental imagery and of
versatility; it can be elaborated by the inclusion of other
physiological data such as records of breathing, speech,
muscular tension, heart rate, skin resistance and the like. It
has been noticed that a subject in one class tends to associate
more readily with someone in the same class than with someone in another class. In this way it is possible to recognize
supplementary pairs (subjects whose alpha type and way of
thinking are similar and who tend to agree in their tactical
habits of behavior, even if they have different strategic aims;
such couples are mutually attractive but tend to make the
same sort of mistakes) and complementary pairs (subjects
who differ in their EEG and in their ways of thinking and
have different tactics even when in stratetic agreement; such
couples are not readily attracted to one another but tend to
limit or correct one another's mistakes). It is intended to
apply this method to the study of more complex situations
and larger groups.

*social
interaction
alpha
patterns
ANS*

J 23. Pinney, E.L.: Reading and arithmetic scores and EEG alpha
blocking in disadvantaged children. *Dis Nerv Syst, 29:388,*
1968.

One hundred children (6 to 15 years old) with behavior disorders were recorded for EEG alpha blocking and were given
the Wide Range Achievement Test (WRAT) to determine
the relationship between alpha blocking and intellectual development. Thirty-three of the subjects showed no alpha
blocking response. WRAT scores and alpha blocking were
correlated for those subjects performing at or above grade
level but not for those performing below grade level. Approximately 78 percent of the subjects were performing below grade level.

*intelligence
children
behavior
problems
alpha
blocking*

MENTAL TASKS

J 24. Livanov, M.N., Gavrilova, N.A., and Aslanov, A.S.: Intercorrelations between different cortical regions of human brain during mental activity. *Neuropsychologia, 2:*261, 1964.

This investigation attempts to detect which changes occur in the interrelations of bioelectrical activity of different points of the brain cortex during mental activity and to determine the regularity of these changes. The electrical activity of half of the recorded brain areas at rest take independent courses, but during mental activity it is seen that throughout the cortex correlations in a low percentage of the time appear and correlations in the high percentage of the time appear against this background. These correlations localize in the anterior portions of the frontal lobes and in the motor analyzer areas; their direction agrees with the morphological paths, suggesting a reflection of functional connectors of the cortex. Distinct changes of correlations require a sufficiently difficult mental task, and the entire process described above has a wave-like character.

mental tasks
topography
EEG
patterns

J 25. Chapman, R.M., Armington, J.C., and Bragdon, H.R.: A quantitative survey of kappa and alpha EEG activity. *Electroencephalogr Clin Neurophysiol, 14:*858, 1962.

One hundred subjects were given three mental arithmetic tasks of various difficulty and a resting condition while being recorded for temporal kappa and occipital alpha under eyes-opened and eyes-closed conditions. The mental arithmetic tasks included counting from 1 to 10, adding 8's serially, and adding 27's serially. Both kappa and alpha activity were greater in the eyes-closed conditions. Mental arithmetic produced a decrease in alpha activity in the eyes-closed conditions but not the eyes-opened conditions. The mental tasks produced increases in kappa activity in both eyes-opened and eyes-closed conditions.

mental tasks
alpha
patterns
kappa
rhythm
eye opening

J 26. Kennedy, J.L., Gottsdanker, R.M., Armington, J.C., and Gray, F.E.: A new electroencephalogram associated with thinking. *Science, 108:*527, 1948.

A frontal rhythm in the alpha frequency range was discovered while measuring electro-oculograms in subjects while reading. Subjects were given a variety of mental tasks to perform while having EEG's made from temporal and occipital electrode placements to determine the effects of these tasks on the new rhythm, "kappa," and the correlation of this rhythm with occipital alpha activity. The tasks included mental multiplication, nonsense syllable learning, finger maze learning, memory and an auditory discrimination. Periods of active thought were accompanied by an increase in kappa activity. Intrusions of kappa activity into periods when subjects were supposed to keep their minds blank were associated with subjective reports of intruding thoughts. Only eighteen out of thirty-two subjects tested demonstrated a kappa rhythm. The authors concluded that the properties of the temporal rhythm were different from alpha and that kappa is associated with active thought for some individuals.

mental tasks
kappa
rhythm
alpha
responses

J 27.   Giannitrapani, D.: Electroencephalographic differences between resting and mental multiplication. *Percept Mot Skills, 22:*399, 1966.

Twenty subjects were recorded for EEG while either resting with eyes closed or solving mental multiplication problems with eyes closed. Mean frequency of the EEG was significantly higher in problem solving than in the resting condition. The frontal and left temporal electrode sites showed significantly higher frequency differences between resting and problem solving than did other electrode placements. Differences were found between the left and right hemispheres for the frontal as well as the temporal electrode placements. The differences were enhanced by problem solving.

mental tasks
EEG
frequency
topography
hemispheric
dominance

J 28.   Giannitrapani, D.: Mental arithmetic changes in the EEG. *Electroencephalogr Clin Neurophysiol, 28:*418, 1970 (abstr).

Thirty-two right-handed male subjects between the ages of eleven and thirteen were given the task of performing sequential subtractions while their EEG's were being recorded. Performance produced bilateral reductions in occipital activity in the 8 to 13 Hz range, bilateral increases in prefrontal

mental tasks
children
EEG
frequency
hemispheric
dominance

3 to 5 Hz and 25 to 33 Hz activity, bilateral increases in laterofrontal 27 to 33 Hz activity, and bilateral increases in temporal 21 to 33 Hz activity. The laterofrontal and temporal increases in beta activity were strongest on the right side. The author indicated that the right hemisphere may be important in mental arithmetic and that arithmetic may be somewhat independent of the verbal activity associated with the left hemisphere.

J 29. Lorens, S.A., Jr., and Darrow, C.W.: Eye movements, EEG, GSR, and EKG during mental multiplication. *Electroencephalogr Clin Neurophysiol, 14:*739, 1962.

Various autonomic response measures were taken for eight male and two female subjects ranging in age from nineteen to thirty-two while performing mental arithmetic tasks. Eye movement rates were found to increase significantly during performance while the presence of the alpha rhythm was reduced due to the blocking response. None of the autonomic measures were found to be quantitatively related.

mental tasks
eye
* movements*
alpha
* amplitude*
ANS

J 30. Simonova, O., and Legewie, H.: EEG changes under different conditions. *Electroencephalogr Clin Neurophysiol, 27:* 627, 1969 (abstr).

Eight subjects were tested for EEG changes in eyes-opened, eyes-closed and mental activity conditions. The eyes-opened conditions resulted in the greatest reduction of alpha from the resting EEG. Mental activity tended to produce a medium level of alpha in the EEG by increasing the eyes-opened alpha and decreasing the eyes-closed alpha. The synchronization of alpha in the eyes-opened conditions was found to be independent of visual components of the tasks.

mental tasks
eye opening
alpha
patterns

J 31. Volavka, J., Matousec, M., and Roubicek, J.: Mental arithmetic and eye opening. An EEG frequency analysis and GSR study. *Electroencephalogr Clin Neurophysiol, 22:*174, 1967.

Twelve subjects were recorded for EEG and skin resistance under eyes-open, eyes-closed, mental arithmetic and rewarded mental arithmetic conditions. Subjects had significantly more GSR changes in the reward condition. A frequency analysis of the EEG from the parietotemporal leads revealed that the

mental tasks
eye opening
EEG
* frequency*
GSR

eyes-opened condition was associated with the greatest attenuation of all frequencies. Theta and alpha activity was greatest in the eyes-closed condition. Mental arithmetic was associated with an increase in the amplitude and a decrease in variability of the beta frequencies in both rewarded and unrewarded conditions. No significant differences were found between the rewarded and unrewarded mental arithmetic conditions.

J 32.   Glass, A., and Kwiatkowski, A.W.: Power spectral density changes in the EEG during mental arithmetic and eye-opening. *Psychol Forsch, 33*:85, 1970.

Fifteen medical students were recorded for occipital and parietal EEG during mental multiplication and while opening eyes. A frequency analysis revealed differential effects for the two conditions. Eye-opening produced greater reduction in 10 Hz activity than did mental arithmetic. The eyes-opening produced significant reductions in 10 Hz, 12.5 Hz and 15 to 25 Hz activity. Mental arithmetic produced reductions in 7.5 Hz, 10 Hz and 15 to 30 Hz activity.

mental tasks
alpha
  blocking
eye opening
spectral
  analysis

J 33.   Glass, A.: Intensity of attenuation of alpha activity by mental arithmetic in females and males. *Psychol Behav, 3*:217, 1968.

Fifty male and eleven female subjects, with mean ages of 22.9 and 19.4 years respectively, were given twenty mental arithmetic problems (multiplication and addition) while eyes-closed EEG alpha was being analyzed. Females were found to have lower resting alpha amplitude than males. Mental arithmetic resulted in a significantly larger reduction in alpha amplitude for females than for males both on an absolute scale and proportional to resting alpha levels.

mental tasks
alpha
  blocking

J 34.   Bente, D., Broeren, W., Hartung, M.L., and Schmitt, W.: Electroencephalographic-psychological test correlation studies. *Arzneim Forsch, 19*:439, 1969.

Results from two groups of eighteen and thirty-seven subjects concerning correlations between EEG activity and psychological information using a frequency-integration-profile

mental tasks
psychologic
  testing

EEG analysis method are given. Specific significant correla- *EEG*
tions between alpha rhythms and psychological test findings *analysis*
were observed.   *EEG*
                                                            integration

J 35.   Glass, A.: Comparison of the effect of hard and easy mental
         arithmetic upon blocking of the occipital alpha rhythm. *Q*
         *J Exp Psychol, 5:*142, 1966.

Thirty-six medical students were given five hard and five easy *mental tasks*
multiplication problems at two-minute intervals to deter-   *alpha*
mine the effects on occipital EEG alpha blocking. No differ-   *blocking*
ences in the intensity of blocking were found between hard
and easy multiplication. Response latency was negatively correlated with the intensity of blocking for the hard multiplication problems. Response latency for easy problems was negatively correlated with pre-task rate of change in potential
associated with alpha blocking. Hard problems were associated with longer response latencies than were the easy
problems.

J 36.   Glass, A.: Mental arithmetic and blocking of the occipital
         alpha rhythm. *Electroencephalogr Clin Neurophysiol, 16:*
         595, 1964.

Fifty-eight medical students participated as subjects under   *mental tasks*
three experimental series. In the first series, ten subjects *motivation*
were given multiplication problems with a thirty-second time *alpha*
limit. In the second series, thirty-six subjects were given un- *blocking*
limited solution time. In the third series, twelve subjects
were either motivated by promise of financial reward for
correct responding or were not promised reward in a control
condition. The amplitude and the latency of the alpha blocking response were analyzed from occipital, parietal and
temporal EEG leads. The rate of change, prior to task and
prior to solution, was found to be significantly correlated
with error probability. Pre-task rate of change was negatively
correlated with response latency in a partial correlation. The
increased motivational state resulted in increased amplitude
changes in alpha blocking.

COGNITION

J 37. Galin, D., Ornstein, R., Kocel, K., and Merrin, E.: Hemispheric localization of cognitive mode by EEG. *Psychophysiology, 8:*248, 1971 (abstr).

Studies with brain-injured patients indicate that there is lateral specialization of cognitive functions. Language and mathematical processing depend heavily upon the left hemisphere while the processing of spatial relationships depends more upon the right. Studies of patients with surgical section of the corpus callosum have shown that learning, memory, perceiving and conceptualizing continue separately in each hemisphere. During verbal tasks the integrated power in the left hemisphere was less than in the right, and during spatial tasks the integrated power in the right hemisphere was less than in the left. The results were not affected by whether the eyes were opened or closed, or by eye movement, or by whether the task involved motor output. Dividing cognition into these two major modes (verbal-analytical and spatial-synthetic) was suggested by observations on brain-injured, neurosurgical and "split-brain" patients. We have been able to distinguish between these two cognitive modes as they occur in normal subjects by using simple scalp recording.

cognition
hemispheric dominance
mental tasks
perceptual tasks

J 38. Johnson, L.C., Ulett, G.A., Sines, J.O., and Stern, J.A.: Cortical activity and cognitive functioning. *Electroencephalogr Clin Neurophysiol, 12:*861, 1960.

Twenty-eight male subjects were tested for performance on five different cognitive tasks: memory of stories, paired-associate learning, digit span memory, serial 7's counting and mental arithmetic. Performance was evaluated under normal and photic induced alpha blocking conditions. The desynchronization of the EEG had no significant effect on task performance or memory overall. Individual subjects responded with varying degrees of cognitive impairment during the photic stimulation.

cognition
mental tasks
photic flicker
alpha blocking
memory

J 39. Grunewald, G., Simonova, O., and Creutzfeldt, O.D.: Differential EEG-alterations during visuomotor and cognitive tasks. *Arch Psychiatr Nervenkr, 212:*46, 1968.

Subjects were given a series of six visuomotor tasks (e.g. maze drawing) and two cognitive tasks while recording EEG's from parietocentral and occipitotemporal electrode pairs. Subjects with a high incidence of alpha in the resting EEG showed the greatest decrease in 8.5 to 12.5 Hz activity in the occipitotemporal leads during task performance, while low alpha subjects showed some increase in alpha during performance. Hertz activtiy (8.5 to 12.5) decreased in the parietocentral leads for all subjects during performance. Task performance resulted in an increase in 12.5 to 16 Hz activity in the occipitotemporal leads for all subjects. Occipitotemporal alpha showed the most increase in the visuomotor tasks while the smallest decreases in parietocentral alpha were associated with the performance of cognitive tasks.

cognition
motor performance
alpha blocking
alpha enhancement

J 40.   MacNeilage, P.F.: EEG amplitude changes during different cognitive processes involving similar stimuli and responses. *Psychophysiology, 2*:280, 1966.

Subjects were given three tasks involving the same set of stimuli, a tape recording of sixty-one single-digit numbers. The tasks involved adding four-digit sequences, writing every fourth digit, or writing all 7's and 9's as they occurred. Alpha blocking and EEG frequency changes analyzed from the records taken from the subjects showed no pattern differences between conditions even though different cognitive processes were assumed to be involved in the different tasks.

cognition
motor performance
alpha blocking
EEG frequency

J 41.   Berlyne, D.W., and McDonnell, P.: Effects of stimulus complexity and incongruity on duration of EEG desynchronization. *Electroencephalogr Clin Neurophysiol, 18*:156, 1965.

Eighty-eight male students having alpha present more than 25 percent of the time while resting were presented with stimulus patterns varying in content complexity. Subjects were either in a motivated (remember the content for later testing) or an unmotivated condition during the presentations. The alpha blocking response of all subjects decreased in duration as the session progressed. Increased complexity of pattern resulted in increased duration of the blocking re-

cognition
motivation
alpha blocking
visual perception

sponse. Specific parameters of complexity which resulted in significant changes in blocking were irregularity, amount of information, incongruity and randomness of distribution. Increased motivation did not result in any change in blocking and no differences were found between first and second presentations of each pattern.

J 42.   Glanzer, M., Chapman, R.M., Clark, W.H., and Bragdon, H.R.: Changes in two EEG rhythms during mental activity. *J Exp Psychol, 68:*273, 1964.

Twelve subjects were given a series of tasks involving different levels of mental activity while being recorded for EEG. The alpha rhythm was recorded from the parieto-occipital EEG while the kappa rhythm (8 to 13 Hz in frontal areas) was being recorded from the temporal pair. One group of tasks involving low mental effort was labeled "mental orientation" and involved a series of mental addition tasks. The more integrative tasks were labeled "conceptual" and involved recognition of pattern changes. The addition tasks were associated with increased kappa activity as a function of increased difficulty. The pattern recognition tasks were associated with decreased alpha activity as a function of increased difficulty. The authors speculated that the two indices of mental activity, increased kappa and decreased alpha, may be functions of different sense modalities involved in the mental tasks.

cognition
mental tasks
alpha
* patterns*
kappa
* rhythm*

J 43.   Christie, B., Delafield, G., Lucas, B., Winwood, M., and Gale, A.: Stimulus complexity and the EEG: Differential effects of the number and variety of display elements. *Can J Psychol, 26:*155, 1972.

Thirty-three undergraduates participated in five experiments showing that (1) number and variety of parts in a visual display affect judgments of complexity; (2) alpha waves decrease with increased complexity, and (3) evidence for the actual effect of variety was not conclusive. These two dimensions of stimulus complexity and variety of elements may cause different EEG effects.

cognition
pattern
* recognition*

MEMORY

J 44.   Surwillo, W.W.: Frequency of the EEG during acquisition
        in short-term memory. *Psychophysiology, 8:*588, 1971.

Twenty-five male children, ranging in age from nine to   *memory*
seventeen, were selected on the basis of having correct re-   *children*
call of number lists up to five numbers in the WISC back-   *reaction*
ward memory test and an artifact-free EEG. Two to five-digit   *time*
lists were presented to the subjects from pre-recorded tapes *alert*
while their EEG's were recorded from bilateral parietal and   *EEG*
occipital electrode placements. A reaction time task was   *frequency*
given to the subjects as a control condition for alertness
without involving memory. Subjects showed significant increases in EEG frequency in the memorization of 4- and 5-
digit lists with respect to the reaction time control condition.

J 45.   Koukkou, M., and Lehmann, D.: EEG and memory storage
        in sleep experiments with humans. *Electroencephalogr Clin
        Neurophysiol, 25:*455, 1968.

Twenty-one subjects between the ages of nineteen and   *memory*
twenty-eight were selected on the basis of having well-de-   *sleep*
veloped alpha in their waking EEGs. Short sentences were   *recall*
presented to the subjects at least one minute following the   *alpha en-*
appearance of the first sleep spindle. Free recall and recogni-   *hancement*
tion were tested after subjects were awakened. Correct free
recall was associated with the longest durations of alpha
elicited by the stimuli, recognition was associated with
medium duration alpha, and failure to recall was associated
with the shortest durations of recall. The authors suggested
that the wakefulness pattern represented by the presence of
alpha reflects time available for long-term storage in memory.

LEARNING

J 46.   Darrow, C., and Gullickson, G.R.: The role of brain waves
        in learning and other integrative functions. *Recent Adv Biol
        Psychiatr, 10:*249, 1967.

The question of lack of specific relationship between specific *learning*
emotional factors and EEG responses is explored. Authors   *review*
suggest that the effects of sensory, motor and ideational pro- *theory*

cesses are below threshold to produce markedly visible EEG
changes, and thus a specific local modulation of the un-
specific generalized EEG carrier rhythm may heterodyne
with adjacent unmodulated samples and trigger differential
signals to associative and affective mechanisms. Specifically
the authors and others had found that more anterior EEG
waves tended to precede relatively posterior cortical waves
during arousal. Thus they postulated several reasons to explore EEG phase relationships: that timing of cerebral
events relates to rapidity of nerve conduction, to cellular excitability, and to metabolism; that the priority of incidence
among impulses may determine the direction and nature of
cellular responses to excitation and that the interaction between rhythmic impulses may, by heterodyning or harmonic
interaction, determine excitability. The authors present results indicating that during high-level attentive, perceptual
and ideational activity it is as if the predominant areas of
excitability or initiative go back and forth, i.e. as diphasic
reversals. The authors postulate that local cortical interaction is the mechanism by which waking alpha monitors for
significant evidence of change in the incoming information
projected on the cortex. The local diphasic effects represent a
mechanical direction of attention. Therefore, situations give
differential stimulus requirements to initiate cortical mass
action, i.e. orienting responses of blocking or activation, and
thus the EEG and alpha reflect processes important for sensory modulation and alerting mechanisms. It was concluded
that variation of EEG phase is useful for timing and integrative brain functions.

J 47. Tani, K., and Yoshii, N.: Efficiency of verbal learning during
sleep as related to the EEG pattern. *Brain Res, 117:277,*
1970.

One hundred and three students were engaged as subjects in
an investigation of the retention of verbal information presented during sleep. Sixty control subjects were presented
with two paired associated word lists mixed together. The
stimulus items from each list were then presented separately
to determine the retention of response words. Forty-three
experimental subjects were presented with one of the two

*learning
memory
sleep
alpha en-
hancement*

lists through a loudspeaker inside a pillow while asleep. Upon awakening, the subjects were given the stimulus words from both lists and asked to recall the associates. EEG's were recorded during the sleep learning process. Subjects were found to retain a significant amount of material when presentation of a word pair elicited alpha in the EEG. Alpha occuring before or after the presentation of the words was not associated with significant retention.

J 48.   Freedman, N.L., Hafer, B.M., and Daniel, R.S.: EEG arousal decrement during paired-associate learning. *J Comp Physiol Psychol, 61:*15, 1966.

Ten normal subjects with measurable alpha in their resting EEG's were separated into two groups equated for alpha incidence. The experimental group was given a series of eight nonsense syllables to be paired with four response keys available to the subject. A typical trial consisted of the auditory presentation of a nonsense syllable, a five-second decision period, a key press response, a reinforcement tone (right, wrong, will not say), and a five-second intertrial interval. The control group was not informed as to the meanings of the tones and were yoked to the experimental subjects for the stimuli. The incidence of alpha increased during the trials for the experimental subjects while it decreased for the yoked control subjects. In the anticipation interval between trials, alpha incidence increased and low frequency activity decreased for both groups. No relationships between EEG parameters and correctness of response were found.

learning
conditioning
alpha enhancement

SECTION K

PSYCHOPATHOLOGY

NEUROSES

K 1.   Strauss, H.: Clinical and electroencephalographic studies: The electroencephalogram in psychoneurotics. *J Nerv Ment Dis, 101:*19, 1945.

One hundred neurotic patients were recorded for EEG under resting and hyperventilating conditions. Bipolar recordings were obtained from bilateral frontal and occipital electrode placements. The EEG's were analyzed in terms of characteristics of the alpha rhythm: incidence (0% to 25%, 26% to 50%, 51% to 75% and 76% to 100%), burst length (less than 3 seconds, greater than 3 seconds, and both), and quality of the EEG (regular alpha, predominant beta, and mixed frequencies with sharp and irregular alpha). Neurotic patients were found to have a greater incidence of mixed frequency EEG's than normal. The incidence of alpha was more often in the 0 to 50 percent range than normal. Burst length was more often in the less than three-second category. Hyperventilation was found to frequently produce changes in mixed frequency EEG's to a pattern with regular alpha in the 75 to 100 percent incidence category with burst length greater than three seconds.

neuroses
alpha
  patterns
hyperventi-
  lation

K 2.   Pine, I., and Pine, H.M.: Clinical analysis of patients with low voltage EEG. *J Nerv Ment Dis, 117:*191, 1953.

Out of two thousand hospital patients, seventy-four were found to have low voltage EEG's with low incidence and amplitude alpha. The patients with low voltage EEG's were given clinical analyses. Forty-eight of the subjects were diagnosed as having primary psychiatric disorders including psychoneurosis with tension headache. The high incidence of psychiatric disorders in this group was interpreted as clinically significant.

neuroses
alpha
  patterns
voltage
tension
  headache

K 3. Aslanov, A.S.: Some specific features of cortical spatial distributions of the biopotentials in patients with obsessional neurosis. *Zh Nevropatol Psikhiatr, 68:*1019, 1968.

Spatial synchronization of cortical biopotentials was examined in patients suffering from obsessional neurosis using fifty points of the cerebral cortex for recording and a computer for analysis. The amount of unidirectional changes in the fluctuation of the biopotentials from moment to moment for a prescribed time period was utilized to calculate coefficients of correlation. Results showed that the number of leads with high coefficients was much higher and that the level of synchronization continued to fluctuate in patients as compared to normals. Mental arithmetic caused an increase in spatial synchronization. The anterior frontal areas proved to be preferred areas of localization for high correlations. Pathodynamic structures underlying the neurosis were assumed to determine the extent and makeup of spatial synchronization of the biopotentials.

neuroses
EEG
 synchrony
topography
mental tasks

K 4. Dongier, M., Dongier, S., Angel-Villegas, G., and Angel-Villegas, A.: Confrontations des donees des examens psychologiques et de l'electroencephalogramme chez 100 nervoses. *Electroencephalogr Clin Neurophysiol (Suppl), 6:*315, 1957.

One hundred neurotic patients were recorded for EEG to determine the characteristics associated with their disorders. Nine of the subjects had low voltage EEG's with an absence of alpha and the dominant frequency being in the beta range. The most characteristic pattern was rhythmic rolandic beta activity which occurred in forty-one of the subjects. Thirty-six of the subjects had theta in their EEG's and seven had posterior delta activity. Beta activity was related to aggressive tendencies while psychopathic personality was related to the incidence of subharmonic alpha.

neuroses
EEG
 frequency
voltage
personality
beta

K 5. Volvka, J., Matousek, M., and Roubicek, J.: EEG frequency analysis and neurotic symptoms in a normal population. *Bratisl Lek Listy, 49:*659, 1968.

One hundred and eight subjects, randomly selected from a normal population, were tested for neurotic symptoms with

neuroses
EEG
 patterns

clinical interviews and a questionnaire. EEG records were analyzed to determine relationships between neurotic characteristics and frequency characteristics of the EEG. Anxiety was associated with increased beta activity and decreased amplitudes of delta, theta and alpha activity. A ratio of beta/alpha proved to be the most effective indicator of anxiety. Subjects scoring high on the neuroticism scale of the questionnaire were found to have higher beta and beta/alpha ratios than subjects scoring low.

measure-
ment
techniques

K 6.   Yasui, M., Higashi, Y., and Yamamoto, Y.: The relationship between neurotic complaints and EEG findings. *J Wakayama Med Soc, 21:*141, 1970.

The relationship between EEG characterics and the presence of neurotic complaints such as palpitation, abdominal symptoms and generalized discomfort was evaluated in 434 EEG tracings of patients aged thirty-one to seventy years. Patients were seen in a public health center. No specific relationships between symptoms and abnormal or borderline abnormal EEG patterns were found. A higher percentage of normal EEG's of patients with neurotic complaints was found in the older subjects. The authors suggest that an exaggeration of self-concern that results in neurotic complaints may play a role in preventing aging processes in the brain.

neuroses
EEG
patterns
aging

K 7.   Ulett, G.A., Gleser, G.C., Winokur, G., and Lawler, A.: The EEG and reaction to photic stimulation as an index of anxiety proneness. *Electroencephalogr Clin Neurophysiol, 5:* 23, 1953.

Frequency analysis of both the resting EEG and the intermittent photic driving of the EEG was used to develop measures for identification of anxiety-prone individuals. One hundred and ninety-one subjects were used. A number of significant correlations were found. Anxiety proneness appeared to be related to the amount of fast and slow low-amplitude alpha, to the pattern of EEG response at the fundamental driving frequency, to the amounts of frequency harmonics occurring to 5 to 10 Hz, and to the degree of subjective dysphoria occurring with the photic stimulation.

neuroses
visual
stimulation
photic
flicker
anxiety

K 8.   Johnson, L.C., and Ulett, G.A.: Stability of EEG activity
        and manifest anxiety. *J Comp Physiol Psychol, 52*:284, 1959.

        Forty-four young adult males were given three EEG record-   *neuroses*
        ing sessions over a nine-month period to determine relation-   *anxiety*
        ships of EEG pattern changes to questionnaire-measured   *alpha*
        manifest anxiety. EEG amplitude and alpha incidence were   *patterns*
        lower in the first recording session than in the second. Sub-
        jects with high manifest anxiety scores showed significantly
        lower EEG amplitude and alpha incidence on the first session
        than other subjects, but no differences were found in the
        second and third recordings. The authors indicated that
        manifest anxiety may be related to the reactions of subjects
        to new situations.

K 9.   Cohn, R.: The influence of emotion on the human electro-
        encephalogram. *J. Nerv Ment Dis, 104*:351, 1946.

        Two types of anxiety patients were described on the basis of   *neuroses*
        personality, autonomic and EEG patterns observed. One   *anxiety*
        type of patient would fit a reactive type classification in   *personality*
        which the anxiety can be related to specific life situations.   *alpha*
        These patients had a low incidence and amplitude of alpha   *patterns*
        with low amplitude, high frequency, random activity in the   *EEG*
        EEG. A normal pattern of alpha in the EEG appeared within   *patterns*
        twenty seconds of the initiation of deep breathing. A second   *hyperventi-*
        type of patient was described as having a more severe and   *lation*
        chronic type of anxiety. These patients showed a rhythmic,   *beta*
        high amplitude beta frequency between 18 and 22 Hz in
        frontal leads of the EEG and normal occipital alpha with
        beta superimposed. These subjects did not respond to hyper-
        ventilation.

K 10.   Gologub, E.B., and Fanagorskaya, T.P.: Evaluation of work-
        ing ability of man under normal conditions and in neurotic
        states. *Electroencephalogr Clin Neurophysiol, 27*:450, 1969
        (abstr) .

        Subjects, who were described as having a neurotic condition   *neuroses*
        due to overtraining, were recorded for EEG in resting and   *depression*
        depressed conditions to determine the associated pattern   *alpha*
        changes. In the depressive condition the EEG was low volt-   *patterns*

age and low frequency with a relatively high incidence of alpha. In the resting condition the EEG was low voltage, high frequency in the background, and a low incidence of alpha.

K 11.   Volavka, J., Grof, P., and Mrklas, L.: The influence of medication and clinical state on the EEG in periodic endogenous depression. *Electroencephalogr Clin Neurophysiol, 23:*490, 1967 (abstr).

This study separates the EEG effect of medication from that of the changing clinical state in periodic endogenous depression. Eight women suffering from periodic endogenous depression were observed over a period of two years. Their treatment was carried out according to a preset schedule. An antidepressant drug or a placebo was administered during the depressive phases. The subjects were taking either an antidepressant, a placebo or nothing while they were symptom free. The EEG and clinical examinations were made during depressive phases and during remissions, both with and without antidepressants. A broad-band frequency analysis of the EEG's was carried out and the output data were subjected to analysis of variance. The antidepressant medication significantly increased the quantity of theta and delta activity, independently of the clinical state. During the depressive phases a significant increase of alpha and beta activity, independent of medication, was shown.

neuroses
depression
drugs
frequency
  analysis
alpha
  abundance
theta
beta
delta

K 12.   Gastaut, H., Dongier, S., and Dongier, M.: Electroencephalography and neurosis: Study of 250 cases. *Electroencephalogr Clin Neurophysiol, 12:*233, 1960.

Two hundred and fifty psychiatric patients were given tests to determine personality characteristics and were recorded for EEG to determine relationships between EEG and personality patterns. Forty-five of the subjects were studied over the course of prolonged psychotherapy. Personality and EEG correlations which were statistically significant included low frequency alpha with low emotionality; high alpha variability with hysterical personality and affective immaturity; high amplitude alpha with weak ego; low amplitude EEG with

neuroses
personality
alpha
  patterns

strong ego; theta with lower anxiety; arched rolandic rhythms with anxiety; hypermotivity and open aggressiveness; rolandic beta with obsessive personality and open aggressiveness; and diffuse beta with hysterical personality. Other correlations between EEG and personality patterns which did not reach significance were discussed.

K 13. Timsit, M., and Koninkx, N.: Statistical approach to the correlations between clinical data and electroencephalographic data in the neuroses. *Acta Neurol Belg, 68:*769, 1968.

One hundred and forty-eight neurotic patients were recorded for EEG to determine the relationships between twelve clinical, personality variables and fourteen EEG parameters. Introversion and obsession were associated with polyrhythmic EEG's, photic driving responsiveness and a medium amount of alpha blocking to stimulus presentations. Hysteria and psychopathic personality were associated with a variable alpha rhythm, excess theta and posterior slow wave activity. Beta, slow alpha and mu rhythms proved of suggestive value only in neurosis.

neuroses
personality
EEG
  patterns
variability

K 14. Rodriguez, S.F.: The electroencephalogram in neurosis. *Arch Neurobiol (Madr), 29:*43, 1966.

One hundred and fifty-four neurotic patients were recorded for EEG under conditions of intermittent photic stimulation and resting to determine the relationships between EEG patterns and symptoms. Patients were diagnosed as having anxiety, hysteria, obsessions, phobias and hypochondrical symptoms and ideas. The EEG was rated for variability, amplitude and synchronization in the analysis. The three EEG measures were found to be independent except in patients with chronic anxiety. The EEG's of patients with anxiety crises, hysteria and reactive depression were characterized by low voltage, high frequency alpha, a high incidence of beta activity, and marked changes with intermittent photic stimulation. Obsessions, phobias and hypochondriasis were associated with an EEG pattern with slow dominant rhythms and instability during hyperventilation.

neuroses
photic
  stimulation
alpha
  responses
alpha
  patterns

K 15. Muller, H.F., and Shamsie, S.J.: Classification of disorders of behavior in adolescents and electroencephalographic data. *Can Psychiatr Assoc J, 13 :*363, 1968.

Seventy-eight teenage girls admitted to the hospital for be- *neuroses*
havior disturbances were classified according to the diag- *social*
nostic groups proposed by Jenkins. They underwent EEG   *interaction*
examinations, the characteristics of which were statistically *EEG*
compared with the clinical features. The overinhibited girls *patterns*
showed faster activity in temporal areas, a stronger reaction
to eye opening and more positive spikes during chlorpromazine induced sleep than the others. The unsocialized aggressive patients had a larger amount of generalized slow activity
and a greater difference between the occipital and temporal
peak frequencies. The socialized aggressive group had more
normal and better regulated EEG's than the other two
groups. These results were plausible when related to the
personality characteristics of the patients. It appears that
Jenkins' groups represent biological as well as psychosocial
syndromes in which certain types of electrical brain activity
indicate predispositions to certain types of behavior, and perhaps also a vulnerability to certain types of environmental
pathology.

K 16. Rudkowska, A., and Szydlik, H.: Electroencephalographic
picture in neurotic crises of puberty. *Psychiatr Pol,* 2:575,
1968.

Eighteen of thirty-two patients with neurotic crises of *neuroses*
puberty and exhibiting mental immaturity in the fields of *behavior*
affect, activity, adaption to social environment and personal *problems*
problems were categorized for body build as either infantile *EEG*
or infantile dysplastic on the basis of body weight, size, *maturation*
physical proportions and sexual maturity. The EEG's were *EEG abnor-*
abnormal and showed physiological traits of adolescence or *malities*
earlier. Therefore, it was concluded that there is reason to
link bioelectric maturation and other forms of maturation;
in particular, slow bioelectric maturation and retarded
somatic and mental maturation were found to be connected
in some cases.

K 17. Scollo, L.G.: A note on cataplexy with simultaneous EEG
recordings. *Eur Neurol, 4:*57, 1970.

A case of cataplexy with simultaneous EEG recording in a
thirty-seven-year-old man is reported in which the patient
suffered attacks of weakness, facial twitching and wild
dreams. The dreams frequently accompanied the onset of
sleep. The EEG correlated with the clinical picture in that
the normal alpha rhythm underwent flattening and then a
typical paradoxical sleep pattern occurred. All night sleep
EEG showed immediate onset of REM sleep with zero latency. In addition there was instability with a prevalence of the
light sleep phase over deep sleep, prolonged awakening and
an increase in the amount of REM sleep. Under medication
with imipramine (30 mg/day) the patient experienced no
cataplectic attacks and could return to work.

neuroses
cataplexy
alpha
  patterns
drugs

BEHAVIOR PROBLEMS

K 18.   Brudo, C.S., and Darrow, C.W.: A preliminary study of percent-time alpha in the EEG and the human movement response in the Rorschach. *Electroencephalogr Clin Neurophysiol, 5:*481, 1953 (abstr).

Ten children with behavior problems and eleven normal
control subjects were recorded for EEG and administered
the Rorschach to determine the relationships between alpha
incidence and the human movement response. Rank order
correlations between alpha incidence and movement responses were significant for all children. No differences between the groups were found.

behavior
  problems
children
alpha
  abundance

K 19.   Martinius, J., and Hoovey, Z.: Automatic analysis of inter-
occipital synchrony in the EEG of children with behavior
disturbances. *Electroencephalogr Clin Neurophysiol, 31:*
412, 1971 (abstr).

School children with behavioral disturbances and normal
control subjects with matched alpha incidence and amplitude were recorded for EEG from occipital leads to determine the phase relations between the two hemispheres. The
spread of inter-occipital alpha phase relationships was greater for the disturbed group as a whole than for the controls.
Individual EEG characteristics did not differentiate the two
groups.

behavior
  problems
children
alpha phase

K 20.   Wiener, J.M., Delano, J.G., and Klass, D.W.: An EEG study of delinquent and nondelinquent adolescents. *Arch Gen Psychiatr, 15:*144, 1966.

Group 1 subjects consisted of eighty males (13 to 15 years old) judged delinquent with a history of persistent anti-social behavior. Group 2 consisted of seventy volunteers from the local community, matched by age and without evidence of antisocial behavior. No one was included in either group who had signs, symptoms or history of organic brain disturbance or mental retardation. The EEG's of group 1 subjects were similar to those of group 2 in all categories studied. The higher incidence in thirteen- and fourteen-year-old subjects in both groups as compared with those fifteen to eighteen years of age suggests that positive-spike activity may represent an age-linked phenomenon. An attempt to relate amounts of slow-wave activity to behavior in adolescents must take into account not only the quantity of slow-wave activity commonly present in this age group, but also differences in the quantity of such activity occurring at different ages within the second decade. The findings in group 2 subjects with respect to alpha, delta and gamma activity in addition to the positive-spike bursts indicate that the EEG of asymptomatic male subjects, however, does show trends of change with increasing age within the second decade. No difference between delinquent and nondelinquent subjects was found in the present study.

behavior problems
EEG patterns

K 21.   Verdeaux, G.: Electroencephalography in criminology. *Med Leg Domm Corpor (Paris), 3:*39, 1970.

The results of many years of investigation into EEG differences between delinquents and normals are presented. Alpha activity averaged about 10 cps in the normal subjects while it was 8 cps in 40 percent of the delinquents; no reason for this was observed. Only irregularities could be seen in the theta frequencies, but activity below 4 cps in the posterior region occurred more frequently in the delinquents. EEG classification by pathology was done in 1964 and yielded four groups as follows: (1) alpha of low amplitude, rare theta and absence of slow activity; (2) high alpha and large amounts of theta which occur most in hyperpnea of adolescents; (3)

behavior problems
EEG patterns
alpha abundance
alpha amplitude
theta

alpha of high amplitude, slow waves posteriorly and altered hyperpnea as seen in immature EEG's; and (4) irregular alpha, diffuse theta and moderate blocking. Most of the selected normal subjects were in groups 1 and 2 while most delinquents fell into groups 3 and 4. It was also found that those delinquents in the first group had the best chance for readjustment to society.

K 22. Olson, W.H., Gibbs, F.A., and Adams, C.L.: Electroencephalographic study of criminals. *Clin Electroencephalogr, 1:*92, 1970.

An EEG study of 104 criminals awake and asleep confirms the previous findings that there is no significant difference between the awake recordings of criminals and normal control subjects; however, sleep recordings reveal a marked difference. An abnormal sleep pattern, namely mittens, the only EEG abnormality thus far recognized that correlates with psychosis, occurred during sleep in 47 percent of 104 criminals that were studied. The incidence in a control group matched for age is 3 percent. In this group of criminals the incidence of classical forms of epileptic discharge (high voltage negative spike) and of abnormalities correlating with nonepisodic neurological disorder (diffiuse or focal slowing) was zero. A small but significant number of criminals (3%) had a non classical form of paroxysmal dysrhythmia (14 and 6 per second positive spikes). The present study, though based on a small sample, presents objective evidence that psychosis and criminality are related and that a small but significant percentage of criminals have a non classical form of epilepsy.

behavior problems sleep wakefulness EEG abnormalities

K 23. Taterka, J.H., and Katz, J.: Study of correlations between electroencephalographic and psychological patterns in emotionally disturbed children. *Psychosom Med, 17:*62, 1955.

One hundred and ninety-five children with severe emotional and behavioral disturbances and forty-four normal control children were given a complete psychological, psychiatric and physical test sequence including Rorschach, Bender Gestalt, human figure drawing and WISC tests. The EEG's of these

behavior problems children psychologic testing

subjects were analyzed for abnormalities and the characteristics of the alpha rhythm. Abnormal EEG's were found in 81.6 percent of the disturbed children and only 27.3 percent of the controls. The characteristics of the alpha rhythm were unrelated to group differences. Those children having high alpha incidence were more accurate in form perception in the Rorschach test.

EEG abnormalities
alpha
patterns

K 24.   Wikler, A., Dixon, J.F., and Parker, Jr., B.: Brain function in problem children and controls: Psychometric, neurological, and electroencephalographic comparisons. *Am J Psychiatry, 127:5,* 1970.

Psychometric, neurological and EEG studies were made of twenty-four children with scholastic-behavioral problems but no classical evidence of neurological disease and of twenty-four matched controls. Differences between the two groups were significant in all three measures, giving evidence of brain dysfunction in the groups with scholastic-behavioral problems. Two subgroups, hyperactive and nonhyperactive, each with characteristics suggesting a different syndrome, are described.

behavior
problems
children
psychologic
testing
EEG
patterns

K 25.   Bonkalo, A.: Electroencephalography in criminology. *Can Psychiatr Assoc J, 12:*281, 1967.

Some practical and theoretical aspects of the use of electroencephalography in criminology are reviewed. Examples are given of various factors in the EEG pattern and in certain activation techniques showing correlation with certain attributes of personality structure. Briefly presented are EEG studies of psychopathic populations and those of convicted criminals, including murderers. The relatively high incidence, among murderers, of clinical epileptics and persons with EEGs showing epileptic implications is discussed, as well as the significance of the 14 and 6 cycles per second positive spike complex which is still a controversial issue. In spite of widely divergent findings, it is generally agreed that there is a relatively high incidence of abnormal EEG's among criminal and delinquent populations, though without a specific and consistent EEG pattern characterizing these

behavior
problems
personality
EEG
patterns

groups; that the most often seen abnormalities are the presence of excessive theta activity, focal temporal lobe pathology, and instability of the patterns, often epileptic in nature; that the age factor needs special consideration in the EEG appraisal of criminal or delinquent populations; and that aggressive behavior, continuous or episodic, appears to be the common denominator in the personality structure of these populations.

K 26. Milstein, V., Stevens, J., and Sachdev, K.: Habituation of the alpha attenuation response in children and adults with psychiatric disorders. *Electroencephalogr Clin Neurophysiol, 26:*12, 1969.

Two hundred and forty-one subjects were recorded for EEG in resting and photic stimulation conditions. Thirty-one adult schizophrenics, ten adult psychopaths and eighty-three children with behavior disturbances were compared with hospital patient and normal control subjects for the characteristics of the alpha blocking response to photic stimulation. With manual techniques of data reduction, state hospital schizophrenics were found to have a faster blocking latency and a longer duration blocking response than normal controls and medical center schizophrenics. With automatic data analysis techniques schizophrenics were found to have faster blocking latencies than psychopaths and normal controls. Children with behavior disturbances were found to have longer response latencies and longer blocking durations than matched controls. Normal children were found to have faster blocking responses and a more gradual curve of the blocking habituation response than normal adults.

behavior problems children schizophrenia photic flicker alpha blocking

CHILDHOOD DISORDERS

K 27. Hartlage, L.C., and Green, J.B.: EEG abnormalities and WISC subtest differences. *J Clin Psychol, 28:*170, 1972.

One hundred and eleven children were classified on the basis of EEG records into normal, diffusely abnormal, and right and left hemisphere abnormal groups. Analyses of variance were computed among groups for each WISC subscale, as well as for overall, verbal and performance IQ's. Only one comparison, which involved the Digit Symbol subscale, pro-

childhood disorders children EEG patterns hemispheric dominance

duced significant differences among groups. It was concluded that interpretation of Wechsler Scales according to criteria found appropriate for adults is not appropriate for children.

K 28. Churchill, J.A., and Rodin, E.A.: Asymmetry of alpha activity in children. *Dev Med Child Neurol, 10*:77, 1968.

An association between asymmetry of alpha activity in children's EEG and the occipital positions of their heads at birth was found. The majority of children from left occipital positions had higher amplitude alpha activity from left hemisphere leads suggesting relative depression of right hemisphere activity. Conversely, alpha amplitudes were higher over the right hemisphere in the majority of children with right occipital births. The findings suggest that one hemisphere may be injured more than the other at birth, the one at greater risk being determined by the head position.

childhood disorders
brain damage
alpha symmetry

K 29. Akiyama, Y., Parmelee, A.H., and Flescher, J.: The electroencephalogram in visually handicapped children. *J Pediatr, 65*:233, 1964.

EEG's and charts of thirty-eight (14 blind, 24 partially sighted) children were reviewed with abnormalities such as spikes, slow waves and absence of alpha activity in the occipital area noted. No correlations were developed between EEG abnormality and intellectual potential or seizures. The lack of visual sensory input was postulated to inhibit occipital alpha and foster parietal alpha-like rhythms. Age was an important factor in development of abnormal EEG's. It is stressed that these abnormal EEG's do not necessarily indicate a need for therapy or a poor prognosis.

childhood disorders
visual perception

K 30. Hutt, S.J., Hutt, C., Lee, D., and Ounstead, C.: A behavioral and electroencephalographic study of autistic children. *J Psychiatr Res, 3*:181, 1965.

Ten children with autism were recorded for EEG in four situations; in an empty room: colored blocks in the room, a passive adult female in the room and an adult female actively engaging the child in design building. Behavioral measures included visual fixations, locomotion, manipula-

childhood disorders
autism
EEG frequency

tion and number of gestures. Subjects were separated into stereotyping and nonstereotyping groups for behavior analysis. All of the subjects showed a greater incidence and complexity of gesturing behavior in the empty room than in other conditions. Subjects with no stereotypic behavior showed a decrease in the incidence of gesturing behavior as the environment became more complex. The subjects with stereotypic behavior had significantly more gesturing behavior in the more complex environments than the other group. The EEG did not differentiate the two groups. Six of the subjects had normal EEG's with a high voltage, dominant slow rhythm. One subject had irregular dominant alpha with a secondary bilateral beta, one had unstable theta, one had paroxysmal delta and one had only bilateral beta. The children showed a lower incidence of desynchronization of the dominant rhythm in the empty room compared to other conditions.

alpha synchrony

K 31.   Hermelin, B., and O'Connor, N.: Measures of the occipital alpha rhythm in normal, subnormal, and autistic children. *Br J Psychiatry, 114:*603, 1968.

Ten children with mongolism, ten children with autism and ten normal control children, ranging in age from five to fifteen, were selected on the basis of having an incidence of alpha greater than 35 percent of the time in the EEG. Subjects were tested for EEG characteristics in five experimental conditions: in the dark with silence, intermittent flashes of light, constant light, intermittent tone and constant tone. EEG's were recorded telemetrically from a single occipital electrode placement. Normal subjects had a lower mean frequency of alpha than the other two groups. Mongol subjects were less aroused by the intermittent light than the other groups and showed less attenuation of the alpha rhythm. Autistic subjects adapted more rapidly to constant light than the other groups but were more aroused by the constant tone. None of the groups showed adaptation to the tone conditions.

childhood disorders
autism
mongolism
visual stimulation
auditory stimulation
alpha frequency
alpha blocking
adaptation

K 32.   Hermelin, B.M., and Venables, P.H.: Reaction time and alpha blocking in normal and severely subnormal subjects. *J Exp Psychol, 67:*365, 1964.

Six mongol imbeciles, six nonmongol imbeciles and six normal control subjects were given auditory reaction time tasks involving the presentation of a forewarning light at varying intervals before the auditory stimulus. The forewarning stimulus was presented either in a discrete burst prior to the reaction tone or started before the tone and overlapped with it in an attempt to produce alpha blocking responses which would terminate prior to the response or continue until the response occurred. Although reaction time did not vary as a function of the alpha blocking latency or duration, patterns of blocking differentiated between the groups. The mongol subjects had long blocking responses to all forewarning stimuli regardless of condition. The non-mongol imbeciles reacted to the discrete forewarning stimuli in the same manner as to the overlapping stimuli with more rapid recovery than the mongol subjects. The normal subjects showed a reduction of the blocking responses in the noncontinuous forewarning condition. Mongols had the slowest reaction times while normals had the fastest.

childhood disorders
mongolism
imbeciles
alpha
   blocking
reaction
   time

SCHIZOPHRENIA

K 33. Rodin, E., Grisell, J., and Gottlieb, J.: Some electroencephalographic differences between chronic schizophrenic patients and normal subjects. *Recent Adv Biol Psychiatr, 10*:194, 1968.

Twenty-five chronic schizophrenic patients and twenty-five normal control subjects were recorded for EEG from bilateral parietal and occipital electrode placements for automatic frequency analysis. Schizophrenic subjects were found to have lower voltage EEG's at all frequencies with alpha being lower on both sides of the head and beta activity being significantly lower on the right side. Schizophrenic subjects had a 10 Hz alpha peak as opposed to an 11 Hz peak for the control subjects. Five of the schizophrenic patients had no alpha peak. Two tests of proprioception were given to sixteen of the patients: placing an arm in a box and flexing it to a position which matched a picture or flexing the visible arm to a position equal to the arm in the box which was positioned by the experimenter. The amount of alpha in the resting EEG was found to be positively correlated with

schizo-
   phrenia
alpha
   abundance
propriocep-
   tion

performance in the tests of proprioception with the same result, a significant positive correlation between amount of EEG alpha and performance.

K 34.   Jus, K., Investigations on slow alpha rhythm in schizo-phrenia. *Pol Med J, 2:*397, 1963.

One hundred and seventy-three schizophrenic patients were recorded for EEG to determine the relationship of frequency patterns to clinical symptoms and prognosis. One hundred and twenty-six of the patients had measurable alpha which was markedly irregular in the majority of cases. Subjects with an alpha rhythm 12 to 13 Hz were not clinically different from subjects with an alpha rhythm 8 to 9 Hz. Confusional stupor was associated with a combination of slow alpha and theta in the EEG. Catatonic schizophrenics were found to have abundant alpha 10 to 12 Hz.

schizo-phrenia alpha frequency

K 35.   Gjessing, L.R., Harding, G.F., Jenner, F.A., and Johannessen, N.B.: The EEG in three cases of periodic catatonia. *Br J Psychiatry, 113:*1271, 1967.

Three schizophrenic subjects with periodic catatonia were recorded for EEG over forty-six sessions to determine the changes in frequency pattern through different stages of the psychosis. The psychotic phase of the reaction was found to be associated with an increase in alpha frequency and a decrease in alpha amplitude. The curves representing the changes in both the frequency and amplitude of alpha were found to covary with blood levels of 4-hydroxyl-3-methoxy-mandelic acid and normetadrenaline. No systematic changes were found for theta or beta frequency ranges.

schizo-phrenia catatonia alpha frequency alpha amplitude

K 36.   Marjerrison, G., Krause, A.E., and Keogh, R.P.: Variability of the EEG in schizophrenia: Quantitative analysis with a modulus voltage integator. *Electroencephalogr Clin Neuro-physiol, 24:*35, 1968.

Ninety-eight schizophrenics (28 chronic and 60 acute) and twenty-four normal volunteers were recorded for occipital EEG integrated amplitude and variability to determine para-

schizo-phrenia alpha patterns

meters differentiating the groups. No differences were found in EEG amplitude between the groups. Chronic schizophrenic patients were found to have a lower variability of EEG than the acute schizophrenics and control subjects. There were no differences between subjects receiving medication and those not being medicated. The difference in variability of EEG was attributed to a lower incidence of alpha blocking in the chronic schizophrenics.

EEG integration alpha responses

K 37. Davis, P.A.: Evaluation of the electroencephalograms of schizophrenic patients. *Am J Psychiatry, 96:*851, 1940.

One hundred and thirty-two schizophrenic patients were recorded for EEG to determine pattern characteristics which would differentiate them from normal population patterns. On an individual basis there was little to distinguish schizophrenic EEG patterns from normal. As a group, the schizophrenic patients showed greater variability, a lower amount of EEG synchronization, and less stability of frequencies than normal. The EEG's from the schizophrenic patients were classified as either normal, dysrhythmic (as in convulsive disorders), or choppy (low voltage, irregular, fast activity dominant). The latter category was found to be associated with a typical response to psychotherapy.

schizophrenia variability EEG synchrony

K 38. Bruck, M.A.: EEG-synchrony and voltage in schizophrenia. *Psychiatr Q, 41:*683, 1967.

One hundred and four schizophrenic patients and 133 normal control subjects were recorded for EEG to determine the differential characteristics of alpha synchrony between scalp locations. Parieto-occipital and occipito-occipital electrode pairs were recorded bilaterally and the phase relations between contralateral electrode pairs were analyzed. Schizophrenics having EEG abnormalities were found to have greater synchronization than control subjects with abnormal EEG. Schizophrenic subjects with normal EEG's were found to have correlated synchrony ratios between parieto-occipital and occipito-occipital pairs where no such correlation was found for control subjects.

schizophrenia alpha synchrony alpha phase

K 39.   Puskina, W.G., and Talavrinov, V.A.: Spatial synchroniza-
        tion of alpha activity in the cerebral cortex in the paranoid
        form of schizophrenia. *Zh Nevropatol Psikhiatr, 67:*76, 1967.

Fifty-four paranoid schizophrenic patients and ten normal
control subjects were recorded for EEG to analyze the phase
relationships between alpha appearing at different scalp
electrode locations. Recordings from the paranoid schizophrenics were separated on the basis of the stage of the disorder at the time of recording: early (paranoidal), middle
(paranoid) and late (paraphrenic) phases. Recordings from
paranoidal stages showed higher synchronization in the right
hemisphere and lower synchronization in the left hemisphere
than normal control subjects. Synchronous alpha was significantly lower in the paranoid and paraphrenic stages.

*schizo-
phrenia
alpha
synchrony
alpha phase*

K 40.   Giannitrapani, D.: Schizophrenia and EEG activity. *Electro-
        encephalogr Clin Neurophysiol, 31:*635, 1971.

Ten schizophrenic and ten normal subjects were recorded
for EEG from sixteen monopolar electrodes to compare EEG
log amplitude scores. The schizophrenics showed a dominant
frequency at 9 cps, but the mean dominant frequency of the
controls was 11 cps. Maturation may account for these findings. Activity diverged significantly between schizophrenics
and controls at 11, 13, 19 and 29 cps; the 19 and 29 cps bands
are first and second harmonics of the 9 cps band, the dominant frequency for schizophrenics. A similar relation between 19 and 29 cps bands for normals was not observed.
A similarity in log amplitude of homologous brain areas was
seen in the schizophrenics, but not in the controls.

*schizo-
phrenia
EEG
frequency
EEG
amplitude*

K 41.   Colony, H.S., and Willis, S.E.: Electroencephalographic
        studies of one thousand schizophrenic patients. *Am J
        Psychiatry, 113:*163, 1956.

One thousand schizophrenic patients were categorized as
either acute, chronic or latent by diagnosis and were recorded for EEG to determine the relative incidence of
normal, fast dominant or slow dominant patterns. Of the 822
acute schizophrenics, 515 had normal EEG's, 272 had fast

*schizo-
phrenia
EEG
frequency*

dominant records and 35 had slow dominant records. Of the ninety-eight chronic schizophrenics, sixty had normal EEG's, twenty-seven had fast dominant and eleven had slow dominant activity. Of the eighty-one latent schizophrenics, fifty had normal EEG's, twenty-six had fast dominant and four had slow dominant activity.

K 42. Igert, C., and Lairy, G.C.: Interet pronostique de l'EEG au cours de l'evolution des schizophrenes. *Electroencephalogr Clin Neurophysiol, 14:*183, 1962.

Sixty-two female schizophrenic patients were repeatedly recorded for EEG during the course of therapy to determine patterns predictive of therapeutic success. A normal EEG pattern was found in 46 percent of the subjects with pure alpha, well localized in the occipital leads and no beta or theta superimposed on the recordings. These subjects showed little or no change in EEG pattern from session to session or across treatment and were said to have little "plasticity." This group had histories of a gradual development of their disorder and had an unfavorable prognosis. EEG abnormalities and records with poorly defined and localized alpha with mixed beta and theta rhythms were found in 54 percent of the subjects. These subjects showed discontinuous histories of their disorder and a greater degree of reactivity to treatment. The prognostic differentiation of schizophrenics on the basis of EEG pattern was found to be most accurate for young patients.

*schizo-
phrenia
EEG
patterns
alpha
patterns
alpha
responses*

K 43. Davis, P.A.: Comparative study of the EEG's of schizophrenic and manic-depressive patients. *Am J Psychiatry, 99:* 210, 1942.

EEG's were categorized as types A (predominantly alpha), B (predominantly beta and little alpha), MF (alpha and beta about equal), MS (alpha and theta mixed) and M (mixed frequencies). EEG's from schizophrenic and manic-depressive patients were categorized and compared. Schizophrenics were found to have MF and B patterns most often while manic-depressive patients were found to have A patterns more often.

*schizo-
phrenia
psychoses
EEG
patterns*

K 44.   Kennard, M.A., and Schwartzman, A.E.: A longitudinal
        study of electroencephalographic frequency patterns in
        mental hospital patients and normal controls. *Electroen-
        cephalogr Clin Neurophysiol, 9:*263, 1957.

Fifteen schizophrenic patients, fifteen nonpsychotic controls   *schizo-*
and fifteen normal controls were repeatedly measured for   *phrenia*
EEG across the course of psychiatric treatment. Frequency   *EEG*
analyses of the EEG's showed that severely disturbed patients   *patterns*
had irregular and disorganized patterns with poorly defined   *EEG*
dominant frequencies. Those subjects which showed signs of   *frequency*
responding to psychiatric treatment had associated changes
in the EEG toward a more normal, organized and alpha
dominant pattern. Subjects who showed signs of deterioration or lack of improvement had EEG patterns which were
more irregular in frequency organization than the other
patients.

K 45.   Goldstein, L., Sugerman, A.A., Stolberg, H., Murphree,
        H.B., and Pfeiffer, C.C.: Electro-cerebral activity in schizo-
        phrenics and non-psychotic subjects: Quantitative EEG am-
        plitude analysis. *Electroencephalogr Clin Neurophysiol, 19:*
        350, 1965.

One hundred and one schizophrenic male patients and 104   *schizo-*
nonpsychotics were measured for EEG amplitude and vari-   *phrenia*
ability. Schizophrenics showed less variability in amplitude   *EEG*
than the control subjects, the lower variability being associ-   *amplitude*
ated with higher arousal as indicated by behavioral criteria.   *EEG*
The variability measure was found to be independent of   *variability*
incidence and amplitude of alpha. Activities such as chang-   *arousal*
ing position or opening eyes, while producing changes in the
variability of the control group EEG's, had little effect on the
variability measure for the schizophrenic subjects.

K 46.   Kennard, M.A., and Levy, S.: The meaning of the abnormal
        electroencephalogram in schizophrenia. *J Nerv Ment Dis,
        116:*413, 1952.

One hundred schizophrenic patients from a state hospital   *schizo-*
population were recorded for EEG to determine the types of   *phrenia*

abnormalities and general characteristics of the EEG patterns. The majority of abnormal records were characterized by high voltage beta activity in the frontal areas. Forty-seven of the patients had irregular and dysrhythmic records, the degree of irregularity being related to length of hospitalization. Ten of the patients had normal EEG's with a high alpha index.

EEG abnormalities
beta

K 47. Berkhout, H.J., Crandall, P., Rickles, W.R., and Walter, R.D.: Spectral characteristics of EEG activity accompanying deep spiking in a patient with schizophrenia. *Electroencephalogr Clin Neurophysiol, 28:*90, 1970 (abstr).

One schizophrenic patient was measured for EEG characteristics accompanying spike activity with a focus in the right septal area. The spike activity was found to be associated with a change in the phase of both alpha and beta activity and an increase in beta amplitude.

schizophrenia
EEG abnormalities
EEG phase

K 48. Abenson, M.H.: EEG's in chronic schizophrenia. *Br J Psychiatry, 116:*421, 1970.

Two hundred and ten chronic schizophrenic patients and one hundred normal control subjects were recorded for EEG to determine parameters which differentiated the two groups. Although no specific pattern was found which characterized the schizophrenic patients, schizophrenics were found to have significantly more EEG abnormalities such as delta waves, spikes, sharp waves, sharp and polyrhythmic bursts of theta and continuous theta discharges. The alpha rhythm was lower in amplitude and incidence in the schizophrenic EEG's and was less responsive to hyperventilation and photic stimulation than for the control EEG's. The incidence of alpha in the schizophrenic EEG's was positively correlated with length of hospitalization. Beta and fast choppy activity occurred more often in the EEG's of the schizophrenic patients.

schizophrenia
EEG abnormalities
alpha patterns
alpha responses
hyperventilation
photic flicker

K 49. Barnes, T.C., Gerson, I.M., and Siverson, J.: The electroencephalogram in schizophrenia. *World Congress of Psychiatry, Mexico City,* 1971.

When schizophrenics are stimulated by flashing light between 1 and 25 cps, some respond with hallucinations but
most find it agreeable and see colors. Patients who have alpha
activity usually follow the alpha frequency. Forty-nine of 160
schizophrenics and 26 nonschizophrenics had increased alpha
after the eyes were opened and then closed; 35 of 160 schizophrenics and 16 nonschizophrenics increased their alpha
during hyperventilation. This is thought to suggest a hidden
or suppressed alpha due possibly to mental activity or anxiety. As a result, the potential of schizophrenics to produce alpha is a more useful measure than alpha percentage. A
further investigation into alpha activity and artistic ability
gave no significant results concerning a relation between
these two parameters, but abnormal EEG's and abnormal
drawings were found to be correlated. No particular abnormal EEG was found to be related to schizophrenia, but
the presence of theta activity indicated to the authors a regression observed in the drawings like those of children.

*schizo-
phrenia
photic
flicker
alpha
abundance
eye opening
hyperventi-
lation*

K 50. Salamon, I., and Post, J.: Alpha blocking and schizophrenia.
       I. Methodology and initial studies. *Arch Gen Psychiatr, 13:*
       367, 1965.

Twenty schizophrenic subjects and twenty control subjects
were recorded for EEG in resting and photic stimulation conditions. Fifteen-second bursts of light were presented to subjects during an alpha burst and the alpha attenuation was
measured as a total number of waves of 50 percent or higher
amplitude of the highest in the resting condition. Schizophrenic subjects were found to have more alpha in the resting condition and less alpha blocking in the photic stimulation condition than control subjects. The amount of alpha
in the resting condition was found to be correlated with
alpha in the photic stimulation condition for those patients
which showed a poor blocking response and patients taking
medications. No similar correlation was found for control
subjects or patients with a normal blocking response.

*schizo-
phrenia
photic
stimulation
alpha
abundance
alpha
blocking*

K 51. Burdick, J.A.: Arousal measurement in schizophrenics and
       normals. *Activ Nerv Sup (Praha), 10:*369, 1968.

Twenty-four schizophrenic patients and twenty-four control subjects matched for age, sex and race were tested for EEG changes under the arousal condition of anticipation of cold pressor stress. Spontaneous GSR bursts, heart rate and integrated occipital EEG variability in the occipital area were analyzed for the two groups. Schizophrenic patients showed more reactivity in GSR and heart rate than the control group, but no differences were found for EEG variability. The indices of arousal correlated higher for the schizophrenic group than for the control group.

schizophrenia
arousal
variability
ANS

K 52. Fedio, P., Mirsky, A.F., Smith, W.J., and Parry, D.: Reaction time and EEG activation in normal and schizophrenic subjects. *Electroencephalogr Clin Neurophysiol, 13:*923, 1961.

Twenty male schizophrenic patients and twenty normal control subjects were given an auditory reaction time task under four conditions of arousal. In the first case, the reaction tone was presented either during an alpha burst or when alpha was absent. In the second, a warning bell preceded the reaction stimulus by either two or four seconds and the warning bell was presented during an EEG alpha burst. Alpha was monitored from a monopolar occipital electrode placement. Normal control subjects responded faster when the reaction stimulus was presented in the absence of alpha and when a warning bell was used than when the reaction stimulus was presented during an alpha burst. Schizophrenic subjects responded more slowly when the warning bell preceded the reaction stumulus by four seconds than in other conditions. Reaction time was unrelated to alpha and no differences were found between the groups for alpha blocking.

schizophrenia
arousal
auditory stimulation
reaction time
alpha responses

K 53. Blum, R.H.: Alpha-rhythm responsiveness in normal, schizophrenic, and brain damaged persons. *Science, 126:*749, 1957.

Twenty-four normal, forty schizophrenic and twenty brain-damaged subjects were recorded for occipital EEG in six conditions to determine the relationships between responsiveness to stimulation and disorder. The tasks included the presentation of pictures, photic flashes at three different frequencies, alpha-triggered photic stimulation and auditory

schizophrenia
alpha responses
sensory stimulation

word association. The normal subjects were more responsive   *brain*
to all forms of stimulation than the schizophrenic or the   *damage*
brain-damaged subjects. The latter groups did not differ
significantly in responsiveness.

K 54. Nideffer, R.M., Deckner, C.W., Cromwell, R.L., and Cash,
T.F.: The relationship of alpha activity to attentional sets
in schizophrenia. *J Nerv Ment Dis, 152:*346, 1971.

Eleven male schizophrenics and ten normal control subjects   *schizo-*
were recorded for EEG while performing an auditory reac-   *phrenia*
tion time task. Recordings were made in an eyes-closed base-   *reaction*
line segment and alternating eyes-opened and eyes-closed   *time*
performance conditions. In the reaction time task a warning   *attention*
stimulus was presented 0.0, 0.4, 1.0 or 2.0 seconds prior to   *alpha*
the reaction stimulus. No significant differences in response   *blocking*
speed were found between the two groups. Schizophrenics   *eye opening*
were found to respond faster in the eyes-closed conditions
than in eyes-opened conditions while the opposite was true
for the control subjects. The incidence of the alpha rhythm
was more related to eye conditions for schizophrenics than
for control subjects. Control subjects were found to respond
fastest with longer preparatory intervals while schizophrenics
responded fastest with short preparatory intervals.

K 55. Puskina, W.G.: The dependence of motor latency upon the
state of alpha activity of the optical cortex in normal persons and in paranoid schizophrenics in the course of therapy.
*Psychiatr Neurol Med Psychol (Leipz), 19:*421, 1967.

Paranoid schizophrenic patients and normal control sub-   *schizo-*
jects were given a reaction time task in which the reaction   *phrenia*
stimulus was activated by the alpha rhythm at different   *reaction*
points in the cycle of the burst of waves: at the peak, falling *time*
point and at its spontaneous disappearance. Paranoid schizo-   *phase of*
phrenics were found to have longer reaction times under all   *wave*
conditions than the normal control subjects. Reaction time   *period*
differences between the stimulus conditions did not differentiate the groups.

K 56. Cromwell, R.L., and Held, J.M.: Alpha blocking latency and reaction time in schizophrenics and normals. *Percept Mot Skills, 29*:195, 1969.

Seven male schizophrenic patients and eight male hospital aides were selected on the basis of having an incidence of alpha greater than 50 percent of the time and no abnormalities in the EEG. Subjects were given a combined auditory and visual reaction time task with the reaction stimuli being presented during a burst of EEG alpha as recorded from right and left parietal and right, left and central occipital electrode placements. No differences in reaction time were found between the two groups. Schizophrenic subjects had faster alpha blocking responses to the stimuli and showed no change during the experiment, while normal subjects increased in the speed of blocking across the trials. When the alpha blocking responses were divided into categories of complete and incomplete blocking, reaction time was found to be correlated with blocking latency for each category separately but not when combined. This held true for all EEG channels in the schizophrenic group but only the occipital channels for the normal group. No differences in the incidence of the two types of blocking responses were found.

schizo-phrenia
reaction time
alpha blocking

K 57.   Marjerrissen, G., and Keogh, R.P.: The neurophysiology of schizophrenia—field dependency and electroencephalogram (EEG) responses to perceptual deprivation. *J Nerv Ment Dis, 152*:390, 1971.

Six schizophrenics and six nonpsychotic volunteers subjected to forty-five-minute periods of perceptual deprivation and a control, resting, perceptually structured state were employed to determine integrated EEG amplitudes, variability and mean alpha frequency. Results were interpreted according to the hypothesis that the integrated EEG indicates cortical activation, and indicated that both field dependency and diagnostic grouping related to the integrated EEG measures. Changes in alpha frequency related to field dependency but not to diagnosis. This was interpreted to indicate that field-dependent subjects tended to become more aroused during perceptual deprivation and field-independent subjects were less aroused in this condition. Changes in alpha frequency

schizo-phrenia
spatial orientation
perceptual depriva-tion
EEG integration
alpha frequency

did not correlate with changes in the integrated EEG. The EEG changes observed are discussed in relation to mechanisms of general arousal, to cortical inhibition and to clinical responses of schizophrenics to perceptual deprivation.

K 58. Serafetinides, E.A., Willis, D., and Clark, M.I.: The EEG effects of chemically and clinically dissimilar antipsychotics— molindone vs. chlorpromazine. *Int Pharmacopsychiatr, 6:* 77, 1971.

EEG studies were conducted in thirty-five out of forty-four *schizo-* chronic schizophrenic patients, both men and women, who *phrenia* participated in a three-month, double-blind, placebo-con- *drugs* trolled study of MOL and CPZ. It was found that the CPZ *theta* subjects, who showed the greatest clinical improvement, showed also the greatest EEG changes (slower and more abundant alpha, emergence of theta), whereas MOL, although different from PL in the amount of slow alpha present, did not show a significant increase in the theta rhythm. In this respect the EEG changes paralleled the clinical changes. The possibility of an electroclinical association between alerting behavioral effects of some antipsychotics (MOL, Haloperidol) and the absence of theta was suggested.

MISCELLANEOUS PSYCHOPATHOLOGY

K 59. Frey, T.S.: Electroencephalographic alpha frequency and mental disease. *Acta Psychiatr Sci, 70:*67, 1970.

This article is a general overview of the EEG as a tool for *miscellane-* diagnosing mental disorders. Specific examples of EEG ab- *ous psycho-* normalities and possible disorders as well as general trends *pathology* indicative of problems are presented. The author feels *alpha* strongly that the EEG should be used at least as a yardstick *frequency* to measure the need for further testing or as an additional piece in the jigsaw of diagnosis.

K 60. Stoller, A.: Slowing of the alpha-rhythm of the electroencephalogram and its association with mental deterioration and epilepsy. *J Ment Sci, 95:*972, 1949.

Twenty subjects were selected for investigation on the basis of having a dominant EEG frequency of 6 to 8 Hz. An additional group of fifteen subjects was selected on the basis of having demonstrated signs of mental deterioration. The slow rhythm group was found to have an incomplete or absent alpha blocking response, frontal bursts of 2 to 7 Hz activity, but no signs of mental deficiency. The group having mental deterioration had a lower incidence of alpha than normal subjects but no other EEG characteristics as a group.

*miscellane-
ous psycho-
pathology
mental de-
terioration
alpha
patterns
theta*

K 61. Roubicek, J., Klos, J., and Tschudin, A.: EEG and clinical study in aggressive oligophrenics, *Psychopharmacologia, 26:* 71, 1972.

Treatment of fifteen imbeciles with indenopyridine was administered for six to sixteen weeks. Within two weeks both verbal and behavioral aggression was considerably reduced and the effect was more pronounced in males. Drug adaptation occurred in females. EEG patterns tended toward hypersynchronization along with slowing and increased amplitude of alpha. Theta activity was enhanced. No change in alpha blocking occurred.

*miscellane-
ous psycho-
pathology
imbeciles
drugs
alpha
synchrony
alpha en-
hancement
theta*

K 62. Synek, V.: The possibilities of the activation and differentiation of low-voltage electroencephalogram. *Int Pharmacopsychiatry,* 2:99, 1969.

Forty psychiatric patients were given a variety of treatments in an attempt to activate alpha in their EEG's. Seventeen of the subjects had EEG's characterized as flat while none of the remaining subjects had an alpha rhythm of greater amplitude than 20 microvolts. Subjects were given a test sequence involving the presentation of a blocking stimulus, hyperventilation and photic driving to activate alpha. Dosages of bemegride, pentobarbital, meprobamate, dexphenmetrazine were also administered during the experiment. No activation response was found in 25 percent of the subjects under any of the treatments. These subjects were characterized as having organic brain lesions and vertebrobasilar insufficiency. Of the remaining subjects the following conditions produced

*miscellane-
ous psycho-
pathology
alpha en-
hancement
drugs
photic
flicker*

activation of alpha: blocking, 10 percent; hyperventilation, 10 percent; photic driving, 37.5 percent; bemegride, 22.5 percent; pentobarbital, 37.5 percent; meprobamate, 50 percent; and dexphenmetrazine, 30 percent.

K 63. Fink, M., Itil, T., and Clyde, D.: The classification of psychoses by quantitative EEG measures. *Recent Adv Biol Psychiatr, 8:*305, 1966.

One hundred and twenty-four psychiatric patients with a wide variety of diagnoses were recorded for EEG with the left fronto-occipital electrode pair used for analysis to determine the relationships between diagnostic categories and EEG pattern. Records were made for resting and hyperventilation conditions. Schizophrenic patients were differentiated from depressive patients by higher incidence of delta and theta activity and a lower incidence of high frequency beta activity. Alpha was found not to be a significant factor in the differentiation of categories. Beta dominant records were found predominantly in depressive and older schizophrenic patients. Theta dominant records were found predominantly in younger schizophrenic patients.

miscellaneous psychopathology depression aging hyperventilation EEG patterns theta

K 64. Volvka, J., Grof, P., and Mrklas, L.: EEG frequency analysis in periodic endogenous depressions. *Psychiatr Neurol Basel, 153:*384, 1967.

Eight female depressive patients, ranging in age from thirty-two to sixty-four, were selected for analysis on the basis of having a history of periodicity in their disorder with alternating phases of depression and complete remission. EEG's were recorded periodically for each subject during depression and remission with placebo or antidepressant medication: imipramine, proheptatriene or prothiadine. Depression was found to be associated with an increase in beta and alpha activity from the EEG patterns in remission. Antidepressant medication was associated with increased theta and delta activity independent of the depressive state.

miscellaneous psychopathology depression drugs alpha enhancement

K 65. Harding, G., Jeavons, P.M., Jenner, F.A., Drummond, P., Sheridan, M., and Howellis, G.W.: The electroencephalogram in three cases of periodic psychosis. *Electroencephalogr Clin Neurophysiol, 21:*59, 1966.

Three subjects with manic depressive psychosis were repeatedly recorded for EEG at different phases in their periodic mood swings to determine relationships between mood and EEG patterns. Bipolar recordings from left and right parieto-occipital electrode placements were analyzed for the incidence of alpha, beta, delta and theta with visual inspection and for detailed characteristics of alpha with a low frequency wave analyzer. The general findings were that depression was associated with relatively high alpha incidence and amplitude while elation was associated with decreased alpha and increased beta activity with alpha having a higher mean frequency.

miscellaneous psychopathology
psyschoses
mood
alpha
patterns

K 66. Cohen, M., Klein, D., and Struve, F.: Relationship between electroencephalographic and sociometric variables among psychiatric patients. *Am J Psychiatry, 127:*97, 1970.

This paper relates the social interactions of hospitalized psychiatric patients to their EEG patterns. The study group consisted of 295 nonchronic patients between the ages of fifteen and thirty-eight. Individual social behavior patterns were measured by responses to sociometric questionnaires. EEG tracings were obtained from all patients during the fourth or fifth week of hospitalization, during which time the patients received no psychotropic drugs. Ninety percent of the EEG records were obtained under waking, drowsy and sleeping conditions. A total of 255 patients were categorized as having (1) an abnormal, (2) a 14 and 6 positive spike or (3) a normal record. The results show a relationship between the EEG patterns of psychiatric patients and the degree and quality of their social behavior. Patients with normal EEG's are liked by an average of $2\frac{1}{2}$ more persons than dislike them, whereas patients with EEG abnormalities of 14 and 6 EEG pattern are liked by only one more person than dislike them. There is a tendency for patients with minimal social interaction and no friends (isolates) to have abnormal EEG's and for extremely disliked patients (rejectees) to have a 14 and 6 EEG pattern. Patients who are

miscellaneous psychopathology
social interaction
EEG patterns

well liked by others (populars) tend to have normal EEG's. The authors caution that diagnosis has been omitted as a variable in this study. However, it is necessary to consider that the population consisted of relatively young, voluntary, nonchronic patients and the results may be specific to such a psychiatric population.

K 67. Dasberg, H., and Robinson, S.: Electroencephalographic variations following anti-psychotic drug treatment. *Dis Nerv Syst, 32:472,* 1971.

Thirty psychiatric patients (18 to 59 years old; 16 male and 14 female) were recorded for EEG for a period of two months prior to the administration of antipsychotic drugs and for two months during drug therapy to determine the relationships between EEG changes and clinical improvement. Nine of the subjects showed a gradual decrease in alpha frequency accompanied by increases in alpha amplitude and incidence, a reduction in beta activity and the appearance of sporadic theta activity (type N EEG change). Nine of the subjects showed no EEG changes during the experiment (type R EEG). Three of the subjects showed only marginal changes (type R-N EEG). Two of the subjects had EEG changes like group N but additional diffuse theta and delta activity (type Ab EEG). Seven of the subjects developed paroxysmal activity (type P EEG). Those subjects with type R EEG's showed no improvement while thirteen of the remaining subjects were found to be clinically improved. Slowing of the alpha frequency was found to be the most predictive of overall clinical improvement and reduction in beta variability was associated with reduction in anxiety independent of overall clinical improvement.

miscellaneous psychopathology drugs EEG frequency

K 68. Secareanu, A., and Sirbu, A.: A dynamic EEG study in delerium tremens. *Electroencephalogr Clin Neurophysiol, 30:* 364, 1971 (abstr).

Fifteen chronic alcoholic patients were recorded for EEG through stages of recovery. The acute stage was associated with an EEG pattern which was dysrhythmic with slow waves and random incidence of alpha or with dominant

miscellaneous psychopathology alcoholism

theta and random incidence of delta particularly in posterior *EEG*
electrode placements. Eleven of the patients who showed a *patterns*
favorable pattern of recovery had an EEG pattern of dominant, low voltage alpha with some posterior dysrhythmia
after one month of treatment and a normal EEG pattern
after one year. Four of the patients with slower recovery
had prolonged confusion following the acute stage associated
with more evident alpha and random theta and delta activity.
Normalization of the EEG began at two to three months
after the acute stage of alcoholism.

K 69.   Barnes, T.C., and Gerson, I.M.: Effects of flickering light on
        EEG of schizophrenics. *Behav Neuropsychiatr*, 2:25, 1970.

Fifty schizophrenic patients were recorded for EEG activity   *miscellane-*
to see if flashing light would cause any abnormal responses   *ous psycho-*
or unreactive brain conditions in the EEG of schizophrenics.   *pathology*
Seventeen were found to have abnormal EEG's while four-   *schizo-*
teen showed good pattern regularity. Alpha ranged from   *phrenia*
8 to 13 cps and from 35 to 90 μv, and all of those with   *photic*
enough alpha responded to eye opening. Eighteen patients   *flicker*
exhibited increased alpha beyond former levels when they   *harmonics*
closed their eyes. Twenty-one of the thirty-six schizophrenics   *arousal*
whose EEG's followed the flashing light with respect to frequency showed normal harmonic response by doubling or
halving the stimulus frequency. The results are interpreted
as following the theory of hyperarousal rather than that of an
inert brain. It was also noted that the association defect seen
in schizophrenia must operate at a higher level than that of
the sensory mechanism involved in response to photic stimulation as studied here.

SECTION L

DRUGS

DRUG EVALUATIONS

L 1.   Dongler, M., Ausloos, G., and Delaunoy, J.: The problem of practical utility of electroencephalography in the psychopharmacology of neuroleptics. *Ann Med Psychol (Paris), 1:* 239, 1970.

This article focuses on practical questions of researcher and practitioner concerning EEG's and neuroleptic drugs. It is pointed out that the definition of neuroleptic drugs could include EEG criteria such as wave synchronizing or slowing of alpha waves but that such criteria could not be used to fully classify these neuroleptic agents since a simple change of dosage could alter such a classification. Also, clinical efficacy cannot be evaluated by EEG effects alone because the small and gradual changes of behavior typical of the relief from psychotic symptoms are not clearly mirrored in EEG activity.

drug evaluations
EEG synchrony
alpha abundance

L 2.   Itil, T.M.: Electroencephalography and pharmacopsychiatry. *Clin Psychopharmacol Mod Probl Pharmacopsychiatr, 1:*163, 1968.

The article classifies psychotropic drugs into six main groups on the basis of effects of the drugs on the EEG. The groups also agree with other classifications based on the clinical effects of these drugs. Tranquilizers, neuroleptics, thymoleptics and major neuroleptics are the first four groupings, all of which cause, in varying degrees, slow activity, synchronization and rhythmic patterns in EEG's while inducing psychomotor inhibition clinically. The other two groups of drugs, anticholinergic hallucinogens and indole hallucinogens, produce disorganization and desynchronization in the EEG and are thought to cause clinical effects such as thought disorders and perceptual disturbances. Frequency analysis and digital computer methods were used to substantiate visual EEG

drug evaluations
EEG patterns

analysis. The thought that this EEG classification of drugs and psychiatric populations may be useful in therapy design was based on the assumption that sudden behavior changes and EEG changes are linked.

L 3. Hynek, K.: Some notes on the effect of psychotropic drugs and mental diseases of the reactivity of alpha rhythms. *Activ Nerv Sup (Praha), 14:*181, 1972.

Two hundred and fifty-five hospitalized patients and twenty-six healthy subjects were studied for their alpha activity in the parietal leads. Amplitude, frequency and incidence of alpha waves was measured in ten-second segments during rest, before and after examination, after Berger's reaction and after photostimulation. Alpha frequency and amplitude declined after treatment with every drug group and this decline occurred more often after photic stimulation than after the Berger reaction. The amplitude of the alpha rhythm changed more than either frequency or incidence. Individual drug groups did not have very different effects on the alpha activity; in fact the effects of the basic psychic problems were more influential. The article gives further details on specific reactions of the alpha rhythm to the various drugs and mental illnesses.

drug
  evaluations
neuroses
alpha
  patterns

L 4. Burdick, J.: Drug effect and possible time trends of the quantitative wakeful EEG. *Acta Physiol Acad Sci Hung, 37:* 133, 1970.

Due to possible diurnal changes in the EEG which could confound present analysis by integration and the gross nature of unfiltered integrated EEG, this two-part experiment was run to present a better parameter, alpha filtered integrated EEG, which does not suffer these problems. In part 1, two subjects were recorded over time for wakeful, drug-free, unfiltered integrated EEG and time trends. Time trends for voltage level and variability seemed to be present. Part 2 studied one subject similarily, except for drug treatment and the use of filtered (alpha) integrated EEG. Time trends were again noted. The author feels that his results demonstrate that integrated alpha frequency is sensitive enough for sta-

drug
  evaluations
alpha
  frequency
EEG
  patterns
  wakefulness

tistical methods to differentiate drug effect. Also, artifacts are less in the alpha range and therefore, artifact editing time can be reduced.

L 5.   Künkel, H.: Quantitative EEG analysis of central drug effects. *Arzneim Forsch, 19:435,* 1969.

The efficiency of a quantitative EEG analysis technique utilizing mean frequency, variability of frequency and integral frequency of alpha and theta activity is demonstrated in experiments using changes of EEG activity in follow-up and acute tests under the influence of drugs. Very small deviations from initial values can be detected by this method and an added degree of efficiency is possible when the experiments involve analysis of variance.

drug evaluations EEG analysis

L 6.   Bruck, M.A.: EEG voltage as an indicator of drug-induced changes in schizophrenia. *Am J Psychiatry, 124:*1591, 1968.

Average voltage values were determined in forty-one pretreatment EEG's of chronic schizophrenic patients. The basic EEG values were significantly correlated with changes in behavioral ratings which occurred after eight weeks of treatment with psychotropic drugs. Thus, the EEG served as a yardstick for predicting the degree of behavior changes in schizophrenics under drug therapy: the less ill a patient was initially, the more improvement in terms of psychological scores could be expected from drugs.

drug evaluations schizo- phrenia EEG patterns

L 7.   Lester, D.: A new method for the determination of the effectiveness of sleep-inducing agents in humans. *Compr Psychiatry, 1:*301, 1960.

Judgments of the sleep continuum from the EEG correlated positively with a frequency count of the brain waves exceeding one third of the amplitude of the alpha rhythm. A method is described which automatically reduces the EEG sleep record so that the relative effectiveness of sleep-inducing and sleep-maintaining drugs in humans may be measured.

drug evaluations hypnotics sedatives sleep

L 8. Henrie, J.R., et al.: Alteration of human consciousness by nitrous oxide as assessed by electroencephalography and psychological tests. *Anesthesiology, 22:247,* 1961.

Nitrous oxide (30%) was administered to eighteen normal subjects and effects on consciousness were evaluated by means of retention tests, subjective, introspective reports and EEG changes. Marked impairment of verbal and visual retention was found. Variations were marked. Correlation of effects by different tests was low. The introspective reports reflected impaired perception. No consistent EEG changes occurred. Changes in alpha activity did not correlate with impairment of performance on the mental tests. Several subjects showed paroxysmal bursts of diffuse theta activity when changed from gas to air.

drug evaluations
conscious-ness
anesthesia
mental tasks
alpha patterns
theta
subjective reports

HALLUCINOGENIC DRUGS

L 9. Rodin, E.A., Domino, E.F., and Porzak, J.P.: The marijuana-induced "social high." Neurological and electroencephalographic concomitants. *JAMA, 213:*1300, 1970.

Ten healthy freshman medical students who had previous extensive experience with marijuana smoking were allowed to inhale the compound in the laboratory until they had reached their usual high. The observed overall effects were mild or minimal. In the electroencephalogram, there occurred a slight but statistically significant shift toward slower alpha frequencies. There were no significant changes in cerebral evoked responses. Results of the neurological examination remained normal. Vibratory sense appreciation improved slightly. Mental status examination showed a slight decrease in intellectual efficiency, some excess jocularity and a slight loosening of associations. Bender-Gestalt drawings were executed slightly more poorly after drug inhalation than before. It is concluded that the subjective pleasure and relaxation which are experienced as a result of marijuana smoking are accompanied by a very slight decrease in highest cortical functions.

hallucino-genic drugs
marijuana
alpha frequency
subjective states

L 10. Gastaut, H., Ferrer, S., and Castells, C.: Action de la diéthylamide de l'acide d'lysergique (LSD 25) sur les fonctions

psychiques et l'électronencéphalogramme. *Confin Neurol,*
*13:*102, 1953.

The effect of a single oral dose of 40 to 60 μg LSD 25 was   *hallucino-*
investigated in twelve normal subjects. The responses were   *genic drugs*
classified as autonomic, psychic and electroencephalographic.   *LSD*
In four instances only one or two of these responses were ob-   *EEG*
served, while in seven cases all three responses were elicited.   *patterns*
In one case LSD 25 had no effect. Hyperactivity and instability of the entire autonomic nervous system followed the ingestion of LSD 25. Perception and global activity were exag-
gerated. Affect became labile, and there was a tendency to
euphoria, or, less frequently, anxiety. Psychological tests
(Cattell, Rorschach, Lahy) revealed that attention and abstract thinking were impaired. Looseness of thought also
occurred. In the electroencephalogram alpha rhythm was increased by 0.5 to 4.0 cycles per second. In half the cases central beta rhythm was initiated, or if already present, was
accentuated. Stimulation by means of a flickering light
caused an increase in occipital potentials in seven instances,
irradiation to the frontal regions occurring in five cases. The
various effects described are considered to be an expression of
neuronic hyperexcitability and a reduction in the "filtering"
of impulses through nervous centers. The therapeutic consequences of these observations are discussed.

L 11.   Fink, M., Volavka, J., Dornbush, R., and Crown, P.: Effects
of THC-Δ-9, marijuana, and hashish on EEG, mood, and
heart rate of volunteers. *Psychopharmacologia, 26:*126, 1972.

Following the smoking of THC-Δ-9, marijuana and hashish,   *hallucino-*
EEG changes occurred rapidly. Changes included increased   *genic drugs*
alpha abundance and decreased beta and theta activity.   *alpha*
These changes were accompanied by subjective feelings of   *abundance*
euphoria and by tachycardia. Chronic administration of
these agents produced similar effects, becoming somewhat
attenuated.

L 12.   Shirahashi, K.: Electroencephalographic study of mental disturbances experimentally induced by LSD 25. *Folia Psy-*
*chiatr Neurol Jap, 14:*140, 1960.

Six normal male adults with regular, well-developed alpha activity were given 50γ of LSD 25 to study the EEG changes associated with the mental symptoms which are induced by LSD 25. The alpha rhythm continued except for the periods when visual phenomena appeared. In some cases alpha frequency did increase 1 to 2 cps but it was concluded that overall the EEG frequency was influenced very little. Although low voltage fast waves did appear temporarily during flight-of-idea symptoms, etc., findings of others indicating much low voltage, fast activity were not supported. Alpha rhythms were suppressed during visual manifestations caused by the LSD 25 and even more remarkable suppression occurred when the objects visualized took on figurative form. Variations in average amplitude of the alpha waves were divided into three types: two-topped, valley and subtype. It is suggested that these correspond to the psychotic reactions of manic depressive psychosis, schizophrenia and the intermediate respectively.

hallucinogenic drugs
LSD
alpha abundance
alpha frequency
beta

L 13.   Denber, H.C.B., and Merlis, S.: Studies on mescaline. I. Action in schizophrenic patients. *Psychiatr Q, 29:421, 1955.*

The intravenous injection of 0.5 grams of mescaline sulfate in twenty-five schizophrenic patients produced a varied clinical picture, with a predominance of emotional over ideational reactions. Within one hour the alpha activity decreased or disappeared in twenty patients, increased in four and showed relatively little change in one patient. There is no relationship between clinical phenomena and brain waves. Following a course of electric conculsive treatments, mescaline reactivated the psychosis in ten to twelve patients. The treatment produced only a quantitative change in symptoms and did not affect the structure of the psychosis.

hallucinogenic drugs
alpha abundance

L 14.   Merlis, S., and Hunter, W.: Studies on mescaline. II. Electroencephalogram in schizophrenics. *Psychiatr Q, 29:430, 1955.*

The post-electric-shock electroencephalograms of eight schizophrenic patients were studied following the intravenous injection of 0.5 grams of mescaline sulfate in each. A symmetrical suppression of high-voltage, slow wave activity

hallucinogenic drugs
alpha abundance

was noted in tracings taken at the first and fourth hours. At the twenty-fourth hour, the patterns had returned to pretest levels in six of eight patients. It has been demonstrated that the high voltage bursts and slow wave activity appearing after electric convulsive treatment originated in the diencephalon. Since mescaline suppresses these slow waves, the diencephalon would appear to be one of its areas of action.

L 15.   Denber, H.C.B.: Studies on mescaline. III. Action in epileptics. *Psychiatr Q, 29:*433, 1955.

The intravenous injection of mescaline sulfate in epileptic patients caused an increase, a decrease or a disappearance of alpha activity as shown on the electroencephalogram. There is either a sharp decrease or disappearance of delta waves. Spike-wave patterns disappear for variable periods following the administration of mescaline. Lethargy, drowsiness and somnolence are the main clinical symptoms produced by mescaline in epileptic patients. All patients denied having auditory or visual hallucinations. Two expressed paranoid ideas, and two had somatic delusions. One patient developed an acute psychotic reaction. Further evidence is offered to support the concept that mescaline acts upon the diencephalon.

*hallucino-
genic drugs
alpha
abundance*

L 16.   Rynearson, R.R., Wilson, M.R., Jr., and Bickford, R.G.: Psilocybin-induced changes in psychologic function electroencephalogram, and light-evoked potentials in human subjects. *Mayo Clin Proc, 43:*191, 1968.

Twenty-two volunteers were monitored for effects of 10 mg of psilocybin and four showed definite changes in evoked potential which were related with visual symptoms. Both alpha and theta activity frequencies decreased during drug effect. Other results under drug conditions showed the following: no gross change in summated electroretinographic data; slowed reaction time and increased pupil size, pulse rate and blood pressure; and no specific pattern to perceptive, affective and cognitive changes, as well as no correlation between these and evoked potential or other physiologic changes.

*hallucino-
genic drugs
visual
evoked
response
alpha
frequency
theta*

L 17. Schiefer, I., Bähr, G., Boiselle, I., and Kiefer, B.: EEG observations in 9 children with LSD intoxication. *Klin Padiatr, 184*:307, 1972.

LSD, in doses between 150 and 600 micrograms, was administered to nine children ranging in age between 2 and 9½ years. EEG recordings were begun thirty hours after administration. Instead of EEG desynchronization as occurs in adults, EEG's showed increased synchrony along with decreased frequency bilaterally in the parieto-occipital regions. EEG's were normal five months later.

*hallucino-
genic drugs
LSD
children
synchrony*

L 18. Deliyannakis, E., Panagopoulos, C., and Huott, A.D.: The influence of hashish on human EEG. *Clin Electroencephalogr 128*:140, 1970.

The EEG's of twenty-seven hashish addicts were recorded at rest and during various combinations of tobacco and tobacco-hashish mixtures. The addicts were soldiers, ranging in age from twenty to twenty-five years, who had been hashish smokers for one to nine years (average 53 months). EEG's were run on twenty-five addicts and one control subject smoking tobacco-hashish mixtures, and on two addicts smoking only tobacco. During hashish smoking, seven addicts showed no change from resting EEG's which were normal in three cases and within normal limits in four. Two subjects had normal resting EEG's but there was an instability of the alpha rhythm in one; during hashish smoking, a stabilization and increase of the amplitude and the total amount of alpha rhythm were noted. In three subjects with normal resting EEG's there was an alpha rhythm blocking effect noted during hashish inhalation or right after it. Long-lasting alpha rhythm blocking as well as instability and general pattern of intermittent disorganization of the tracing was noted in nine cases. In seven of these a general decrease in amplitude was also noted. Five of the nine subjects had normal resting EEG's and four were within normal limits but with increased amount of theta wave activity in the temporal and posterior areas. Finally, in four cases, there was a rather marked decrease of the slow waves which were found in the temporal and the posterior areas of the resting EEG's. These slow waves were symmetrical in one case and asymmetrical in

*hallucino-
genic drugs
EEG
patterns*

three. In the first case an amplitude decrease accompanied
the diminution of the slow waves. In all of the above groups
of reaction patterns, except for the last, there were subjects
with and without any objective clinical evidence of hashish,
such as hallucinations, delusions and confusion. Thus, while
the correlation between clinical and EEG manifestations due
to hashish was not absolute, it existed in the great majorit;
of cases. Confusion was generally accompanied by an increased amount and stabilization of alpha rhythm, while
hallucinations, delusions, dizziness and headaches were accompanied by disorganization of the tracing or tendency to
it.

L 19. Volavka, J., Zaks, A., Roubicek, J., and Fink, M.: Electro-
       graphic effects of diacetylmorphine (heroin) and naloxone
       in man. *Neuropharmacology, 9*:587, 1970.

Pre-heroin, post-heroin and post-naloxone EEG's were taken   *hallucino-*
of sixty-three addicts using 20 to 40 mg/2 cc/2 min, for   *genic drugs*
heroin and 2 to 2 mg naloxone eight to thirty-two minutes   *heroin*
later. Results were consistent with established theories of   *alpha*
association of EEG and behavior in humans after psycho-   *patterns*
active drugs. That is, the early response (4 minutes into the
experiment) was increased alpha amplitudes, alpha frequency decrease and occasional alpha spindling increases,
while the late response (5 to 32 minutes after injections began) was a decrease in alpha abundance, an increase in theta
and delta activity and paroxysmal EEG activity.

L 20. Roubicek, J., Zaks, A., and Freedman, A.M.: EEG changes
       produced by heroin and methadone. *Electroencephalogr Clin
       Neurophysiol, 27*:667, 1969 (abstr).

Intravenous heroin yields increased alpha abundance, slow-   *hallucino-*
ing of alpha frequency, theta activity (occasionally in bursts)   *genic drugs*
and occasional delta bursts. Periods of desynchronization oc-   *heroin*
cur. Chronic methadone yields similar changes to which   *alpha*
adaptation occurs after two to three months at dosages of 100   *patterns*
mg/day. The behavioral and EEG effects of intravenous
heroin after methadone vary with the dose of heroin (25 to
75 mg) and the time after last dose of methadone. The EEG

changes often appear dissociated from the behavioral changes. These observations will be related to observations of the percent methadone maintenance treatment of opiate addiction.

PSYCHOACTIVE DRUGS

L 21. Saletu, B., Saletu, M., Itil, T.M., and Marasa, J.: The relationship between somatosensory evoked potential and quantitatively analyzed EEG during psychotropic drug treatment. *Psychophysiology, 9:*276, 1972 (abstr).

One widely debated area in neurophysiology concerns the relationship between evoked potential (EP) and EEG background activity. While some authors report relationships, others doubt them. The authors have investigated the drug-induced changes in Somatosensory Evoked Potential (SEP) measurements in correlation with both EEG Digital Computer Period Analysis and Analog Power Spectrum Analysis measurements. Twenty-seven chronic schizophrenic patients were recorded after eight weeks of placebo administration, and during the twelfth week of treatment with major tranquilizers. Simple correlation analysis showed that a drug-induced increase in SEP latency was correlated with decreases in EEG average frequency, frequency deviation and fast beta activity, as well as with increases in alpha activity and amplitude variability (period analysis measurements). In regard to power spectrum analysis data, an increase of power in the theta and alpha bands was correlated with an increase of SEP latency and amplitude, whereas an increase of power in the beta bands was related to an amplitude decrease.

psychoactive drugs tranqui-lizers schizo-phrenia alpha patterns EEG patterns spectral analysis

L 22. Fink, M.: Quantitative electroencephalography and human psychopharmacology. I. Frequency spectra and drug action. Neuropsychopharmakologie, 2. Symposium, Nurnberg 1961. *Med Exp (Basel), 5:*364, 1961.

One method of quantifying the psychotropic drug-induced changes in the scalp-recorded human EEG is by electronic frequency analysis. Different spectral responses for imipramine and for a chlorpromazine-procyclidine mixture are de-

psychoactive drugs tranqui-lizers

scribed. The technique provides numerical data for compara-   *spectral*
tive drug studies and is a method for screening new psycho-   *analysis*
tropic compounds in man.

L 23.   Korein, J., Fish, B., Shapiro, T., Gerner, E.W., and Levidow,
L.: EEG and behavioral effects of drug therapy in children.
Arch Gen Psychiatry, 24:552, 1971.

The results of a double-blind study evaluating the EEG and   *psychoactive*
behavioral effects of chlorpromazine hydrochloride and   *drugs*
dyphenhydramine hydrochloride on twenty-nine children in-   *tranqui-*
dicate that EEG findings alone can show whether or not a   *lizers*
child is receiving medication. There was also a significant   *children*
correlation between the more marked clinical behavior   *alpha*
changes and the more marked EEG changes. The EEG effects   *patterns*
of both drugs included slow alpha waves and generalized
slowing. In the case of diphenhydramine hydrochloride, high
voltage four- to six-cycle-per-second activity was uniformly
produced by the relatively high doses used in this study.

L 24.   Herman, M.N., Rowan, A.J., and Goldensohn, E.S.: EEG
changes occurring during L-dopa treatment. *Electroencepha-*
logr Clin Neurophysiol, 31:418, 1971 (abstr).

Animal studies have shown that L-dopa produces activation   *psychoactive*
with desynchronization of the EEG. The influence of L-dopa   *drugs*
on the EEG of human beings, however, has not been docu-   *L-dopa*
mented adequately. Accordingly, a controlled study was   *EEG*
undertaken utilizing patients enrolled in the L-dopa study   *frequency*
group of Columbia University. Twenty-five patients in the   *EEG abnor-*
drug trial group who had EEG studies before and during   *malities*
L-dopa treatment were selected for study. A significant decline in the dominant frequency occurred during L-dopa
treatment (p = 0.05). This was clearly correlated with the
presence of a pre-existing organic dementia but not with
such factors as drowsiness or other anti-Parkinsonian drugs.
Seven patients showed focal slow waves or paroxysmal activity. Six, three of whom had previous thalamotomies, developed the foci while receiving L-dopa.

L 25.   Marjerrison, G., Boulton, A.A., and Rajput, A.H.: EEG and urinary non-catecholic amine changes during L-dopa therapy of Parkinson's disease. *Dis Nerv Syst, 33*:164, 1972.

Forty cases of Parkinson's disease were recorded for EEG before and after therapy with L-dopa to determine the related changes. The treatment was found to reduce the incidence of diffuse theta and delta activity and to increase the incidence of alpha. The integrated amplitude of the EEG, initially higher than normal, decreased during treatment, and the coefficient of variability, initially lower than normal, increased during therapy.

psychoactive drugs L-dopa EEG integration variability

L 26.   White, R.P.: Electrographic and behavioral signs of anticholinergic activity. *Recent Adv Biol Psychiatr, 8*:127, 1966. (Published by Plenum Publishing Corp, New York, J. Wortis, Ed.)

Some of the behavioral and EEG effects of atropine and scopolamine in rabbits, dogs, monkeys and man are presented. These results are compared with the reports of others on the actions of the newer anticholinergic hallucinogens such as JB-329 (Ditran®). It was concluded that reported differences between the belladonna alkaloids and the newer agents were principally quantitative in nature. These differences may be related to known differences among the interactions of acetylcholine receptors with drugs and differences in potency to lower brain acetycholine among the compounds. The newer anticholinergic psychotomimetics, however, evidently produce more gradual EEG's and psychological changes as the dose is increased, induce richer hallucinogenic episodes, and have less intense autonomic side-effects, which make them superior tools for neuropsychiatric research.

psychoactive drugs anticholinergic EEG activation

L 27.   Itil, T.M.: Quantitative EEG changes induced by anticholinergic drugs and their behavioral correlates in man. *Recent Adv Biol Psychiatr, 8*:151, 1966. (Published by Plenum Publishing Corp., New York, J Wortis, Ed.)

Quantitative EEG analysis clearly demonstrated EEG changes induced by the intravenous anticholinergic drugs

psychoactive drugs

Ditran and atropine. The changes were shown to depend on *anti-* the anticholinergic agent given, on the dosage and on the *cholinergic* type of resting EEG pattern prior to drug induction. Elec- *EEG* troencephalographic changes showed a close relationship *patterns* with behavioral alterations. When a patient experienced a confusional-delirious state, there was a marked decrease in EEG alpha activity, an increase of delta-theta activity and some increase of beta activity. When patients demonstrated sleep and subcoma-like states, there was a decrease of EEG alpha and beta activity and an increase in slow activity. Appearance of hypermotor activity after Ditran was associated with a marked increase of fast activity in the electroencephalogram. The correlations between EEG and behavior changes were more distinct when the Ditran-induced delirious state was subsequently altered by the intravenous administration of additional drugs. The addition of chlorpromazine altered the Ditran delirium to a stuporous and coma-like state, associated with further increase of EEG slowing and a decrease of fast activity. When yohimbine, neostigmine sulfate or THA was given, the changes in consciousness induced by Ditran were reversed. This was accompanied in the electroencephalogram by a decrease of slow activity and an increase of fast activity. THA reversed also the psychopathological alterations. These changes in the electroencephalogram were related to a recurrence of alpha activity. The central mode of action of anticholinergic drugs was discussed according to these findings, and the possible clinical-therapeutic use of these EEG and behavioral correlations was suggested.

L 28.   Fenton, G.W., Hill, D., and Scotton, L.: An EEG measure of the effect of mood change on the thiopentone tolerance of depressed patients. *Br J Psychiatry, 114:*1141, 1968.

A technique is described for measuring sedation thresholds *psychoactive* using some distinct EEG patterns. The threshold dose de- *drugs* creases in those individuals who show recovery or marked *sedatives* improvement after E.C.T. Neurotic depression caused a *neuroses* higher threshold than endogenous illness, but age difference *mood* between the groups studied may account for this finding.

L 29.   Johnson, G., Maccario, M., Gershon, S., and Korein, J.: The effects of lithium on electroencephalogram, behavior and serum electrolytes. *J Nerv Ment Dis, 151*:273, 1970.

Lithium carbonate was used in the treatment of five psychotics. Minimal EEG changes occurred with acute administration. Following chronic administration EEG changes occurred including alterations of alpha activity, diffuse slowing, accentuation of focal abnormalities and changes in responses evoked by photic stimulation. Clinical changes were not related to EEG changes.

psychoactive drugs
EEG patterns

L 30.   Serafetinides, E.A., Willis, D., and Clark, M.L.: Haloperidol, clopenthixol, and chlorpromazine in chronic schizophrenia. II. The electroencephalographic effects of chemically unrelated antipsychotics. *J Nerv Ment Dis, 155*:366, 1972.

Electroencephalographic (EEG) studies were conducted in forty chronic schizophrenic men and women participating in a three-month haloperidol (HAL), clopenthixol (CX) and chlorpromazine (CPZ) double-blind placebo-controlled study. Of these forty patients, thirteen were on HAL, nine on CX, eight on CPZ and ten on placebo (PL). Despite some suggestive differences, the overall EEG measures of these drugs were similar, paralleling in this respect their similarity in overall clinical effectiveness despite their chemical differences.

psychoactive drugs
schizo- phrenia
alpha abundance
alpha frequency
theta
beta

L 31.   Robinson, S., Dasberg, H., and Winnik, H.Z.: Clinical and electroencephalographic effects of anafranil treatment in depression. *Dis Nerv Syst, 33*:268, 1972.

The drug Anafranil® was used in the treatment of depressive states. Follow-up EEG's showed polyrhythmic activity typical of tricyclic antidepressants but also caused a remarkable slowing of alpha activity. The latter was interpreted as enhancing the anti-anxiety effect of the drug.

psychoactive drugs
alpha frequency

L 32.   Lettich, E., and Margerison, J.H.: The use of data from low frequency analysis to illustrate serial EEG changes in depressed patients during treatment with iproniazid. *J Ment Sci, 106*:1111, 1960.

Obvious slowing of the dominant frequency and reduction of alpha (8 to 13 cps) amplitude is seen in all cases of depressed patients treated with iproniazid. This usually begins in the third week after drug administration, an interesting fact in view of the time lag reported in clinical response to this drug. Also, reduction of iproniazid dosage by half after six weeks is followed by increased EEG frequency.

psychoactive drugs
neuroses
alpha frequency

L 33.   Itil, T., Shapiro, D., and Fink, M.: Differentiation of psychotropic drugs by quantitative EEG analysis. *Agressologie, 9:* 267, 1968.

Three psychotropic drugs were evaluated with respect to EEG activity which was assessed on a visual basis and later by digital period analysis. Chlorpromazine caused immediate slow wave activity following a temporary increase in percent time of alpha synchronized and rhythmic pattern activity. Also, there was a decrease in superimposed fast beta brainwaves after chlorpromazine. An initial increase and then disappearance of alpha waves, the appearance of disorganized-desynchronized slow wave activity and superimposed fast beta activity were all results of imipramine. The third drug studied, chloridiazepoxide, was characterized by rhythmic spindle-like fast activity mainly in the anterior regions of the brain. Digital period analysis further supports these observations and gives added information concerning the late onset of slowing, high frequency and amplitude variability after imipramine, less frequency variability after chlordiazepoxide and a slowed alpha activity after chlorpromazine. In nine subjects it was observed that the effects of these three drugs and saline could be differentiated by electronic frequency analysis of the EEG. Chlorpromazine and chlordiazepoxide had quite different frequency distributions but were similar in frequency and amplitude variability. The effects of saline were clear in all frequency ranges except the very fast, and seemed to agree with clinical findings of anxious and restless behavior which are probably due to the lack of expected drug effects. Saline and chlorpromazine were easily separated, while the increased fast activity after imipramine and chloriazepoxide made their differentiation rather difficult.

psychoactive drugs
EEG frequency
alpha abundance
desynchronization

L 34.   Fink, M., Itil, T.M., and Shapiro, D.M.: EEG patterns with minimal alterations in consciousness in man. *Electroencephalogr Clin Neurophysiol, 28:*102, 1970 (abstr).

Seventeen normal drug-free asymptomatic female volunteers, between twenty and thirty-five years of age, received either 100 mg or 50 mg amobarbital, 10 mg dextroamphetamine, 40 mg fenfluramine or placebo at weekly intervals during their intermenstrual periods. EEG electrode combinations from conventional scalp electrodes were recorded on magnetic tape and analyzed using digital computer period analytic programs. A reaction time task to a 1000 cps tone was introduced approximately every twelve minutes to maintain an equivalent state of alertness. The EEG samples immediately following alerting were analyzed. The results are as follows: (1) There were no differences in the EEG variables in pre-drug samples, although there was a sequence effect with more alpha and beta-1 activity and less delta and theta activity in the first record than in the succeeding four sessions. (2) The baseline cross variables which discriminated the differences among the drugs at different times were the average frequency deviation, and percent alpha and delta activities. The first derivative variables were the average frequency and percent alpha and beta-2 frequencies. (3) Differences between the two barbiturate dosages and placebo and between dextroamphetamine, placebo and the barbiturate dosages were defined by these variables individually. Fenfluramine was distinguished from dextroamphetamine and placebo, and least from 50 mg amobarbital.

psychoactive drugs alert EEG patterns

L 35. Fink, M., Shapiro, D.M., and Itil, T.M.: EEG profiles of fenfluramine, amobarbital and dextroamphetamine in normal volunteers. *Psychopharmacologia, 22:*369, 1971.

A series of drug treatments were given to fifteen adult female subjects (20 to 35 years) who were free of stimulants to determine effects on the EEG. Bifrontal and right occipito-central electrode pairs were used for recording prior to and four hours after drug ingestion. Constant levels of alertness were maintained by using auditory reaction time tasks and re-scheduling subjects who exhibited slow reaction times. Using a period analysis program, computer processing of the

psychoactive drugs reaction time alert

EEG showed that fenfluramine and 100 mg amobarbital enhanced delta activity while dextroamphetamine decreased it.
Alpha activity was increased by dextroamphetamine but
decreased by fenfluramine and amobarbital. Throughout all
five sessions, beta activity increased.

L 36.   Fink, M.: Electroencephalograms, the mental state, and
        psychoactive drugs. *Pharmacol Physicians, 3:*1, 1969.

Nine patterns of frequency change were suggested by com-   *psychoactive*
puter analysis of EEG's after administration of psychoactive   *drugs*
drugs. It was also found that drugs indicating similar effects   *EEG*
on the EEG had similar clinical usefulness. Specifically,   *frequency*
barbiturates and nonbarbiturates (minor tranquilizers) increased fast activity with increased amplitude while major
tranquilizers (phenothiazines, butyophenones and thioxan-
thene) slowed the EEG frequency with three subgroups
causing different EEG and behavior changes. The sympatho-
mimetic indole compound hallucinogens (LSD and mescaline) increased fast activity with decreased amplitude as did
amphetamines. Atropine and the other anticholinergic de-
liriants increased both slow and fast activity with decreased
amplitude. Lastly, chlorpromazine antagonizes behavior and
EEG characteristics of indole hallucinogens, but it causes
stupor and possibly coma when used after anticholinergic
drugs. In this last case, the EEG slows and shows high voltage
activity, a pattern similar to deep sleep. The author feels
that this use of EEG allows not only drug classification but
also allows prediction of clinical usefulness.

SMOKING

L 37.   Phillips, C.: The EEG changes associated with smoking.
        *Psychophysiology, 8:*64, 1971.

This report compared computer analysis of EEG data record-   *smoking*
ed under both resting and work conditions following smok-   *alpha*
ing to appropriate control data in six male twenty-five to   *frequency*
thirty-five-year-old nurses. Following digitizing, a power
spectral analysis was performed which revealed significant
reductions in the peak alpha frequency component up to

twenty minutes following smoking, during a visual task. Eyes-open resting data show a similar but not significant loss after nine minutes. No indications of increased fast activity were found. Results are related to comparable work on animals and humans. A suggestion is made as to the relevance of these changes.

L 38. Brown, B.B.: Some characteristic EEG differences between heavy smoker and non-smoker subjects. *Neuropsychologia,* 6:381, 1968.

Heavy smokers were easily distinguishable from non-smokers by minimal content of alpha activity, higher frequency of alpha and an abundance of rhythmic and synchronous, high amplitude 12 to 15 cps activity. Responses of the EEG to visual stimuli eliciting the visual evoked response (VER) were also significantly different between heavy smokers and nonsmokers. EEG pattern and responsiveness differences between heavy smokers and nonsmokers indicate differences in central neuronal activity, constitutional in origin. EEG frequency distributions of average smokers and former heavy smokers proved to be roughly intermediate between those of the nonsmokers and heavy smokers. EEG responses to colored photic flicker of these intermediate groups tended to resemble those of the respective extreme groups (heavy smoker, nonsmoker).

smoking alpha patterns

L 39. Brown, B.B.: Additional characteristic EEG differences between smokers and non-smokers. In Dunn, W.L., Jr. (Ed.): *Smoking and Behavior: Motives and Incentives.* Washington, V.H. Winston & Sons, 1973, pp. 67-81.

Subjects with varying degrees of cigarette smoking activity were compared to nonsmokers to study EEG characteristics. Alpha frequency, beta amplitude and theta regularity were parameters showing particular differences, indicating substantial long-term differences in EEG synchronizing mechanisms. Smokers seem predisposed to do so and the habit seems to maintain a balance between brain synchronizing and desynchronizing mechanisms and associated behavior patterns.

smoking EEG patterns

L 40. Murphree, H.B., Pfeifer, C.C., and Price, L.M.: Electroencephalographic changes in man following smoking. *Ann NY Acad Sci, 142*:245, 1967.

This paper reports progress on work to study quantitative electroencephalographic effects of smoking. It has been found that drug effects on the central nervous system as seen in the EEG depend upon the subject's condition or state prior to administration. In the case of smoking, it was observed that reflex effect in the EEG could occur after smoking but before any pharmacological effects can be seen in the blood, and that smoking seems to be a stimulant rather than a tranquilizer in most cases. Slight stimulating effects reflected by reduced variance of the EEG can be seen even before any reduction of alpha or total EEG activity.

smoking
EEG
patterns

L 41. Ulett, J.A., and Itil, T.M.: Quantitative electroencephalogram in smoking and smoking deprivation. *Science, 164:* 969, 1969.

Electronic and digital computer analysis were made of the EEG's of eight young heavy smoker males following twenty-four hours of smoking deprivation. Results showed a significant increase in the slow frequencies which was reversed by resumption of smoking.

smoking
EEG
frequency

L 42. Itil, T.M., Ulett, G.A., Hsu, W., Klingenberg, H., and Ulett, J.A.: The effects of smoking withdrawal on quantitatively analyzed EEG. *Clin Electroencephalogr, 2:*44, 1971.

EEG's were recorded at the end of a twenty-four-hour period of smoking deprivation and again after smoking three cigarettes in thirty-two young chronic cigarette smokers. Using frequency and computer analysis, EEG changes were an increase in slow activity while ten minutes after smoking EEG's returned to resting levels. Results are interpreted as an EEG sign of decreased vigilance, and its reversibility is analogous to the psychosomatic complexity of drug addiction.

smoking
withdrawal
EEG
frequency

L 43. Hauser, H., Schwarz, B.E., Roth, G., and Bickford, R.G.: Electroencephalographic changes related to smoking. *Electroencephalogr Clin Neurophysiol, 10:*576, 1958 (abstr) .

In a study of the effects of smoking on healthy young adults using the EEG and frequency analysis, it was found that 85 percent of smokers and 70 percent of nonsmokers increased alpha frequency by 1 to 2 Hz upon smoking. The change occurred early and was persistent. Four of five subjects who smoked nicotine-free and cotton-simulated cigarettes showed a similar increased alpha frequency. Changes were not associated with cardiovascular changes. It was concluded that the effect on alpha was a psychophysiologic response and more related to the act of smoking than to effects of ingredients of cigarettes.

smoking
alpha
frequency

MISCELLANEOUS DRUGS

L 44. Friedlander, W.J.: The relation of metrazol EEG-convulsant threshold and alpha index. *Electroencephalogr Clin Neurophysiol, 14:*751, 1962.

In order to substantiate past studies which indicated that flat EEG's and epilepsy are not compatible, the authors compared the alpha index measured from the right anterior parieto-occipital bipolar lead and the "convulsive threshold" measured by the Metrazol EEG threshold of thirty patients suffering from a variety of problems and thirty controls. No correlation between the parameters could be found, but it is suggested that epileptics have more alpha than nonepileptics regardless of Metrazol response.

miscellane-
ous drugs
alpha
patterns

SUPPLEMENTAL REFERENCES

BECAUSE OF THE TENDENCY for research to update techniques, methods and concepts, the references abstracted were confined chiefly to scientific reports appearing after 1960. Many earlier reports do, however, contain important background information about EEG alpha activity. These are given in the following list, and, when combined with the abstracts constitute nearly all scientific reports containing information on EEG alpha.

Adrian, E.D., and Matthews, B.H.C.: The Berger Rhythm: Potential changes from the occipital lobes in man. *Brain, 57:355,* 1934.

Adrian, E.D., and Matthews, B.H.C.: The interpretation of potential waves in the cortex. *J Physiol, 81:440,* 1934.

Adrian, E.D., and Matthews, B.H.C.: Observations on the electrical activity of the cortex. *J Physiol, 80:1,* 1934.

Adrian, E.D.: Cortical rhythms. *J Nerv Ment Dis, 81:55,* 1935.

Adrian, E.D.: The electrical activity of the cortex. *Proc R Soc, 29:197,* 1935.

Adrian, E.D., and Yamagiwa, K.: The origin of the Berger Rhythm. *Brain, 58:323,* 1935.

Adrian, E.D.: The localization of activity in the brain. *Proc R Soc Lond (Biol), 126:433,* 1939.

Adrian, E.D.: Electro-encephalogram. *Cambridge Univ M Soc Mag, 18:57,* 1941.

Adrian, E.D.: Brain rhythms. *Nature, 153:360,* 1944.

Adrian, E.D.: The mental and the physical origins of behaviour. *Int J Psycho-anal, 27:1,* 1946.

Adrian, E.D.: Cerebral function. *Br Med J, 2:349,* 1948.

Aird, R.B., and Zealer, D.S.: The localizing value of asymmetrical electroencephalographic tracings obtained simultaneously by homologous recording. *Electroencephalogr Clin Neurophysiol, 3:487,* 1951.

Aird, R.B., and Garoutte, B.: Studies on the "cerebral Pacemaker." *Neurology, 8:581,* 1958.

Aird, R.B., and Gastaut, Y.: Occipital and posterior electroencephalographic rhythms. *Electroencephalogr Clin Neurophysiol, 11:637,* 1959.

Alberti, J.L.: Psychoelectric phenomena in the electroencephalogram. *Ann Inst Psiocol Univ Buenos Aires, 3:521,* 1941.

Altschul, S., and Wikler, A.: Electroencephalogram during a cycle of addiction to ketobemidone hydrochloride. *Electroencephalogr Clin Neurophysiol, 3:149,* 1951.

Andermann, K.: Electroencephalographic evidence of personality changes produced by ataraxic drugs in mentally disturbed patients. *Med J Aust, 2:1,* 1957.

Anliker, J.: Variations in alpha voltage of the electroencephalogram and time perception. *Science, 140:1307,* 1963.

Arellano, A.P., and Jeri, V.R.: Scalp and basal electroencephalogram during the effect of reserpine. *Arch Neurol Psychiatr, 75:525,* 1956.

Armington, J.C., and Mitnick, L.L.: Electroencephalogram and sleep deprivation. *J Appl Physiol, 14:247,* 1959.

Babiyan, S.M.: Dynamics of the EEG changes in the formation of conditioned reflexes in man. *Bull Exp Biol Med, 49*:11, 1960.

Bagchi, B.K.: The adaptation and variability of response of the human brain rhythm. *J Psychol, 3*:463, 1937.

Bagchi, B.K.: The origin of cortical potentials. *Sci Culture, Calcutta, 5*:1939.

Bagchi, B.K.: The origin and nature of the brain Rhythm. *Calcutta Med J, 36*:334, 1939.

Bagchi, B.K.: The electrical rhythm of the human brain. *Sci Culture, Calcutta, 5*:658, 1940.

Bakes, F.P.: Effect of response to auditory stimulation on the latent time of blocking of the Berger Rhythm. *J Exp Psychol, 24*:406, 1939.

Barker, W., and Burgwin, S.: Brain wave patterns accompanying changes in sleep and wakefulness during hypnosis. *Psychosom Med, 10*:317, 1948.

Barker, W., and Burgwin, S.: Brain wave patterns accompanying changes in sleep and normal sleep. *Arch Neurol Psychiatr, 62*:412, 1949.

Barlow, J.S.: Rhythmic activity induced by photic stimulation in relation to intrinsic alpha activity of the brain in man. *Electroencephalogr Clin Neurophysiol, 12*:317, 1960.

Barnes, T.C.: Physiological conditions affecting the electrical activity of the brain. *Anat Rec, 89*:544, 1944.

Barnes, T.C.: Brain waves. *Hahnemannian Monthly, 80*:78, 1945.

Barnes, T.C.: Electrical pulsations in human brain. *Trans NY Acad Sci, 7*:87, 1945.

Barnes, T.C.: Somatic conditions affecting brain waves. *Fed Proc, 4*:5, 1945.

Barnes, T.C.: Electroencephalographic studies of mental fatigue. *J Psychol, 22*:181, 1946.

Barnes, T.C.: Students' brain waves taken before and after classes. *Anat Rec, 94*:380, 1946.

Barnes, T.C., and Brigger, H.: II. Students electroencephalograms taken at 8 AM and 5 PM. *Fed. Proc, 5*:5, 1946.

Barnes, T.C., and Amoroso, M.C.: The effect of age of the human brain on the electroencephalogram during hyperventilation. *Anat Rec, 99*:622, 1947.

Barnes, T.C.: Psychological and physiological factors in electroencephalography. *Am Psychol, 2*:337, 1947.

Barnes, T.C.: Electroencephalographic validation of the Rorschach, Hunt, and Bender Gestalt Tests. *Am Psychol, 5*:322, 1950.

Barratt, E.S.: Relationship of psychomotor tests and EEG variables at three developmental levels. *Percept Mot Skills, 9*:63, 1959.

Bartoshuk, A.K.: Electromyographic reactions to strong auditory stimulation as a function of alpha amplitude. *J Comp Physiol Psychol, 52*:540, 1959.

Bates, J.A.V.: A technique for identifying changes in consciousness. *Electroencephalogr Clin Neurophysiol, 10*:279, 1958.

Beckett, P.G.S., et al.: The electroencephalogram in various aspects of mental deficiency. *Am J Dis Child, 92*:374, 1956.

Beevers, C.A., and Furth, R.: The encephalophone: A new method for investigating electroencephalographic potentials. *Electronic Eng, 15*:420, 1943.

Behague, P., et al.: Study of a population of 440 truck drivers. Relationship between the EEG and results of various psychotechnical tests. *Rev Neurol, 101*:397, 1959.

Bender, M.B.: The eye-centering system. *Arch Neurol Psychiatr, 73*:685, 1955.

Bental, E.: Dissociation of behavioural and electroencephalographic sleep in two brothers with enuresis nocturna. *J Psychosom Res, 5*:116, 1961.

Berger, H.: About the EEG of man. *J Psychol Neurol, 40*:160, 1930.

The Alpha Syllabus

Berger, H.: On the human electroencephalogram. *Arch F Psychiatr, 94*:16, 1931.

Berger, H.: On the EEG of man. *Arch F Psychiatr, 97*:6, 1932 and *Arch F Psychiatr Nervenkr, 98*:231, 1932.

Berger, H.: The EEG in man and its significance for psychophysiology. *Z Psychol, 126*:1, 1932.

Berger, H.: About the electroencephalogram of humans. *Arch F Psychiatr, 101*:452, 1933.

Berger, H.: About the human EEG. *Arch F. Psychiatr, 100*:301, 1933.

Berger, H.: On the human electroencephalogram. *Arch Psychiatr, 102*:538, 1934.

Berger, H.: On the EEG of man. *Naturwissenschaften, 23*:121, 1935.

Berger, H.: On the human electroencephalogram. *Arch F Psychiatr, 103*:444, 1935.

Berger, H.: On the human electroencephalogram. *Arch Psychiatr, 104*:678, 1936.

Berger, H.: About the human EEG. *Arch F Psychiatr, 106*:577, 1937 and *Arch F Psychiatr, 106*:165, 1937.

Berger, H.: The human electroencephalogram and its interpretations. *Boll Soc Ital Biol Sper, 13*:263, 1937.

Berger, H.: The human EEG and its psychophysiological interpretation. *XIme Int Congr Psychol, Paris, 1*:220, 1937.

Berger, H.: The human EEG and its psychophysiological interpretation. *Ind Psychotechnol, 7-8*:222, 1937.

Berger, H.: On human EEG. *Arch F Psychiatr, 108*:407, 1938 and *Allg Z Psychiatr, 109*:254, 1938.

Bergman, P.S.: Cerebral blindness. An analysis of twelve cases, with special reference to the electroencephalogram and patterns of recovery. *Arch Neurol Psychiatr, 78*:568, 1957.

Bernhard, C.G., and Skoglund, C.R.: Alpha frequency and age. *Scand Arch Physiol, 82*:178-184, 1939.

Bernhard, C.G.: Research on the frequency of the alpha waves of EEG's of children. *Acta Psychiatr KBH, 14*:223-231, 1939.

Bernhard, C.G. and Skoglund, C.R.: On blocking time (due to light stimuli) of cortical alpha rhythm in children. *Acta Psyhciatr KBH, 18*:159-170, 1943.

Bert, J., et al.: Alpha-rhythm reactivity to eyes opening during diverse perceptual situations. *Ann Med Psychol (Paris), 117*:819-830, 1959.

Bjerner, B.O.: Alpha depression and lowered pulse rate during delayed actions in a serial reaction test. A study in sleep deprivation. *Acta Physiol Scand (Suppl), 65*:93, 1949.

Bjerner, B.O.: Alpha depression and lowered pulse rate during delayed actions in a serial reaction test. *Acta Physiol Scand (Suppl), 65*:93, 1949.

Blum, J.S., et al.: A behavioral analysis of the organization of the parieto-temporo-pre-occipital cortex. *J Comp Neurol, 93*:53-100, 1950.

Blum, R.H.: Photic stimulation, imagery, and alpha rhythm. *J Ment Sci, 102*:160-167, 1956.

Blum, R.H.: Alpha-rhythm responsiveness in normal, schizophrenic, and brain-damaged persons. *Science, 126*:749-750, 1957.

Bokonjic, N., and Trojaborg, W.: The effect of meprobramate on the electroencephalogram during treatment, intoxication and after abrupt withdrawal. *Electroencephalogr Clin Neurophysiol, 12*:177, 1960.

Borehan, J.L., et al.: A relation between a psychomotor response and the phase of the alpha rhythm. *J Physiol, 109*:17, 1949.

Borenstein, P., et al.: Contribution to the study of reserpine in psychiatry. Clinical and electroencephalographic results. *Ann Med Psychol (Paris), 114:*545-580, 1956.

Brazier, M.A.B., et al.: Characteristics of the normal electroencephalogram. II. The effect of varying blood sugar levels on the occipital cortical potentials in adults during quiet breathing. *J Clin Invest, 23:*313-317, 1944.

Brazier, M.A.B., et al.: Characteristics of the normal electroencephalogram. III. The effects of varying blood sugar levels on the occipital cortical potentials in adults during hyperventilation. *J Clin Invest, 23:*319-323, 1944.

Brazier, M.A.B., and Finesinger, J.E.: A study of the occipital cortical potentials in 500 normal adults. *J Clin Invest, 23:*303-311, 1944.

Brazier, M.A.B., and Finesinger, J.E.: Action of barbiturates on the cerebral cortex. *Arch Neurol Psychiatr, 53:*51-58, 1945.

Brazier, M.A.B., and Beecher, H.K.: Alpha content of the electroencephalogram in relation to movements made in sleep, and effect of a sedative on this type of motility. *J Appl Physiol, 4:*819-825, 1952.

Brazier, M.A.B.: EEG studies of flicker in normal man. ERDL Symposium on Flicker. Fort Belvoir, Virginia and Tulane University, April 1957, pp. 199-221.

Bremer, F., and Terzuolo, C.: Role of the cerebral cortex in the process of awakening. *Arch Int Physiol, 60:*228-231, 1952.

Brill, N.Q., et al.: Electroencephalographic studies in delinquent behavior problem children. *Am J Psychiatry, 98:*494-498, 1942.

Browne-Mayers, A.N., and Kane, F.D.: Studies in alpha blocking following electroconvulsive therapy. *J Nerv Ment Dis, 121:*257-261, 1955.

Brown, W.T., and Solomon, C.I.: Delinquency and the electroencephalograph. *Am J Psychiatry, 98:*499-503, 1942.

Bruck, M.A.: A method to determine average voltage in the EEG. *Electroencephalogr Clin Neurophysiol, 12:*525, 1960.

Bucy, P.C., and Case, T.J.: An association between homonymous hemianopsia and unilateral absence of alpha waves. *Trans Am Neurol Assoc, 66:*17-20, 1940.

Bujas, Z., and Petz, B.: Les modifications des ondes alpha au couvs dutravail mental prolonge. *Travail Humain, 17:*201-206, 1954.

Burch, N.R.: Automatic analysis of the electroencephalogram: A review and classification of systems. *Electroencephalogr Clin Neurophysiol, 11:*827, 1959.

Burford, G.E.: Involuntary eyeball motion during anesthesia and sleep: relationship to cortical rhythmic potentials. *Anesth Analg (Paris), 20:*191-199, 1941.

Burge, W.E., et al.: A study of the electrical potential of the cerebral cortex in relation to anesthesia, consciousness and unconsciousness. *Am J Physiol, 116:*19-20, 1936.

Burrow, T.: Preliminary report of electroencephalographic recordings in relation to behavior modifications. *J Psychol, 15:*109-114, 1943.

Burrow, T., and Galt, W.: Electroencephalographic recordings of varying aspects of attention in relation to behavior. *J Gen Psychol, 32:*269-288, 1945.

Busses, E.W., et al.: Psychological functioning of aged individuals with normal and abnormal electroencephalograms. I. A study of non-hospitalized community volunteers. *J Nerv Ment Dis, 124:*135-141, 1956.

Callaway, E., and Yeager, C.L.: Relationship between reaction time and electroencephalographic alpha phase. *Science, 132:*1765-1766, 1960.

Carels, F.: Slow posterior waves in the EEG of a young adult and their quantitative variations with time. *Acta Neurol Psychiatr Belg, 59:*409-413, 1959.

Case, T.J.: Alpha waves in relation to structures involved in vision. *Biol Symposia, 7:* 107-116, 1942.

Cate, J. Ten, et al.: Can the alpha waves of the electroencephalogram originate in brain parts outside the cerebral cortex. *Arch Neerl Physiol, 25:*366-380, 1940.

Cate, J. Ten, and Walter, W.G.: Can alpha waves in the electroencephalogram be produced in the nucleus caudatus. *Psychiatr Neurol Bl. Amsterdam, 45:*364-369, 1941.

Chamberlain, G.H.A., and Russell, J.G.: The EEG's of the relatives of schizophrenics. *J Ment Sci, 98:*654-659, 1952.

Chapple, E.D., and Harding, C.F.: Simultaneous measure of human relations and emotional activity. *Proc Natl Acad Sci, 26:*319-326, 1940.

Chertok, L., and Kramarz, P.: Hypnosis, sleep and electroencephalography. *J Nerv Ment Dis, 128:*227-238, 1959.

Chu, C.P.: The dynamics of the general and local changes in the EEG in elaboration of conditioned motor reflexes in man. *Bull Exp Biol Med, 49:*8-13, 1960.

Chweitzer, A., et al.: The action of mescalin on the alpha waves (Bergers Rhythm) in man. *CR Soc Biol (Paris), 124:*1296-1299, 1937.

Chyatte, C.: A note on the relationship of alpha index to critical flicker frequency *Electroencephalogr Clin Neurophysiol, 10:*553, 1958.

Cohen, J.J., et al.: Lack of alpha reduction in patients with defective revisualization. *Neurology (Minneap), 11:*665-675, 1961.

Cohn, R.: An experimental study of monopolar and bipolar derivations in the human electroencephalogram. *Proc Soc Exp Biol, 55:*240-242, 1944.

Cohn, R.: Influence of harmonic content on wave forms of the human electroencephalogram. *J Neurophysiol, 9:*161-164, 1946.

Cohn, R.: A correlation of symbol organization with brain function (EEG). *Am J Psychiatry, 116:*1001-1008, 1960.

Condero, A., et al.: Critical flicker frequency and cortical alpha. *Electroencephalogr Clin Neurophysiol, 8:*465, 1956.

Cornil, L., and Gastaut, H.: EEG data on the dominance of one hemisphere. *Rev Neurol, 79:*207, 1947.

Cornil, L., and Gastaut, H.: Electroencephalographic study on the sensory dominance of one cerebral hemisphere. *Pr Med, 55:*421-422, 1947.

Corriol, J.: Analysis and comparison of phase in electroencephalography. *Electroencephalogr Clin Neurophysiol, 3:*443, 1951.

Crighel, E., and Nestianu, V.: Electroencephalographic study of cortical reactivity. *Pavlov J Higher Nerv Activ, 8:*529-539, 1958.

Dahl, W.D.: Brain-wave modification by flicker. *Naval Research Reviews (Washington),* June 1962, pp. 15-17.

Darrow, C.W., et al.: Autonomic indications of excitatory and homeostatic effects on the EEG. *J Psychol, 14:*115-130, 1942.

Darrow, C.W.: Physiological and clinical tests of autonomic function and autonomic balance. *Physiol Rev, 23:*1-36, 1943.

Darrow, C.W., et al.: Autonomic significance of "blocking" and "facilitation" in electroencephalogram. *Fed Proc, 5:*21, 1946.

Darrow, C.W.: Psychological and psychophysiological significance of the electroencephalogram. *Psychol Rev, 54:*157-168, 1947.

Darrow, C.W., et al.: Central and peripheral indications of the conditioning, adaptation, anticipation and extinction. *J Nerv Ment Dis, 124:*38-44, 1956.

Darrow, C.W., et al.: Electroencephalographic "blocking" and "adaptation". *Science, 126*:74-75, 1957.

Daumezon, G., and Lairy, G.C.: Dynamics of alpha rhythm in psychopathology. *Ann Med Psychol, 115*:35-51, 1957.

Davis, F.H., and Malmo, R.B.: Electromyographic recording during interview. *Am J Psychiatry, 107*:908-916, 1951.

Davis, H., et al.: Changes in human brain potentials during the onset of sleep. *Science, 86*:448-450, 1937.

Davis, P.A., et al.: The effects of alcohol upon the electroencephalogram. *Q J Stud Alcohol, 1*:626-637, 1941.

Davis, P.A.: Effect on the EEG of changing the blood sugar level. *Arch Neurol Psychiatr, 49*:186-194, 1943.

Dell, P., Bonvallet, M., and Hiebel, G.: Tonus sympathique et activite elecyrique corticale. *Electroencephalogr Clin Neurophysiol, 6*:119, 1953.

Dement, W., and Kleitman, N.: Cyclic variations in EEG during sleep and their relation to eye movements, body motility and dreaming. *Electroencephalogr Clin Neurophysiol, 9*:673, 1957.

Dement, W., and Kleitmen, N.: The relation of eye movements during sleep to dream activity: An objective method for the study of dreaming. *J Exp Psychol, 53*:339-346, 1957.

Dennison, A.C., Jr., et al.: Effect of reserpine upon the human electroencephalogram. *Neurology, 5*:56-68, 1955.

Dodge, P.R., et al.: Studies in experimental water intoxication. *AMA Arch Neurol, 3*:513-529, 1960.

Dondey, M.: EEG terminology and semantics. *Electroencephalogr Clin Neurophysiol, 13*:612, 1961.

Drever, J.: Further observations on the relation between EEG and visual imagery. *Am J Psychol, 71*:270-276, 1958.

Dreyfus-Brisac, C., and Blanc, C.: Electroencephalogram and cerebral maturation. *Encephale, 45*:205-245, 1956.

Dublineau, J., and Soboul, I.: Study of some relationships between type and EEG. *Ann Med Psychol, 114*:17-35, 1956.

Dubner, H.H.: Further studies of factors influencing brain rhythms. *Am J Physiol, 123*:56-57, 1938.

Dynes, J.B.: Objective method for distinguishing sleep from the hypnotic trance. *Arch Neurol Psychiatr, 57*:84-93, 1947.

Ebbecke, U.: Spontaneous oscillations of excitation of the visual field and electrophysiological oscillations (alpha-waves). *Arch Ges Physiol, 250*:421-430, 1948.

Ellingson, R.J., and Lindsley, D.B.: Brain waves and cortical development in newborns and young infants. *Am Psychol, 4*:248-249, 1949.

Ellingson, R.J.: Response to physiological stress in normal and behavior problem children. *J Genet Psychol, 83*:19-29, 1953.

Ellingson, R.J.: Brain waves and problems of psychology. *Psychol Bull, 53*:1-34, 1956.

Ellingson, R.J., et al.: EEG frequency-pattern variation and intelligence. *Electroencephalogr Clin Neurophysiol, 9*:657, 1957.

Engel, G.L., et al.: A simple method of determining frequency spectra in the electroencephalogram. Observations on physiological variations in glucose, oxygen, posture, and acid-base balance on the normal electroencephalogram. *Arch Neurol Psychiatr, 51*:134-146, 1944.

Epstein, A.W.: Relationship of fetishism and transvestism to brain and particularly to temporal lobe dysfunction. *J Nerv Ment Dis, 133*:247-253, 1961.

Essig, C.F., and Fraser, H.F.: Electroencephalographic changes in man during use and withdrawal of barbiturates in moderate dosage. *Electroencephalogr Clin Neurophysiol, 10*:649, 1958.

Faure, J.: The EEG of anxiety states (cortical and basal activity during anxiety). *CR Cong Med Al Neurol, Paris, Masson et Cie, 45*:230-233, 1947.

Faure, J.: A bio-electrical approach to the emotions. *J Physiol (Paris), 45*:589-590, 1950.

Faure, J.: Effect of photic stimulation on the EEG of certain neurotics. *Rev Otoneuroophtalmol, 22*:554-556, 1950.

Faure, J., and Guerin, A.: On the EEG of difficult children. *Rev Neurol (Paris), 99*:209-219, 1958.

Fedio, P., et al.: Reaction time and EEG activation in normal and schizophrenic subjects. *Electroencephalogr Clin Neurophysiol, 13*:923, 1961.

Feldman, H.: The EEG in personality and behavior disorders in children. *Schweiz Arch Neurol Neurochir Psychiatr, 69*:170-212, 1952.

Feng, Y.K., et al.: Immediate effect of acupuncture on electroencephalograms of epileptics. *Chinese Med J, 79*:521-530, 1959.

Ferguson, R.S.: Some physiological responses in neurotics. *J Nerv Ment Dis, 125*:240-246, 1957.

Fessard, A.: Nervous rhythms and oscillations of relaxation. *L'Annee Psychol, 32*:49-117, 1931.

Fessard, A.: Electric signs of cerebral activity in man. *Paris Med, 1*:301-312, 1938.

Finesinger, J.E., et al.: The effect of varying blood sugar levels on the electroencephalogram in the normal adult during normal breathing and hyperventilation. *J Clin Invest, 21*:631, 1942.

Finesinger, J.E., et al.: A study of levels of consciousness based on electroencephalographic data in pentothal anesthesia. *Trans Am Neurol Assoc, 72*:183-185, 1947.

Finley, K.H., and Campbell, C.M.: EEG in schizophrenia. *Am J Psychiatry, 98*:374-379, 1941.

Fischgold, H.: The EEG at the age of 21 years. *Med Paris, 31*:13-16, 1950.

Fischgold, H.: Consciousness and its modifications: system of reference in clinical electroencephalography. *Priemier Congres International de Sciences Neurologique Bruxelles,* 21-28 Juillet 1957. Also *Acta Med Belgica, 11,* 1957.

Fischgold, H., and Mathis, P.: Pharmacologic modifications of "Alpha" rhythm. *Presse Med, 68*:1445-1446, 1960.

Fisher, J., and Friedlander, W.J.: The relation of age to metrazol activated EEG's. *Electroencephalogr Clin Neurophysiol, 7*:357, 1955.

Forbes, T.W., and Andrews, H.L.: Independent control of alpha rhythm and "psychogalvanic" response. *Science, 86*:474-476, 1937.

Ford, A.: Bioelectrical potentials and mental effort. II. Frontal lobe effects. *J Comp Physiol Psychol, 47*:28-30, 1954.

Ford, W.L., and Yeager, C.L.: Changes in the EEG in subjects under hypnosis. *Dis Nerv Syst, 9*:190, 1948.

Foster, A.L.: The relationship between EEG abnormality, some psychological factors and delinquent behavior. *J Proj Tech, 22*:276-280, 1958.

Franek, B., and Thren, R.: Electroencephalographic findings in graded active hypnotic exercises. *Arch Psychiatr Nervenkr, 181*:360-368, 1949.

Franke, L.F., and Koopman, L.J.: Parallels in electrobiologic changes of the hemisphere in pathophysiologic and parapsychologic phenomenon. *Z Gesamte Neurol Psychiatr, 162*:259-288, 1938.

Freestone, N.W.: Brain-wave interpretation of stuttering. *Q J Speech, 28*:446-468, 1942.

Frey, T., and Sjoegren, H.: The electroencephalogram in elderly persons suffering from neuropsychiatric disorders. *Acta Psychiatr (Scand), 34*:438-450, 1959.

Frey, T., and Holmgren, B.: Conditions of psychic insufficiency and the electroencephalogram. *Arch F Psychiatr UZ Neurol, 183*:64-70, 1949.

Friedman, S.B., and Engel, G.L.: Effect of cortisone and adrenocorticotropin on the electroencephalogram of normal adults: quantitative frequency analyses. *J Clin Endocrinol, 16*:839-847, 1956.

Friedlander, W.J.: The effect of cortisone on the electroencephalogram. *Electroencephalogr Clin Neurophysiol, 3*:311, 1951.

Friedlander, W.J.: Electroencephalographic alpha rate in adults as a function of age. *Geriatrics, 13*:29-31, 1958.

Friedlander, W.J.: Demerol as an EEG "activating" agent. *Electroencephalogr Clin Neurophysiol, 12*:914, 1960.

Friedlander, W.J.: The use of benadryl for sleep EEG's. *Electroencephalogr Clin Neurophysiol, 13*:285, 1961.

Friedlander, W.J.: The relation of metrazol EEG-convulsant threshold and alpha index. *Electroencephalogr Clin Neurophysiol, 14*:751, 1962.

Furth, R., and Beevers, C.A.: Encephalophone. New method for investigating electroencephalographic potentials. *Nature, 151*:110-111, 1943.

Gachkel, V., et al.: On the physiopathologic interpretation of a hallucinatory syndrome, trigger role of work, confirmed by the EEG. *Evol Psychiatr (Paris), 28*:695-716, 1956.

Gallagher, J.R., et al.: Relation between the electrical activity of the cortex and the personality in adolescent boys. *Psychosom Med, 4*:134-139, 1942.

Gallais, P., et al.: Preliminary EEG study in the Negro. *Med Trop (Mars), 5*:687-695, 1949.

Gallais, P., et al.: The EEG in the African Negro study of the first 100 records of normal subjects). *Rev Neurol (Paris), 83*:622-624, 1950.

Gallais, P., et al: Introduction to the study of the physiological EEG of the African Negro. *Med Trop (Mars), 11*:128-146, 1951.

Galla, S.G., et al.: Evaluation of the traditional signs and stages of anesthesia: an electroencephalographic and clinical study. *Anesthesiology, 19*:328-338, 1958.

Garcia-Austt, E., et al.: Changes of EEG background activity during photic changes on EEG background activity during photic habituation in man. *Acta Neurol Lat Am, 7*:82-90, 1961.

Garvin, J.S., et al.: Paroxysmal anterior cerebral bradyrhythmia. *AMA Arch Neurol Psychiatr, 73*:573, 1955.

Gastaut, H., and Corriol, J.: On a new method of driving cortical rhythms of intermittent and synchronized photo-acoustic stimulations. *CR Soc Biol (Paris), 42*:349-350, 1948.

Gastaut, H., and Duplay, J.: Preliminary data on the direct electroencephalography of the occipital lobes in man during intermittent stimulation with light. *Rev Neurol, 80*:638-639, 1948.

Gastaut, H., et al.: Study of an unrecognized EEG activity. The rolandic rhythm in arceau. *Mars Med, 89*:296-310, 1952.

Gastaut, H., et al.: Action of the diethylamide of d-lysergic acid (LSD 25) on psychological functions and the EEG. *Confin Neurol, 13*:102-120, 1953.

Gastaut, H., et al.: Relations between electroencephalographic variables and those which express personality and motor-sensory functions. Results of a survey done in a young male, homogenous population. *Rev Neurol, 101*:320-390, 1959.

Gastaut, H., et al.: Comparative EEG and psychometric data for 825 French naval pilots and 511 control subjects of the same age. *Aerosp Med, 31*:547-552, 1960.

Geddes, L.: A note on phase distortion. *Electroencephalogr Clin Neurophysiol, 3*:517, 1951.

Gerard, R.W., and Marshall, W.H.: Cerebral action potentials. *Proc Soc Exp Biol Med, 30*:1123-1125, 1933.

Gerard, R.W., et al.: Brain action potentials. *Am J. Physiol, 109*:38-39, 1934.

Gerard, R.W.: Brain waves. *Sci Monthly, 44*:48-56, 1937.

Gianascol, A.J., and Yeager, C.L.: Simultaneous study of behavior and brain waves. *Science, 132*:470-471, 1960.

Gibbs, F.A., and Davis, H.: Changes in the human electroencephalogram associated with loss of consciousness. *Am J Physiol, 113*:49-50, 1935.

Gibbs, F.A.: Interpretation of the electroencephalogram. *J Psychol, 4*:365-382, 1937.

Gibbs, F.A.: Regulation of frequency in the cerebral cortex. *Am J Physiol, 119*:317, 1937.

Gibbs, F.A., and Grass, A.M.: Cortical frequency spectra in three dimensions. *Am J Physiol, 126*:502, 1939.

Gibbs, F.A., and Knott, J.R.: Changes in the frequency-energy spectrum of the electroencephalogram from birth to 24 years. *Psychol Bull, 39*:600, 1942.

Gibbs, F.A.: Cortical frequency spectra of healthy adults. *J Nerv Ment Dis, 95*:417-426, 1942.

Gibbs, F.A., et al.: An electroencephalographic study on adult criminals. *Trans Am Neurol Assoc, 68*:87-90, 1942.

Glanville, A.D., and Antonittis, J.J.: The relationship between occipital alpha activity and laterality. *J Exp Psychol, 49*:294-299, 1955.

Goldman, G., et al.: The influence of an intermittent stimulation on Berger's Rhythm. *CR Soc Biol (Paris), 127*:1217-1220, 1938.

Goldie, L., and Green, J.M.: Paradoxical blocking and arousal in the drowsy state. *Nature, 187*:952-953, 1960.

Goldfarb, W.: Effect of blood sugar on EEG. *NY State J Med, 45*:1460-1462, 1945.

Golla, F., et al.: Objective study of mental imagery, physiological concomitants. Appendix on new method of electroencephalographic analysis. *J Ment Sci, 89*:216-223, 1943.

Gon, J.J., Van Der, and Hinte, N. Van.: The relation between the frequency of the alpha-rhythm and the speed of writing. *Electroencephalogr Clin Neurophysiol, 11*: 669, 1959.

Goodenough, C.R., et al.: A comparison of "dreamers" and "nondreamers": eye movements, electroencephalograms, and the recall of dreams. *J Abnorm Soc Psychol, 59*: 295-302, 1959.

Goodwin, J.E.: Bilateral synchronicity of alpha activity in man. *Proc Can Physiol Soc, 12*: 1939.

Goodwin, J.E.: The significance of alpha variants in the EEG and their relationship to an epileptiform syndrome. *Am J Psychiatry, 104*:369-379, 1947.

Gottlober, A.B.: The inheritance of brain potential patterns. *J Exp Psychol, 22*:193-200, 1938.

Gottlober, A.B.: The relationship between brain potentials and personality. *J Exp Psychol, 22*:67-74, 1938.

Gottschalk, L.A.: Psychologic conflict and electroencephalographic patterns. *Arch Neurol Psychiatr, 73:*656-662, 1955.

Granada, A.M., and Hammack, J.T.: Operant behavior during sleep. *Science, 133:*1485-1486, 1961.

Green, J.: Some observations on lambda waves and peripheral stimulation. *Electroencephalogr Clin Neurophysiol, 9:*691, 1957.

Gresham, S.C., et al.: Alcohol and caffeine: Effect on inferred visual dreaming. *Science, 140:*1226-1227, 1963.

Gros, C., and Vlahovitch, B.: Electroencephalographic studies on children having measles with no clinical evidence of involvement of the central nervous system. *Pediatrics, 18:*556-560, 1956.

Gruenthal, E., and Remy, M.: Essentials and significance of the human alpha rhythm in the EEG. *Mschr Psychiatr (Basel), 122:*319-324, 1951.

Gruesser, O.J., and Gruetzner, A.: Neurophysiologic basis of periodic after-image phases after short light flashes. *Graefes Arch F Ophtalmol, 160:*65-93, 1958.

Gruttner, R., and Bonkalo, A.: About tiredness and sleep on the basis of cerebral bioelectrical studies. *Arch F Psychiatr, 111:*652-665, 1940.

Gunnarson, S.: Electroencephalographic examinations of imbeciles. *Acta Paediatrica, 32:*240-248, 1945.

Hadidian, Z., and Hoagland, H.: Chemical pacemakers for alpha brain wave frequencies in general paresis. *Am J Psychol, 126:*517-518, 1939.

Hadley, J.M.: Some relationships between electrical signs of central and peripheral activity. I. During Rest. *J Exp Psychol, 27:*640-656, 1940.

Hadley, J.M.: Some relationships between electrical signs of central and peripheral activity. II. During "mental work." *J Exp Psychol, 28:*53-62, 1941.

Hailman, H.F., et al.: Influence of lowered barometric pressure on electroencephalogram. *Proc Soc Exp Biol Med, 54:*74-76, 1943.

Halstead, W.C.: Specialization of behavioral functions and the frontal lobes. *Res Publ Assoc Nerv Ment Dis, 27:*59-66, 1948.

Harlan, W.L., et al.: Electric activity produced by eye flutter simulating frontal electroencephalographic rhythms. *Electroencephalogr Clin Neurophysiol, 10:*164, 1958.

Harris, H.I.: Repression and the electroencephalogram *Psychoanal Q, 21:*402-407, 1952.

Harrison, J.M.: An examination of the varying effect of certain stimuli upon the alpha rhythm of a single normal individual. *Br J Psychol, 37:*20-29, 1946.

Harvey, E.N., et al.: Cerebral processes during sleep as studied by human brain potentials. *Science, 85:*443-444, 1937.

Heath, R.G., et al.: Effect on behavior in humans with the administration of taraxein. *Am J Psychiatry, 114:*14-24, 1957.

Heimann, H., and Spoerri, T.: Electroencephalographic investigation in the hypnotized. *Mschr Psychiatr Neurol, 125:*261-271, 1953.

Henry, C.E.: Electroencephalographic individual differences and their constancy. I. During sleep. *J Exp Psychol, 29:*117-132, 1941.

Henry, C.E.: Electroencephalographic individual differences and their constancy. II. During waking. *J Exp Psychol, 29:*236-241, 1941.

Henry, C.E., and Knott, J.R.: Rhythm of the electroencephalogram. A note on the relationship between "personality" and A. *J Exp Psychol, 28:*362-366, 1941.

Henry, C.E.: Electroencephalograms of normal children. Society for Research in Child Development Monograph, *9:*1-71, 1944.

Henrie, J.R., et al.: Alteration of human consciousness by nitrous oxide as assessed by electroencephalography and psychological tests. *Anesthesiology, 22:*247-259, 1961.

Henssge,: Treatment with alpha wave action current in organic brain diseases. *Phychiatr Neurol Wschr, 41:*72-73, 1939.

Herberg, L.J.: Eye movements in relation to the EEG alpha rhythm, speed of work and intelligence score. *J Natl Inst Personnel Res, 7:*98-103, 1958.

Hess, M.R.: The EEG in tension states. *Ann Med Psychol,* 1949.

Heusler, A.F., et al.: Comparative EEG studies of tranquilizing drugs. *Universitas Medica, 5:*33-47, 1962.

Hill, D., and Watterson, D.: Electroencephalographic studies of psychopathic personalities. *J Neurol Psychiatr, 5:*47-65, 1942.

Hill, D.: Cerebral dysrhythmia, its significance in aggressive behaviour. *Proc R Soc Med, 37:*317-330, 1944.

Hoagland, H.: Electrical brain waves and temperature. *Science, 84:*139-140, 1936.

Hoagland, H.: On the mechanism of the Berger Rhythm in normal man and in general paretics. *Am J Physiol, 116:*77-78, 1936.

Hoagland, H.: Pacemakers of human brain waves in normals and in general paretics. *Am J Physiol, 116:*604-615, 1936.

Hoagland, H.: Some pacemaker aspects of rhythmic activity in the nervous system. *Cold Spring Harbor Symp Quant Biol, 4:*267-284, 1936.

Hoagland, H.: Temperature characteristics of the "Berger Rhythm" in men. *Science, 83:* 84-85, 1936.

Hoagland, H.: Brain metabolism and brain wave frequencies. *Am J Physiol, 123:*102, 1938.

Hoagland, H.: Rhythmic behavior of the nervous system. *Science, 109:*157-164, 1949.

Hodge, R.S., et al.: Juvenile delinquency: An electrophysiological psychological and social study. *Br J Delinquency, 3:*1-18, 1953.

Hoefer, P.F.A., et al.: Periodicity and hypsarrhythmia in the EEG. *AMA Arch Neurol, 9:*424, 1963.

Holmgren, G., and Kraepelin, S.: EEG studies of asthmatic children. *Acta Paediatr UPPS, 42:*432-441, 1953.

Holmberg, G., and Martens, S.: Electroencephalographic changes in man correlated with blood alcohol concentration and some other conditions following standardized ingestion of alcohol. *Q J Stud Alcohol, 16:*411-424, 1955.

Horsten, G.P.M.: Influence of the body temperature on the EEG. *Acta Brevia Neerl, 17:*23-25, 1949.

Hugelin, A.: The physiologic bases of vigilance. *Encephale, 45:*267-292, 1956.

Ingvar, D.H.: Intelligence, personality and brain rhythms in a socially isolated community. *Nature, 185:*484-485, 1960.

Israel, L., et al.: Modifications of electroencephalographic rhythms during relaxation. Analysis of frequency. *Rev Med Psychosom, 3:*133-136, 1960.

Ivanova, M.P.: On the correlation between the duration of the depression of the basic brain electrical rhythms and the latency of motor reaction. *J Higher Nerv Activ (Moscow), 12:*437-442, 1962.

Ivanova, M.P.: Changes of biopotentials in human brain in connection with physical efforts. *J Higher Nerv Activ (Moscow), 12:*202-207, 1962.

Janzen, R., and Kornmueller, A.E.: Cerebral bioelectrical phenomena of the changes of state of consciousness. *Dtsch Z Nervenheilk, 149:*74-92, 1939.

Jasper, H.H., and Carmichael, L.: Electrical potentials from the intact human brain. *Science, 81:*51-53, 1935.

Jasper, H.H.: Cortical and excitatory state and synchronism in the control of bioelectric autonomous rhythms. *Cold Spring Harbor Symp Quant Biol, 4:*320-338, 1936.

Jasper, H.H.: Cortical excitatory state and variability in human brain rhythms. *Science, 83:*259-260, 1936.

Jasper, H.H., and Cruikshank, R.M.: Variations in blocking time of occipital alpha potentials in man as affected by the intensity and duration of light stimulation. *Psychol Bull, 33:*770-771, 1936.

Jasper, H.H., and Cruikshank, R.M.: Visual stimulation and the after image as affecting the occipital alpha rhythm. *J Gen Psychol, 17:*29-48, 1937.

Jasper, H.H., and Raney, E.T.: The physiology of lateral cerebral dominance. *Psychol Bull, 34:*151-165, 1937.

Jasper, H.H.: Charting the sea of brain waves. *Science, 108:*343-347, 1948.

Jenkins, R.L., and Pacella, B.L.: Electroencephalographic studies of delinquent boys. *Am J Orthopsychiatry, 13:*107-120, 1943.

Jensen, A.V., et al.: Changes in brain structure and memory after intermittent exposure to simulated altitude of 30,000 feet. *Arch Neurol Psychiatr, 60:*221-239, 1948.

Jiminez Vargas, J.: Some observations on the EEG manifestations of mental activity and emotional reactions. *Trab Inst NAC Cienc Med, 4:*287-292, 1945.

Jiminez Vargas, J.: Observations on the electroencephalographic manifestations of mental activity and emotional reactions. *Rev Espan Fisiol, 1:*1-8, 1945.

Jirmounskaya, E.A.: The limits of normal variations of particular characteristics in the electroencephalogram. *Nevropat I Psichiatr, 62:*862-865, 1962.

Johnson, L.C., and Ulett, G.A.: Quantitative study of pattern and stability of resting electroencephalographic activity in a young adult group. *Electroencephalogr Clin Neurophysiol, 11:*233, 1959.

Jouvet, M., et al.: Neurophysiologic documents concerning the mechanism of attention in man. *Rev Neurol (Paris), 100:*437-450, 1959.

Jouvet, M., et al.: Comparative electroencephalographic analysis of physiologic sleep in man and cat. *Rev Neurol, 103:*189-205, 1960.

Jung, R.: The electroencephalogram and the clinical application: Methods of recording, registration and interpretation of the EEG. *Nervenarzt, 12:*569-591, 1939.

Jung, R.: The EEG and its clinical application. The EEG of normals, its variations and changes and their meaning for the pathological EEG. *Nervenarzt, 14:*57 and 104, 1941.

Kaada, B.R.: Electrical activity of the brain. *Ann Rev Physiol, 15:*39-62, 1953.

Kaada, B.R., and Bruland, H.: Blocking of the cortically induced behavioral attention (orienting) response by chlorpromazine. *Psychopharmacologia, 1:*372-388, 1960.

Kakegawa, Y.: Electroencephalographic changes during mental efforts. *Folia Psychiatr Neurol Jap, 2:*109-123, 1947.

Kanigowski, Z.: Electroencephalographic alterations in work and mental weariness under the influence of alcohol. *Neurol Neurochir Psychiatr Polska, 2:*309-326, 1952.

Kaplan, H.A., and Browder, J.: Observations on the clinical and brain wave patterns of professional boxers. *JAMA, 156:*1138-1144, 1954.

Karashima, S.: Some observations on the autocorrelation curves and power spectra of electroencephalograms obtained on mentally deficient children. *Nagasaki Igakkai Z, 35:*1089-1109, 1960.

Karp, E., et al.: Critical flicker frequency and EEG alpha: A reliability study. *Electroencephalogr Clin Neurophysiol, 14:*60, 1962.

Karreman, G.: Some types of relaxation oscillations as models of all-or-none phenomena. *Bull Math Biophys, 11:*311-318, 1949.

Kaufman, I.C., and Hoagland, H.: Dominant brain wave frequencies as measures of physiochemical processes in cerebral cortex. *Arch Neurol Psychiatr, 56:*207-215, 1946.

Kawakami, M., and Sawyer, C.H.: Neuroendocrine correlates of changes in brain activity thresholds by sex steroids and pituitary hormones. *Endocrinology, 65:*652-668, 1959.

Kawi, A.A.: Electroencephalography and the sedation threshold (comparative studies on drug-induced phenomena). *Dis Nerv Syst, 21:*508-512, 1960.

Kellaway, P.: The use of sedative-induced sleep as an aid to electroencephalographic diagnosis in children. *J Pediatr, 37:*862-877, 1950.

Kennedy, J.L., et al.: A new electroencephalogram associated with thinking. *Science, 108:*527-529, 1948.

Kennedy, J.L., and Gottsdanker, R.M.: The relation between the kappa electroencephalogram and recall. *Am Psychol, 4:*224, 1949.

Kennard, M.A., et al.: Correlation between electroencephalograms and deep reflexes in normal adults. *Dis Nerv Syst, 5:*337-342, 1945.

Kennard, M.A.: Value of electroencephalogram in the field of psychosomatic medicine. *Diplomate, 19:*115-116, 1947.

Kennard, M.A.: Inheritance of electroencephalogram patterns in children with behavior disorders. *Psychosom Med, 11:*151-157, 1949.

Kennard, M.A.: The value of the electroencephalogram as an index of generalized cortical activity. *Confin Neurol, 9:*193-205, 1949.

Kennard, M.A.: Factors affecting the electroencephalograms of children and adolescents. *Arch Neurol Psychiatr, 63:*822-826, 1950.

Kennard, M.A.: The electroencephalogram in psychological disorders. *Psychosom Med, 15:*95-115, 1953.

Kennard, M.A.: The electroencephalogram and disorders of behavior. A review. *J Nerv Ment Dis, 124:*103-124, 1956.

Kennard, M.A., and Schwartzman, A.E.: A longitudinal study of electroencephalographic frequency patterns in mental hospital patients and normal controls. *Electroencephalogr Clin Neurophysiol, 9:*263, 1957.

Kennard, M.A., et al: Sleep, consciousness, and the electroencephalographic rhythm. *Arch Neurol Psychiatr, 79:*328-335, 1958.

Kessler, L.B.: Alcoholism: A psychological and eletroencephalographic study. *Am Psychol, 4:*275, 1949.

Kibbler, G.O., et al.: Relations of the alpha rhythm of the brain to psychomotor phenomena. *Nature (Lond), 164:*371, 1949.

Kidron, D.P., and Weiss, A.: Maturation defect. Electroencephalographic and psychological correlation. *Psychiatr Neurol (Basel), 135:*378-401, 1958.

Kirstein, L.: Suppression-burst activity during sleep. *Electroencephalogr Clin Neurophysiol, 6:*671, 1954.

Kleitman, N.: Sleep, wakefulness and consciousness. *Psychol Bull, 54:*354-360, 1957.

Klove, H.: Relationship of differential electroencephalographic patterns to distribution of Wechsler-Bellevue scores. *Neurology, 9:*871-876, 1959.

Knauel, H.: Electroencephalography in the diagnosis of children and juveniles with behavior disturbances. *Nervenarzt, 31:*279-281, 1960.

Knott, J.R.: Brain potentials during silent and oral reading. *J Gen Psychol, 18:*57-62, 1938.

Knott, J.R.: Reduced latent time of blocking of the Berger Rhythm to light stimuli.

Proc Soc Exp Biol Med, 38:216-217, 1938.

Knott, J.R., et al.: Brain potentials during sleep. A comparative study of the dominant and non-dominant alpha groups. Contribution to the study of the human EEG. *J Exp Psychol, 24*:157-168, 1939.

Knott, J.R., and Gibbs, F.A.: A fourier transform of the electroencephalogram from one to eighteen years. *Psychol Bull, 36*:512-513, 1939.

Knott, J.R.: Some effects of mental set upon electrophysiological processes of the human cerebral cortex. *J Exp Psychol, 24*:384-405, 1939.

Knott, J.R.: The physiological correlates of intelligence. *39th Year Book of the National Society for the Study of Education, 1*:133, 1940.

Knott, J.R., and Henry, C.E.: The conditioning of the blocking of the alpha rhythm of the human electroencephalogram. *J Exp Psychol, 28*:134-144, 1941.

Knott, J.R., and Hadley, H.D.: Changes in the energy of the alpha band of the electro-encephalogram following stimulation. *Psychol Bull, 39*:600, 1942.

Knott, J.R., et al.: Some electroencephalographic correlates of intelligence in eight year and twelve year old children. *J Exp Psychol, 30*:380-391, 1942.

Knott, J.R., et al.: Construction notes on an American equivalent of the Walter Analyser. *Electroencephalogr Clin Neurophysiol, 3*:91, 1951.

Knowlton, G.C., et al.: Electromylography of fatigue. *Arch Phys Med, 32*:648-652, 1951.

Knox, G.W.: The control of occipital brain wave frequency, voltage, and wave form by means of flashing light stimuli. *Am J Optom, 2*:345-349, 1950.

Kodman, F., et al.: Wakefulness in catatonic schizophrenia. *Confin Psychiatr (Basel), 5*:189-195, 1962.

Kohler, W., and Held, R.: The cortical correlate of pattern vision. *Science, 109*:442, 1949. *Science, 110*:414-419, 1949.

Koopman, L.J.: Quantitative electroencephalography. *Arch Neurol Physiol, 26*:303-322, 1942.

Korenyi, C., et al.: Placebo-controlled electroencephalographic comparison of benzheta-mine with three anorexgenics. *Curr Ther Res, 3*:207-211, 1961.

Kornmuller, A.E.: Bioelectrical phenomena of the cerebral cortex. *Frtsch Neurol Psychiatr, 5:4-9-441, 1933. Dtsch Z Nervenheilk, 130*:44, 1933.

Kornmuller, A.E., and Schaeder, J.A.: Arrangement of electrodes when registering bio-electric potential variations of the cortex. *J Neurophysiol, 1*:287-300, 1938.

Kornmueller, A.E.: Further results about the normal cerebral bioelectrical phenomena in man by derivation from the scalp. Mechanism of cortical stimuli and specific areas of the cerebral cortex. *Z Gesamte Neurol Psychiatr, 168*:248-268, 1940.

Kornmueller, A.E.: Newer results in the cerebral bioelectrical studies in normal men. *Zentralbl Neur Psychiatr, 102*:192, 1942.

Kornmueller, A.E.: Basic phenomena of the EEG, their analysis and evaluation. *Klin Physiol, 1*:27-43, 1960.

Kozhevnikov, V.A., and Soroko, V.I.: Electronic measurement of EEG alpha-rhythm changes appearing upon imposition of stimulation. *Probl Fiziol Akust Moskva, 4*:80-83, 1959.

Krakau, C.E.T., and Nyman, G.E.: On the effect of artificial fever on the alpha activity in man. *Acta Physiol Scand, 29*:281-292, 1953.

Kreezer, G.: Electric potentials of the brain in certain types of mental deficiency. *Arch Neurol Psychiatr, 36*:1206-1214, 1936.

Kreezer, G., and Smith, F.W.: Brain potentials in the hereditary type of mental deficiency. *Psychol Bull, 34*:535-536, 1937.

Kreezer, G.: The dependence of the electroencephalogram upon intelligence level. *Psychol Bull, 34:*769-770, 1937.

Kreezer, G.: The EEG and its uses in psychology. *Am J Psychol, 51:*737-759, 1938.

Kreezer, G.: The human electroencephalogram at different levels of intelligence and for different types of mental deficiency. *Yearbook Am Phil Soc,* 1938, (1937), pp. 238-240.

Kreezer, G.: Intelligence level and occipital alpha rhythm in the mongolian type of mental deficiency. *Am J Psychol, 52:*503-532, 1939.

Kreezer, G.: The relation of intelligence level and the electroencephalogram. *Year Book of the National Society for the Study of Education, 39:*130-133, 1939.

Kreezer, G.L., and Smith, F.W.: The relation of the alpha rhythm of the electroencephalogram and intelligence level in the nondifferentiated familial type of mental deficiency. *J Psychol, 2:*48-51, 1950.

Kropfl, W.J., et al.: Apparatus for scoring selected electroencephalographic rhythms. *Electroencephalogr Clin Neurophysiol, 14:*921, 1962.

Kugler, H., et al.: The EEG picture during accidentally produced dreams. *Rev Neurol, 107:*138-141, 1962.

Kugler, J., and Finckh, R.: The sleep activation of the EEG with a barbiturate free product (thalidomid). *Psychiatr Neurol (Basel), 143:*45-54, 1962.

Lairy, G.C.: The concept of normality in electroencephalography. *Rev Psychol Normale Pathol, 4:*445, 1961.

Lamb, W., et al. Premenstrual tension-EEG, hormonal and psychiatric evaluation. *Am J Psychiatry, 109:*840-848, 1953.

Lansing, R.W., et al.: Reaction time and EEG activation under alerted and non-alerted conditions. *J Exp Psychol, 58:*1-7, 1959.

Larsson, L.E., et al.: Further investigations on the development of the alpha frequency of human brain potentials in normal and pathological conditions. *Acta Paediatr UPPS (Suppl), 76:*62-70, 1949.

Larsson, L.E., et al.: A study of the changes in the alpha frequency of human brain potentials in normal and pathological conditions. *Acta Paediatr, 38:*404-412, 1949.

Larsson, L.E., et al.: Examination of boxers before and after fighting (A) clinical study, (B) electroencephalographic study. *Nord Med, 47:*25-28, 1952.

Larsson, L.E.: Can the non-specific EEG response be an artefact caused by scalp movements? *Electroencephalogr Clin Neurophysiol, 12:*502, 1960.

Laufberger, V.: Conditioned response in the EEG through imagination. *CR Soc Biol (Paris), 144:*467-468, 1950.

Le Gros, Clark W.: The thirty-second Maudsley Lecture: Sensory experience and brain structure. *J Ment Sci, 104:*1-13, 1958.

Lemere, F.: The significance of individual differences in the Berger Rhythm. *Brain, 59:*366-375, 1936.

Lemere, F.: Berger's Alpha Rhythm in organic lesions of the brain. *Brain, 60:*118-125, 1937.

Lemere, F.: Electroencephalograph as a method of distinguishing true from false blindness. *JAMA, 118:*884-885, 1942.

Lennox, W.G., et al.: The brain wave pattern, a hereditary trait. *J Hered, 36:*223-243, 1945.

Lesny, I., and Stein, J.: The effect of sonic stimulation by a constant tone of various frequency on the EEG in children. *CS Neurol, 25:*50-59, 1962.

Lesny, I., and Roessler, M.: Premature electroencephalogram. *CS Neurol, 26:*50-54, 1963.

Lester, D.: A new method for the determination of the effectiveness of sleep-inducing agents in humans. *Compr Psychiatry, 1:*301-307, 1960.

Lettich, E., and Margerison, J.H.: The use of data from low frequency analysis to illustrate serial EEG changes in depressed patients during treatments with iproniazid. *J Ment Sci, 106:*1111-1114, 1960.

Lettich, E., and Margerison, J.H.: Presentation of data from low frequency analysis to illustrate serial changes in the electroencephalogram. *Electroencephalogr Clin Neurophysiol, 13:*606, 1961.

Levy, S., and Kennard, M.A.: The electroencephalographic pattern of patients with psychologic disorders of various ages. *J Nerv Ment Dis, 118:*416-428, 1953.

Levy, S., and Kennard, M.: A study of the electroencephalogram as related to personality structure in a group of inmates of a state penitentiary. *Am J Psychiatry, 109:* 832-839, 1953.

Liberson, W.T.: Study of word association processes. Part I. Depression of alpha activity during administration of the test. *Digest Neurol Psychiatr, 13:*594-601, 1945.

Lindsley, D.B.: Brain potentials in children and adults. *Science, 84:*354, 1936.

Lindsley, D.B., and Rubinstein, B.B.: Relation between brain potentials and some other physiological variables. *Proc Soc Exp Biol Med, 35:*558-563, 1937.

Lindsley, D.B.: Electrical potentials of the brain in children and adults. *J Gen Psychol, 19:*285-306, 1938.

Lindsley, D.B.: Foci of activity of the alpha rhythm in the human EEG. *J Exp Psychol, 23:*159-171, 1938.

Lindsley, D.B.: Longitudinal study of the occipital alpha rhythm in normal children, frequency and amplitude standards. *J Genet Psychol, 55:*197-213, 1939.

Lindsley, D.B.: Bilateral differences in brain potentials from the two cerebral hemispheres in relation to laterality and stuttering. *J Exp Psychol, 26:*211-225, 1940.

Lindsley, D.B.: Psychological phenomena and the electroencephalogram. *Electroencephalogr Clin Neurophysiol, 4:*457, 1952.

Lindquist, T.: Finger tremor and alpha waves on the electroencephalogram. *Acta Med Scand, 108:*580-585, 1941.

Livanov, M.N.: Rhythmical stimuli and the interrelation between the areas of the cerebral cortex. *J Physiol (USSR), 28:*183-194, 1940.

Livanov, M.N.: Spatial analysis of bioelectrical activity of the brain. *J Higher Nerv Activ (Moscow), 12:*399-407, 1962.

Loomis, A., et al.: Electrical potentials of the human brain. *J Exp Psychol, 19:*249-279, 1936.

Low, N.L., and Dawson, S.P.: EEG findings in juvenile delinquency. *Pediatrics, 28:*452-457, 1961.

Lundholm, H., and Lowenback, H.: Hypnosis and the alpha activity of the electroencephalogram. *Character and Personality, 11:*145-149, 1942.

Lytton, G.J., and Knobel, M.: Diagnosis and treatment of behavior disorders in children. *Dis Nerv Syst, 20:*334-340, 1959.

MacKay, D.M.: Some experiments on the perception of patterns modulated at the alpha frequency. *Electroencephalogr Clin Neurophysiol, 5:*559, 1953.

Maggs, R., and Turton, E.C.: Some EEG findings in old age and their relationship to affective disorder. *J Ment Sci, 102:*812-818, 1956.

Mangan, G.L., and Adcock, C.J.: EEG correlates of perceptual vigilance and defense. *Percept Mot Skills, 14:*197-198, 1962.

Marinesco, G., et al.: EEG studies: Normal and hypnotic sleep. *Bull Acad Natl Med (Paris), 117:*273-276, 1937.

Martinson, B.M.: Study of brain potentials during mental blocking. *J Exp Psychol, 24:* 143-156, 1939.

Maslove, N.P.: The electroencephalogram of neurasthenics in the waking state, during sleep and at the time of wakening. *Pavlov J Higher Nerv Activ, 8:*482-488, 1958.

Masland, R.L., et al.: The electroencephalogram following occipital lobectomy. *Electroencephalogr Clin Neurophysiol, 1:*273, 1949.

Mathis, P., and Fischgold, H.: Utilization of "nitonan" as detector of alpha ryhthm in ancient cranio-encephalic traumatism. *Psychiatr Neurol (Basel), 140:*41-50, 1960.

Matthys, E., and Popowycz, V.: Unilateral posttraumatic abolition of the arrest reaction of Berger. *Acta Neurol Belg, 61:*456-459, 1961.

McCranie, E.J., et al.: The electroencephalogram in hypnotic age regression. *Psychiatr Q., 29:*85-88, 1955.

Merrill, G.G., and Cook, E.E.: The electroencephalogram in the Negro. *Electorencephalogr Clin Neurophysiol, 9:*531, 1957.

Metrakos, K., and Metrakos, J.D.: Is the centrencephalic EEG inherited as a dominant? *Electroencephalogr Clin Neurophysiol, 13:*289, 1961.

Meurice, E.: Report on the EEG and psychologic phenomena from the colloquy of Marseille. *Acta Neurol Psychiatr Belg, 56:*253-263, 1956.

Mimura, K.: On the frequency characteristics of the occipital EEG activities. *Brain Nerve, 10:*397-404, 1958.

Mirsky, A.F., and Cardon, P.V.: A comparison of the behavioral and physiological changes accompanying sleep deprivation and chlorpromazine administration in man. *Electroencephalogr Clin Neurophysiol, 14:*1, 1962.

Miyazaki, M., and Torres, F.: Alterations of the alpha rhythm occurring after temporal lobe resections in man. *AMA Arch Neurol, 1:*502-512, 1959.

Monakhow, K.K.: On the spatial distribution of the bioelectrical activity. *Bull Exp Biol Med, 50:*23-28, 1960.

Mond, W.: An index for the determination of the stability of the wave sequence in the occipital recording in EEG. *Psychiatr Neurol, 129:*411-418, 1955.

Monnier, M.: Organization plan, continuity and developmental stages of cerebral electric activities. *Dialectica, 11:*167-178, 1957.

Morin, G., et al.: EEG study of activity induced by rhythmic intermittent photic stimulation in man. *J Physiol (Paris), 40:*199-222, 1948.

Morison, R.S., et al.: On the propagation of certain cortical potentials. *Am J Physiol, 131:*744-751, 1941.

Morrice, J.K.W.: Slow wave production in the EEG, with reference to hyperpnoea, carbon dioxide and autonomic balance. *Electroencephalogr Clin Neurophysiol, 8:*49, 1956.

Moruzzi, G.: The arrest reaction of Berger and the physiological problem of sleep. *Ricerca Sci, 20:*491-495, 1950.

Motokawa, K., and Tuziguti, K.: About the distribution of alpha waves on the cortex of humans during optically excited states. *Jap J Med Sci, 9:*135-144, 1943.

Motokawa, K.: On the mechanism of origin and inhibition of brain potential waves. *Tohoku J Exp Med, 45:*297-308, 1943.

Motokawa, K., and Tuziguti, K.: The difference in phase of alpha waves and local differences in electrical activity of the cerebral cortex of man. *Jap J Med Sci, 10:*23-38, 1944.

Mueller-Limmroth, W., and Caspers, H.: Theories on the mechanism of generation of the spontaneous rhythms in the normal electroencephalogram. *Klin Wochenschr, 34:* 13-14, 1956.

Mundy-Castle, A.C.: Clinical significance of EEG. *S Afr Med J, 27:*298-310, 1953.

Mundy-Castle, A.C., and McKiever, B.L.: A comparative study of the electroencephalograms of normal Africans and Europeans of Southern Africa. *Electroencephalogr Clin Neurophysiol, 5:*533, 1953.

Mundy-Castle, A.C.: The alpha rhythm and rate of visual perception. Preliminary investigation. *J Natl Inst Personnel Res, 6:*38-43, 1955.

Mundy-Castle, A.C.: The electroencephalogram in relation to temperament. *Acta Psychol, 11:*397-411, 1955.

Mundy-Castle, A.C.: The EEG in twenty-two cases of murder or attempted murder. Appendix on possible significance of alphoid rhythms. *J Natl Inst Personnel Res, 6:* 103-120, 1955.

Mundy-Castle, A.C.: The relationship between primary-secondary function and the alpha rhythm of the electroencephalogram. *J Natl Inst Personnel Res, 6:*95-102, 1955.

Obermann, C.E.: Effect on Berger Rhythm of mild affective states. *J Abnorm Soc Psychol, 34:*84-95, 1939.

Obrist, W.D.: The electroencephalogram of normal aged adults. *Electroencephalogr Clin Neurophysiol, 6:*235, 1954.

Obrist, W.D., et al.: Relation of the electroencephalogram to intellectual function in senescence. *J Gerontol, 17:*197-206, 1962.

Offner, F.F.: The EEG as potential mapping: the value of the average monopolar reference. *Electroencephalogr Clin Neurophysiol, 2:*213, 1950.

Okuma, T., et al.: Cortical and subcortical recordings in nonanesthetized and anesthetized periods in man. *Electroencephalogr Clin Neurophysiol, 6:*269, 1954.

Ostow, M.: Psychic function and the electroencephalogram. *Arch Neurol Psychiatr, 64:* 385-400, 1950.

Ostow, M.: A psychoanalytic contribution to the study of brain function. The frontal lobes. *Psychoanal Q, 23:*317-338, 1954.

Ostow, M.: Psychic contents and processes of the brain. *Psychosom Med, 17:*396-406, 1955.

Oswald, I.: Experimental studies of rhythm, anxiety and cerebral vigilance. *J Ment Sci, 105:*269-294, 1959.

Ozaki, T.: On the average time and frequency pattern of photic flicker response in relation to intrinsic alpha activity verified by a new simple method. *Acta Med Nagasaki, 6:*83-90, 1962.

Pampiglione, G.: The phenomenon of adaptation in human EEG. *Rev Neurol, 87:*197, 1952.

Pampiglione, G., and Martin, F.: Periodicity of certain cerebral phenomena. *Schweiz Arch Neurol Neurochir Psychiatr, 71:*277-284, 1953.

Parr, G., and Walter, W.G.: Electrobiology. Normal activity of the human brain. *Electronic Eng, 15:*462-464, 1943.

Penuel, H., et al.: Studies of the electroencephalogram of normal children: comparison of visual and automatic frequency analyses. *Electroencephalogr Clin Neurophysiol, 7:* 15, 1955.

Perkins, F.T.: Genetic study of cerebral action currents. *Science, 79:*418, 1934.

Petersen, I., and Sorbye, R.: Slow posterior rhythm in adults. *Electroencephalogr Clin Neurophysiol, 14:*161, 1962.

Petsche, H., and Marko, A.: Toposcopic studies about the propagation of the alpha rhythm. *Wein Z Nervenheilkd, 12:*87-100, 1955.

Planques, J., and Grezes-Rueff, C.: Electroencephalographic contribution to the report of mental status in the adult. *Ann Med Leg, 33:*253-257, 1953.

Plaza, D.M.: The rapidity and asynchronism of the EEG in some subjects as a stable physical feature of their personality. *Rev Psicol Gen Apl, 11:*243-252, 1956.

Plaza, D.M.: Analytic and comprehensive systematics of the normal human EEG. Psychosomatic personality and EEG. *Rev Psicol Gen Apl, 12:*669-691, 1957.

Popov, C.: The repetitive property of the human brain as studied by the electroencephalogram and the method of after-images. *Nature, 180:*328-329, 1957.

Popov, N.A.: Contribution to the study of the arrest reaction of the alpha rhythm in man. *CR Soc Biol (Paris), 144:*1667-1669, 1950.

Posey, H.T.: The electroencephalogram in mental deficiency. *Am J Ment Defic, 55:*515-520, 1951.

Purpura, D.P.: Observations on the cortical mechanism of EEG activation accompanying behavioral arousal. *Science, 123:*804, 1956.

Ralston, B., and Ajmone-Marsan, C.: Thalamic control of certain normal and abnormal cortical rhythms. *Electroencephalogr Clin Neurophysiol, 8:*559, 1956.

Raney, E.T.: Bilateral brain potentials and lateral dominance in identical twins. *Psychol Bull, 34:*534, 1937.

Rechtschaffen, A., and Maron, L.: The effect of amphetamine on the sleep cycle. *Electroencephalogr Clin Neurophysiol, 16:*438, 1964.

Redlich, F.C., Callahan, A., and Mendelson, R.H.: Electroencephalographic changes after eye opening and visual stimulation. *Yale J Biol Med, 18:*367-376, 1946.

Remond, A., and Offner, F.: Topographic studies of EEG activity in the occipital region. *Rev Neurol, 87:*182-189, 1952.

Remond, A., Conte, C., and Zarindjian, M.: Description of some organizational aspects of alpha rhythm in the waking state. Communication a la Society D-EEG, April 1962. *Rev Neurol, 107:*225-231, 1962.

Remond, A., and Conte, C.: The spatio-temporal organization of EEG responses to intermittent photic stimulation at a frequency of 10 flashes per second. *Rev Neurol, 107:*250-257, 1962.

Remy, M.: Affectivity in the EEG. *Ann Med Psychol (Paris), 107:*341, 1949.

Renfrew, A., Haggar, I., and Watson, M.: Predictability of the electroencephalogram in people. *Arch Neurol Psychiatr, 78:*329-338, 1957.

Richter, K., and Jachnik, D.: EEG findings in abnormal children. *Arch Psychiatr Nervenkr, 201:*605-625, 1961.

Roberts, D.R.: An electrophysiological theory of hypnosis. *Int J Clin Exp Hypnosis, 8:* 43-55, 1960.

Robin, A.A., et al.: Neurophysiological aspects of social behavior. *Int J Soc Psychiatr, 2:*33-38, 1956.

Rodin, E.A., Luby, E.D., and Gottlieb, J.S.: The electroencephalogram during prolonged experimental sleep deprivation. *Electroencephalogr Clin Neurophysiol, 14:*544, 1962.

Rohracher, H.: Cerebral electrical phenomena during mental waste. *Z Psychol, 136:*308-324, 1935.

Rohracher, H.: The electrical phenomena of the brain during psychic processes. *Arch Ital Psicol, 15:*113, 1937.

Rohracher, H.: Behavior of alpha waves in intellectual work. *Arch Psicol Neurol (Milan), 3:*528-538, 1941.

Rohracher, H.: A simple index for evaluation of the alpha waves of the electroencephalogram. *Arch Psychiatr Nervenkr, 134*:487-492, 1950.

Rondpierre, J., Verdeaux, G., and Dules, J.: Electroencephalogram and mental illness. *Ann Med Psychol, 108*:361-363, 1950.

Rosenberg, M.: About "As-if-attacks" and their relations to EEG. *Psychiatr Neurol Med Psychol (Leipzig), 11*:46-50, 1959.

Ross, D.A., and Schwab, R.S.: The cortical alpha rhythm in thyroid disorders. *Endocrinology, 25*:75-79, 1939.

Ross, I.S., and Loeser, L.H.: Electroencephalographic findings in essential hypoglycemia. *Electroencephalogr Clin Neurophysiol, 3*:141, 1951.

Rossen, R., Simonson, E., and Baker, J.: Electroencephalograms during hypoxia in healthy men. Responses characteristic for normal aging. *AMA Arch Neurol, 5*:648-654, 1961.

Roth, D., and Simek, J.: Electroencephalographic finding in essential and symptomatic narcolepsy. *Neurol Psychiatr Cesk, 15*:80-109, 1952.

Roth, M., and Green, J.: The lambda wave as a normal physiological phenomenon in the human EEG. *Nature, 172*:864-866, 1953.

Rubin, M.A.: The distribution of the alpha rhythm over the cerebral cortex of normal man. *J Neurophysiol, 1*:313-323, 1938.

Rubin, M.A.: A variability study of the normal and schziophrenic occipital alpha rhythm. *J Psychol, 6*:325-334, 1938.

Rubin, M.A., and Cohen, L.H.: A variability study of the normal and schizophrenic occipital alpha rhythm. II. The EEG and imagery type. *J Ment Sci, 85*:779-783, 1939.

Rubin, S., and Bowman, K.M.: Electroencephalographic and personality correlates in peptic ulcer. *Psychosom Med, 4*:309-318, 1942.

Ruf, H., and Vattuone, G.: Cerebral potentials during reading. *Arch Psychiatr, 116*:329-338, 1943.

Sager, O., and Herman, M.: Statistical analysis of the EEG from the point of view of amplitudes. *Rev Neurol, 71*:625-633, 1939.

Sarkisov, S.A., and Livanov, M.N.: Characteristics of Berger's rhythm in normal and pathological states. *Nervopatol Psikhiatr, 10*:28, 1941.

Sato, K., and Nakane, K.: Note on the general probability function of the alpha wave amplitudes in electroencephalogram. *Folia Psychiatr Neurol Jap, 3*:44-57, 1948.

Sato, K.: On the relationship between the simple practical method for determining the amplitude of the EEG tracings and the frequency analysis. *Folia Psychiatr Neurol Jap, 8*:232-236, 1954.

Saul, L.J., Davis, H., and Davis, P.A.: Correlations between electroencephalograms and the psychological organization of the individual. *Trans Am Neurol Assoc, 63*:167-169, 1937.

Saul, L.J., Davis, H., and Davis, P.A.: Psychologic correlations with the electroencephalogram. *Psychosom Med, 11*:361-376, 1949.

Saunders, D.R.: Further implications of Mundy-Castle's correlations between EEG and Wechsler-Bellvue variables. *J Natl Inst Personnel Res, 8*:91-101, 1960. (*Cf.* comment by Mundy Castle, pp. 102-105.)

Saunders, M.G.: The measurement of phase shift in electroencephalograph pen recorders. *Electroencephalogr Clin Neurophysiol, 9*:344, 1957.

Schmelvkin, D.G.: Electroencephalogram and its clinical significance; localization of alpha rhythm. *Sov Psikonecrol, 16*:82, 1940.

Schuetz, E., Mueller, H.W., and Schoenenberg, H.: The development of central nervous rhythms in the electroencephalogram of the child. *Z Gesamte Exp Med, 117:*157-170 1951.

Schwarz, B.E., Wakim, K.G., Bickford, R.G., and Lichtenheld, F.R.: Behavioral and electroencephalographic effects of hallucinogenic drugs. *Arch Neurol Psychiatr, 75:*83-90, 1956.

Sem-Jacobsen, C.W., Petersen, M.C., Lazarte, J.A., Dodge, H.W., and Holman, C.B.: Electroencephalographic rhythms from the depths of the frontal lobe in 60 psychotic patients. *Electroencephalogr Clin Neurophysiol, 7:*193, 1955.

Sem-Jacobsen, C.W., Dodge, H.W., Jr., Petersen, M.C., Lazarte, J.A., and Holman, C.B.: Electroencephalographic rhythms from the depths of the parietal, occipital and temporal lobes in man. *Electroencephalogr Clin Neurophysiol, 8:*263, 1956.

Shagass, C.: An attempt to correlate the alpha frequency of the electroencephalogram with intelligence. *Proc Assoc Comm Aviation Med Res NRC (Can),* C-2994, 1942.

Shagass, C.: Conditioning human alpha rhythm to voluntary stimulus. *J Exp Psychol, 31:*367-379, 1942.

Shagass, C., and Johnson, E.P.: Course of acquisition of conditioned response of occipital alpha rhythm. *J Exp Psychol, 33:*201-209, 1943.

Shagass, C.: Attempt to correlate occipital alpha frequency with performance on mental ability test. *J Exp Psychol, 36:*88-92, 1946.

Shagass, C.: Differentiation between anxiety and depression by the photically activated electroencephalogram. *Am J Psychiatry, 112:*41-46, 1955.

Shagass, C., and Kerenyi, A.B.: Neurophysiologic studies of personality. *J Nerv Ment Dis, 126:*141-147, 1958.

Sharpless, S., and Jasper, H.: Habituation of the arousal reaction. *Brain, 79:*655-680, 1956.

Sherman, M.: Frustration reactions of normal and neurotic persons. *J Psychol, 13:*3-19, 1942.

Sherman, M., and Jost, H.: Diagnosis of juvenile psychosis. *Am J Dis Child, 65:*868-872, 1943.

Shmelkin, D.G.: Diagnostic value of alpha rhythm in the EEG in visual disorders. *Nevropatol Psikhiat (Moscow), 55:*171-175, 1955, and *(Cf. ABS. Sov Med, 1*(153): Part B, 1957.

Short, P.L.: The objective study of mental imagery. *Br J Psychol, 44:*38-51, 1953.

Short, P.L., and Walter, W.G.: The relationship between physiological variables and stereognosis. *Electroencephalogr Clin Neurophysiol, 6:*29, 1953.

Silverman, A., et al.: Studies in the processes of aging: electroencephalographic findings in 400 elderly subjects. *Electroencephalogr Clin Neurophysiol, 7:*67, 1955.

Silverman, D., and Morisaki, A.: Reevaluation of sleep electroencephalography. *Electroencephalogr Clin Neurophysiol, 10:*425, 1958.

Silverman, A.J., et al.: Studies on the processes of aging. 4. Physiologic influences on psychic functioning in elderly people. *Geriatrics, 8:*370-376, 1953.

Silverman, D.: EEG of criminals. *Arch Neurol Psychiatr, 52:*38-42, 1944.

Silverman, D., and Rosanoff, W.R.: Electroencephalographic and neurologic studies of homosexuals. *J Nerv Ment Dis, 101:*311-321, 1945.

Silverman, D.: Sleep as a general activation procedure in electroencephalography. *Electroencephalogr Clin Neurophysiol, 8:*317, 1956.

Simon, C.W.: Some immediate effects of drowsiness and sleep on normal human performance. *Hum Factors, 3:*1-17, 1961.

Simon, C.W., and Emmons, W.H.: EEG, consciousness, and sleep. *Science, 124*:1066-1069, 1956.

Sirna, A.A.: An electroencephalographic study of the hypnotic dream. *J Psychol, 20*: 109-113, 1945.

Sisson, B.D., and Ellingson, R.J.: On the relationship between "normal" EEG patterns and personality variables. *J Nerv Ment Dis, 121*:353-358, 1955.

Smith, J.R.: The origin and genesis of rhythm in the electroencephalogram. *Psychol Bull, 34*:534-535, 1937.

Smith, J.R.: The "occipital" and "pre-central" alpha rhythms during the first two years. *J Psychol, 7*:221-226, 1939.

Smith, J.R.: The frequency growth of the human alpha rhythms during normal infancy and childhood. *J Psychol, 11*:177-198, 1941.

Smith, S.M.: Discrimination between electro-encephalograph recordings of normal females and normal males. *Ann Eugen (Lond), 18*:351-353, 1954.

Solomon, P., et al.: Electroencephalographic analyses of behavior problem children. *Am J Psychiatry, 95*:641-658, 1938.

Spiegel, E.A., et al.: The central mechanism of the emotions. *Am J Psychiatry, 108*:426-432, 1951.

Stamm, J.S.: On the relationship between reaction time to light and latency of blocking of the alpha rhythm. *Electroencephalogr Clin Neurophysiol, 4*:61, 1952.

Stevens, J.M., and Derbyshire, A.J.: Shifts along the alert-response continuum during remission of catatonic "stupor" with amobarbital. *Psychosom Med, 20*:99-107, 1958.

Stoller, A.: Slowing of the alpha rhythm of the electroencephalogram and its association with mental deterioration and epilepsy. *J Ment Sci (Lond), 95*:972-984, 1949.

Strauss, H., et al.: EEG studies. Bilateral differences in alpha activity in cases with and without cerebral pathology. *J Mt Sinai Hosp, 9*:957-962, 1943.

Strobos, R.J.: Significance of amplitude asymmetry in the electroencephalogram. *Neurology (Minneap), 10*:799-803, 1960.

Sugar, O.: Asymmetry in occipital electroencephalograms. *Dis Nerv Syst, 8*:141-150, 1947.

Surwillo, W.W.: The relation of response-time variability to age and the influence of brain wave frequency. *Electroencephalogr Clin Neurophysiol, 15*:1029, 1963.

Tarlau, M., et al.: Dysrhythmic migraine with unusual clinical and electroencephalographic features. *Electroencephalogr Clin Neurophysiol, 13*:114, 1961.

Taterka, J., and Katz, J.: Study of correlations between electroencephalographic and psychological patterns in emotionally disturbed children. *Psychosom Med, 17*:62-72, 1955.

Thaler, M.: Relationships among Wechsler, Weigl, Rorschach, EEG findings, and abstract-concrete behavior in a group of normal aged subjects. *J Gerontol, 11*:404-409, 1956.

Therman, P.O.: Bilateral synchronization in the human EEG. *Am J Physiol, 129*:479-480, 1940.

Thiesen, J.W.: Effects of certain forms of emotion on the normal electroencephalogram. *Arch Psychol, 40*:1-85, 1943.

Thomson, M.M., et al.: Brain potential rhythms in a case showing self-induced apparent trance states. *Am J Psychiatry, 93*:1313-1314, 1937.

Toennies, J.F.: Derivation of bioelectrical phenomena from the unopened skull. *J Psychol Neurol (Leipzig), 45*:154-171, 1933.

Toman, J.: Flicker potentials and the alpha rhythm in man. *J Neurophysiol, 4*:51-61, 1941.

Torrents, E.: Analysis of the alpha-waves of the electroencephalogram in man. *CR Soc Biol (Paris), 134*:295-297, 1940.

Travis, L.E.: Brain potentials and the temporal course of consciousness. *J Exp Psychol, 21*:302-309, 1937.

Travis, L.E., et al.: Effect of response on the latency and frequency of the Berger Rhythm. *J Gen Psychol, 16*:391-401, 1937.

Travis, L.E., and Gottlober, A.: How consistent are an individual's brain potentials from day to day? *Science, 85*:223-234, 1937.

Travis, L.E., and Egan, J.P.: Conditioning of the electrical response of the cortex. *J Exp Psychol, 22*:524-531, 1938.

Travis, L.E., and Barber, V.: The effect of tactile stimulation upon the Berger rhythm. *J Exp Psychol, 22*:269-272, 1938.

Travis, L.E., and Egan, J.P.: Increase in frequency of the alpha rhythm by verbal stimulation. *J Exp Psychol, 23*:384-393, 1938.

True, R.M., and Stephenson, C.W.: Controlled experiments correlating electroencephalogram, pulse, and plantar reflexes with hypnotic age regression and induced emotional states. *J Personality, 1*:252-263, 1951.

Tyler, D.B., et al.: The effect of experimental insomnia on the rate of potential changes in the brain. *Am J Physiol, 149*:185-193, 1947.

Uchida, H.: The autocorrelograms of elderly brain waves and their power spectra. *Nagasaki Igkkai Zashi, 38*:516-550, 1963.

Ulett, G.A., et al.: Electrocortical changes during conditioning. *Recent Adv Biol Psychiatr, 8*:106-122, 1960.

Ulett, G.A.: The relationship of the EEG to emotions. *Psychiatr Res Rep, 12*:176-182, 1960.

Ulett, G.A., et al.: Influence of chlordiazepoxide on drug alerted EEG patterns and behavior. *Med Exp, 5*:386-390, 1961.

Uttley, A.M.: The classification of signals in the nervous system. *Electroencephalogr Clin Neurophysiol, 6*:479, 1954.

Van Hof, M.W.: The relation between the cortical responses to flash and to flicker in man. *Acta Physiol Pharmacol Neerl, 9*:210-224, 1960.

Van Leeuwen, W.S., and Kok, L.: Some ways in which EEG changes may be produced by photic stimulation. *Folia Psychiatr Neerl, 4*:519-524, 1953.

Van Wulfften Palthe, P.M.: Electroencephalographic examination in healthy young men (special edition). *Aeromed Acta Soesterberg*, 1956, pp. 207-225.

Veit, H., et al.: A study of the use of record music in the electroencephalography laboratory. *Electroencephalogr Clin Neurophysiol, 11*:582, 1959.

Veit, H., et al.: A study of the use of recorded music in the electroencephalography laboratory. *Electroencephalogr Clin Neurophysiol, 11*:809, 1959.

Verdeaux, G., and Verdeaux, J.: Electroencephalographic study of a large group of first offenders and chronic delinquents during the course of their detention. *Ann Med Psychol, 2*:643-658, 1955.

Verhaegen, P.: The EEG in the autochtonous from congo and the racial differences. *Acta Neurol Psychiatr Belg, 56*:842-852, 1956.

Vesely, L.: Electroencephalic recording of hypnotic states. *Neurol Psychiatr Cesk, 13*:210-219, 1950.

Visser, S.L.: Correlations between the contingent alpha blocking, EEG characteristics and clinical diagnosis. *Electroencephalogr Clin Neurophysiol, 13*:438, 1961.

Vogel, F., and Goetze, W.: Family studies for the genetics of the normal electroencephalogram. *Disch Z Nervenheilk, 178:*668-700, 1959.

Vorontsov, D.S.: What does the electroencephalogram express? *Pavlov J Higher Nerv Activ, 10:*42-54, 1960.

Wada, J.: Behavioral and EEG correlates of modified levels of brain neurohumoral agents. *J Neuropsychiatry, 4:*251-254, 1963.

Wada, T., and Shimizu, T.: Automatic EEG-frequency analyzer: An approach to periodometry of alpha-rhythm with electrotachometric system. *Tohoku J Exp Med, 77:* 187-194, 1962.

Waggoner, R.W., and Bagchi, B.K.: Simultaneous intra-twin and inter-twin electroencephalogram. *Univ Mich Hosp Bull, 9:*102-104, 1943.

Walker, A.E., et al.: Photic driving. *Arch Neurol Psychiatr, 52:*117-125, 1944.

Walsh, E.C.: Autonomy of alpha rhythm generators studied by multiple channel cross-correlation. *Electroencephalogr Clin Neurophysiol, 10:*121, 1958.

Walsh, E.G.: Visual reaction time and the alpha-rhythm, an investigation of a scanning hypothesis. *J Physiol, 118:*500-508, 1952.

Walsh, E.G.: "Visual attention" and the alpha-rhythm. *J Physiol, 120:*155-159, 1953.

Walter, R.D., and Yeager, C.L.: Visual imagery and electroencephalographic changes. *Electroencephalogr Clin Neurophysiol, 8:*193, 1956.

Walter, V.J., and Walter, W.G.: The central effects of rhythmic sensory stimulation. *Electroencephalogr Clin Neurophysiol, 1:*57, 1949.

Walter, W.G., et al.: Analysis of the electrical response of the human cortex to photic stimulation. *Nature, 158:*540-541, 1946.

Walter, W.G., and Walter, V.J.: The electrical activity of the brain. *Ann Rev Physiol, 11:*199-230, 1949.

Watkins, A.L., et al.: Psychiatric and physiologic studies on fatigue. *Arch Physical Med, 28:*199-206, 1947.

Webb, W.B., and Ades, H.W.: Sleep tendencies: Effects of barometric pressure. *Science, 143:*263-264, 1964.

Weil, A.A.: EEG findings in a certain type of psychosomatic headache: dysrhythmic migraine. *Electroencephalogr Clin Neurophysiol, 4:*181, 1952.

Weil, A.A.: Dysrhythmic migraine. *Ohio St Med J, 50:*668-671, 1954.

Weinstein, E.A., et al.: Withdrawal, inattention and pain asymbolia. *Arch Neurol Psychiatr, 74:*235-248, 1955.

Wells, C.E.: Modifications of alpha-wave responsiveness to light by juxtaposition of auditory stimuli. *AMA Arch Neurol, 1:*689-694, 1959.

Wells, C.E.: Response of alpha waves to light in neurologic disease. *Arch Neurol, 6:*478-491, 1962.

Wheeler, E.T., and Koskoff, Y.D.: Certain aspects of personality as related to the electroencephalogram. *Am Psychol, 3:*278, 1948.

Wickler, A., et al.: Electroencephalograms during cycles of addiction to barbiturates in man. *Electroencephalogr Clin Neurophysiol, 7:*1, 1955.

Wikler, A., et al.: Electroencephalographic changes associated with chronic alcoholic intoxication and the alcohol abstinence syndrome. *Am J Psychiatry, 113:*106-114, 1956.

Williams, A.C.: Some psychological correlates of the electroencephalogram. *Arch Psychol, 34:*1-48, 1939.

Williams, A.C.: Facilitation of the alpha rhythm of the electroencephalogram. *J Exp Psychol, 26:*413-422, 1940.

Williams, D., and Parsons-Smith, G.: Cortical rhythms not seen in the electroenceph-alogram. *Brain, 73:*191-202, 1950.

Williams, D.: Cerebral basis of temperament and personality. *Lancet, 2:*1-4, 1954.

Winfield, D.L.: A comparison of oral and rectal chloral induced sleep in clinical elec-troencephalography. *Electroencephalogr Clin Neurophysiol, 7:*424, 1955.

Wissfeld, E., and Neu, O.: About EEG changes in migraine and the importance of oc-cipital delta waves in the EEG. *Nervenarzt, 31:*418-422, 1960.

Wyke, B.D.: Electrical activity of the human brain during artificial sleep. II. Regional differentiation of response to barbiturate sedation. *J Neurol Neurosurg Psychiatr, 14:* 137-146, 1951.

Yuzuriha, T.: The autocorrelation curves of normal brain waves and power spectra. *Psychol Neurol Jap, 62:*902-910, 1960.

Yoshii, N., et al.: The electroencephalogram in juvenile delinquents. *Folia Psychiatr Neurol Jap, 15:*85-91, 1961.

Yoshii, N., et al.: Electroencephalographic conditioning of frequency specific waves in human beings. *Med J Osaka Univ, 13:*37-50, 1962.

PUBLISHERS AND AUTHORS

T HE FOLLOWING publishers and authors are thanked for permission to re-
print abstracts of publications.

Academic Press, Inc.
 Walter, D.O.: *Exp Neurol,* 1963.
Akademie-Verlag GMBH
 Roth, N., and Klingberg, F.: *Acta Biol Med Ger,* 1970.
 Tatsuno, J., et al.: *Acta Biol Med Ger,* 1970.
Almaquist and Wiksell Periodicals Co.
 Eeg-Olofsson, O., and Petersen, I.: *Acta Paediatr Scand,* 1970.
 Eeg-Olofsson, O.: *Acta Paediatr Scand,* 1971.
American Association for the Advancement of Science
 Chapman, R.M., et al.: *Science,* March 1971.
 Daniel, R.S.: *Science,* August 1964.
 Elul, R.: *Science,* April 1969.
 Evans, C.R., and Mulholland, T.B.: *Science,* January 1969.
 Fox, S.S., and Norman, R.J.: *Science,* March 1968.
 Stern, J.A., et al.: *Science,* August 1961.
American Medical Association
 Greenberg, I.M.: *Arch Gen Psychiatry,* 1969.
 Heninger, G., et al.: *Arch Neurol,* 1969.
 Hollister, L.E., and Gillespie, H.K.: *Arch Gen Psychiatry,* 1970.
 Korein, J., et al.: *Arch Gen Psychiatry,* 1971.
 Rodin, E.A., et al.: *JAMA,* 1970.
 Shimazono, Y., et al.: *Arch Gen Psychiatry,* 1965.
 Tucker, G.J., et al.: *Arch Gen Psychiatry,* 1965.
 Wiener, J.M., et al.: *Arch Gen Psychiatry,* 1966.
American Psychiatric Association
 Bruck, M.S., *Am J Psychiatry,* 1968.
 Cohen, M., et al.: *Am J Psychiatry,* 1970.
 Mirin, S.M., et al.: *Am J Psychiatry,* 1971.
 Saletu, B., et al.: *Am J Psychiatry,* 1971.
 Wikler, A., et al.: *Am J Psychiatry,* 1970.
American Psychological Association
 Albino, R., and Burnand, G.: *J Exp Psychol,* 1964.
 Barber, T.X.: *Psychol Bull,* 1965.
 Jasper, H., and Shagass, C.: *J Exp Psychol,* 1941.
 Leavitt, F.: *J Exp Psychol,* 1968.
 Legg, C.F.: *J Exp Psychol,* 1968.
 Miller, H.L.: *Psychol Bull,* 1968.
 Shagass, C.: *J Exp Psychol,* 1942.
 Shagass, C., and Johnson, E.P.: *J Exp Psychol,* 1943.

Stoyva, J., and Kamiya, J.: *Psychol Rev*, 1968.

Travis, L.E., and Egan, J.P.: *J Exp Psychol*, 1938.

Canadian Psychiatric Association

Bonkalo, A., *Can Psychiatr Assoc J*, 1967.

Muller, H.F., and Shamsie, S.J.: *Can Psychiatr Assoc J*, 1968.

Clinical Psychology Publishing Co., Inc.

Hartlage, L.C., and Green, J.B.: *J Clin Psychol*, 1972.

Elsevier Publishing Company

Bagchi, B.K., and Wenger, M.A.: *Electroencephalogr Clin Neurophysiol*, 1957.

Becker, D.: *Electroencephalogr Clin Neurophysiol, Abstract*, 1971.

Bickford, R.G., and Fortescue, P.: *Electroencephalogr Clin Neurophysiol*, Abstract, 1971.

Boddy, J.: *Electroencephalogr Clin Neurophysiol, Abstract*, 1971.

Brazier, M.A.B.: *Electroencephalogr Clin Neurophysiol, Abstract*, 1969.

Brown, B.B.: *Electroencephalogr Clin Neurophysiol*, 1968.

Chapman, R.M., et al.: *Electroencephalogr Clin Neurophysiol*, 1970.

Childers, D.G., and Perry, N.W.: *Brain Res*, 1971.

Churchill, J.A.: et al.: *Electroencephalogr Clin Neurophysiol*, 1966.

Clusin, W.: *Electroencephalogr Clin Neurophysiol, Abstract*, 1969.

Clusin, W.T., and Giannitrapani, D.: *Electroencephalogr Clin Neurophysiol*, 1970.

Cohen, D.: *Electroencephalogr Clin Neurophysiol, Abstract*, 1970.

Daly, D.D., and Yoss, R.E.: *Electroencephalogr Clin Neurophysiol*, 1957.

Doroshenko, V.A., et al.: *Electroencephalogr Clin Neurophysiol, Abstract*, 1970.

Dumermuth, G., et al.: *Electroencephalogr Clin Neurophysiol*, 1971.

Eberlin, P., and Yager, D.: *Electroencephalogr Clin Neurophysiol*, 1968.

Fink, M. et al.: *Electroencephalogr Clin Neuophysiol, Abstract*, 1970.

Frost, J.D., Jr., and Elazar, Z.: *Electroencephalogr Clin Neurophysiol*, 1968.

Gaarder, K., et al.: *Electroencephalogr Clin Neurophysiol*, 1966.

Giannitrapani, D.: *Electroencephalogr Clin Neurophysiol, Abstract*, 1970.

Giannitrapani, D.: *Electroencephalogr Clin Neurophysiol, Abstract*, 1971.

Giannitrapani, D.: *Electroencephalogr Clin Neurophysiol, Abstract*, 1973.

Goldstein, S.: *Electroencephalogr Clin Neurophysiol*, 1970.

Harrison, A., et al.: *Electroencephalogr Clin Neurophysiol*, 1970.

Harter, M.R.: *Electroencephalogr Clin Neurophysiol*, 1967.

Herman, M.N., et al.: *Electroencephalogr Clin Neurophysiol, Abstract*, 1971.

Hjorth, B.: *Electroencephalogr Clin Neurophysiol*, 1970.

Hjorth, B., and Berglund, K.: *Electroencephalogr Clin Neurophysiol, Abstract*, 1971.

Hommes, O.R., and Panhuysen, L.H.H.M.: *Psychiatr Neurol Neurochir*, 1971.

Hoovey, Z.B., et al.: *Electroencephalogr Clin Neurophysiol*, 1972.

Hord, D., et al.: *Electroencephalogr Clin Neurophysiol*, 1972.

Huertas, J., and Westbrook, R.C.: *Electroencephalogr Clin Neurophysiol*, 1970.

Itil, T., et al.: *Electroencephalogr Clin Neurophysiol, Abstract*, 1971.

Jensen, D.R., and Engel, R.: *Electroencephalogr Clin Neurophysiol*, 1971.

Kaiser, E.K., et al.: *Electroencephalogr Clin Neurophysiol*, 1964.

Kasamatsu, A., et al.: *Electroencephalogr Clin Neurophysiol*, 1957.

Keesey, U.T., and Nichols, D.J.: *Electroencephalogr Clin Neurophysiol*, 1969.

Lairy, G.C.: *Electroencephalogr Clin Neurophysiol*, 1967.

Lansing, R.W., and Barlow, J.S.: *Electroencephalogr Clin Neurophysiol*, 1972.

Leader, H.S., et al.: *Electroencephalogr Clin Neurophysiol, Abstract*, 1971.

Lehmann, D.: *Electroencephalogr Clin Neurophysiol, Abstract, 1971.*

Lehmann, D.: *Electroencephalogr Clin Neurophysiol,* Abstract, 1971.

Lehtonen, J.B., and Lehtinen, I.: *Electroencephalogr Clin Neurophysiol,* 1972.

Lifshitz, K., and Gradijan, J.: *Electroencephalogr Clin Neurolphysiol, Abstract,* 1971.

Liske, E., et al.: *Electroencephalogr Clin Neurophysiol,* 1967.

Martin, W.B., et al.: *Electroencephalogr Clin Neurophysiol,* Abstract, 1971.

Martinius, J.W., and Hoovey, Z.B.: *Electroencephalogr Clin Neurophysiol,* 1972.

Metcalf, D.R.: *Electroencephalogr Clin Neurophysiol,* Abstract, 1971.

Mulholland, T., and Runnals, S.: *Electroencephalogr Clin Neurophysiol,* 1962.

Mulholland, T.: *Electroencephalogr Clin Neurophysiol,* 1964.

Mulholland, T.B.: *Electroencephalogr Clin Neurophysiol,* Abstract, 1969.

Needham, C.W., and Dila, C.J.: *Brain Res,* 1968.

Noel, P., and Leroy, C.L.: *Electroencephalogr Clin Neurophysiol,* Abstract, 1969.

Olofsson, O., and Petersen, I.: *Electroencephalogr Clin Neurophysiol,* Abstract, 1972.

Olsen, P.Z., et al.: *Electroencephalogr Clin Neurophysiol,* 1972.

Otomo, E.: *Electroencephalogr Clin Neurophysiol,* 1966.

Otomo, E., and Tsubaki, T.: *Electroencephalogr Clin Neurophysiol,* 1966.

Pasquali, E.: *Electroencephalogr Clin Neurophysiol,* 1969.

Pechstein, J.: *Electroencephalogr Clin Neurophysiol,* 1971.

Peters, J.F., et al.: *Electroencephalogr Clin Neurophysiol,* 1970.

Petersen, I., and Matousek, M.: *Electroencephalogr Clin Neurophysiol,* Abstract, 1972.

Remond, A., et al.: *Electroencephalogr Clin Neurophysiol,* 1969.

Roubicek, J., et al.: *Electroencephalogr Clin Neurophysiol,* Abstract, 1969.

Sacks, B., et al.: *Electroencephalogr Clin Neurophysiol,* 1972.

Shaw, J.C.: *Electroencephalogr Clin Neurophysiol,* Abstract, 1970.

Shipton, J., and Walter, W. Grey: *Electroencephalogr Clin Neurophysiol,* 1957.

Sorel, L.: *Electroencephalogr Clin Neurophysiol,* 1971.

Timsit-Berthier, M., et al.: *Electroencephalogr Clin Neurophysiol,* Abstract, 1971.

Volavka, J., et al.: *Electroencephalogr Clin Neurophysiol,* Abstract, 1967.

Walter, D.O., et al.: *Electroencephalogr Clin Neurophysiol,* Abstract, 1969.

Wennberg, A., and Zetterberg, L.H.: *Electroencephalogr Clin Neurophysiol,* 1971.

Wilson, G.F., and Lindsley, D.B.: *Electroencephalogr Clin Neurophysiol,* Abstract, 1969.

Grune and Stratton, Inc.

Freemon, F.R., and Walter, R.D.: *Compr Psyciatr,* 1970.

Hippokrates Verlag GMBH

Eeg-Olofesson, O.: *Neuropaediatrie,* 1971.

Institute of Electrical and Electronics Engineers, Inc.

Estrin, T., and Uzgalis, R.: *IEEE Trans Bio Med Eng,* 1969.

Sklar, B., et al.: *IEEE Trans Bio Med Eng,* 1973.

Macmillian (Journals) Ltd.

Adrian, E.D., and Matthews, B.H.C.: *Brain,* 1934.

Hockaday, J.M., and Whitty, C.W.M.: *Brain,* 1969.

Lippold, O.: *Nature,* 1970.

Lippold, O.: *Nature,* 1970.

Mulholland, T., and Evans, C.R.: *Nature,* 1965.

Mulholland, T., and Evans, C.R.: *Nature,* 1966.

Weinberg, H.: *Nature,* 1969.

Williams, D.: *Brain,* 1969.
National Institute for Personnel Research
    Griesel, R.D.: *Psychol Africana,* 1968.
New York Academy of Sciences
    Mulholland, T.: *Trans NY Acad Sci,* 1962.
New York State Dept. of Mental Hygiene
    Denber, H.C.B., and Merlis, S.: *Psychiatr Q,* 1955.
    Denber, H.C.B.: *Psychiatr Q,* 1955.
    Merlis, S., and Hunter, W.: *Psychiatr Q,* 1955.
North-Holland Publishing Co.
    Kleiner, B., et al.: *Comput Programs, Biomed,* 1970.
Physicians Postgraduate Press
    Marjerrison, G., et al.: *Dis Nerv Syst,* 1972.
    Wilson, N.J.: *Dis Nerv Syst,* 1968.
Plenum Publishing Corp.
    Itil, T.M.: *Recent Adv Biol Psychiatr,* 1966.
    Liberson, W.T., and Liberson, C.W.: *Recent Adv Biol Psychiatr,* 1966.
    White, R.P., *Recent Adv Biol Psychiatr,* 1966.
Postgraduate Medicine
    Swaiman, K.F.: *Postgrad Med, J Appl Med,* 1971.
Psychonomic Society, Inc.
    Barry, B.J., and Beh, H.C.: *Psychon Sci,* 1972.
    Gaarder, K., et al.: *Psychon Sci,* 1966.
    Gale, A., et al.: *Psychon Sci,* 1972.
Revista De Neuro-Psiquiatria
    Gomez, E.A.: *Rev Neuropsiquiatr,* 1968.
Rivista Di Neurobiologia
    Nigro, A.: *Riv Neurobiol,* 1969.
Schwabe & Co.
    Dumermuth, G.: *Helv Paediatr Acta,* 1969.
    Robert, F., and Karbowski, K.: *Helv Paediatr Acta,* 1971.
Society for Psychophysiological Research
    Brown, B.B.: *Psychophysiology,* 1966.
    Brown, B.B.: *Psychophysiology,* 1970.
    Galin, D., et al.: *Psychophysiology,* Abstract, 1971.
    Galin, D., and Ornstein, R.: *Psychophysiology,* 1972.
    Hart, J.T.: *Psychophysiology,* Abstract, 1968.
    Heinemann, L.G., and Emrich, H.: *Psychophysiology,* 1970.
    Hicks, R.G., and Angner, E.: *Psychophysiology,* Abstract, 1970.
    Honorton, C., et al.: *Psychophysiology,* Abstract, 1970.
    Johnson, L.C.: *Psychophysiology,* 1970.
    Lubin, A., et al.: *Psychophysiology,* 1969.
    Mulholland, T.B., and Peper, E.: *Psychophysiology,* 1971.
    Nowlis, D.P., and Kamiya, J.: *Psychophysiology,* 1970.
    Paskewitz, D.A.: *Psychophysiology,* 1971.
    Paskewitz, D.A., and Orne, M.T.: *Psychophysiology,* Abstract, 1972.
    Pasquali, E.: *Psychophysiology,* 1969.
    Phillips, C.: *Psychophysiology,* 1971.
    Saletu, B., et al.: *Psychophysiology,* Abstract, 1972.

Schwartz, G.E., et al.: *Psychophysiology*, Abstract, 1972.

Silverman, S., and Sherwood, M.: *Psychophysiology*, Abstract, 1972.

Spilker, B., et al.: *Psychophysiology*, 1969.

Stennett, R.G.: *Psychophysiology*, 1966.

Surwillo, W.W.: *Psychophysiology*, 1971.

Travis, T.A., et al.: *Psychophysiology* Abstract, 1972.

S. Karger AG

Fink, M.: *Med Exp*, 1961.

Gastaut, H., et al.: *Confin Neurol*, 1953.

Scollo, L.G.: *Eur Neurol*, 1970.

Serafetinides, E.A., et al.: *Int Pharmacopsychiatry*, 1971.

Spastics International Medical Publications

Churchill, J.A., and Rodin, E.A.: *Dev Med Child Neurol*, 1968.

Springer-Verlag

Birk, J.R.: *Kybernetik*, 1970.

Dieker, H., and Lauschner, E.: *Humangenetik*, 1967.

Emrich, H., and Heinemann, L.G.: *Psychol Forsch*, 1966.

Itil, T.M.: *Psychopharmacologia*, 1969.

Keidel, W.D., et al.: *Naturwissen*, 1971.

Peper, E.: *Kybernetik*, 1970.

Peper, E., and Mulholland, T.: *Kybernetik*, 1970.

Ritter, G.: *Nervenarzt*, 1969.

Vogel, F.: *Humangenetik*, 1970.

Statni Zdravotnicke Nakladatelstvi

Mulholland, T.B.: *Activ Nerv Sup (Praha)*, 1968.

Rosadini, G., and Rossi, G.F.: *Activ Nerv Sup (Praha)*, 1969.

Thieme Verlag

Barolin, G.S.: *Fortschr Neurol Psychiatr*, 1968.

Tohoku University School of Medicine

Mizuno, T., et al.: *Tohoku J Exp Med*, 1970.

University of Michigan, Ann Arbor

Wenger, M.A., and Bagchi, B.K.: *Behav Sci*, 1961.

Verlag Dr. Schwappach & Co.

Pechstein, J.: *Fortschr Med*, 1970.

Williams & Wilkins Co.

Merlis, S., and Denber, H.C.B.: *J Nerv Ment Dis*, 1956.

Serafetindes, E.A., Willis, D., and Clark, M.L.: *J Nerv Ment Dis*, 1972.

DESCRIPTOR EQUIVALENTS AND EXPLANATIONS

IN ORDER TO REDUCE the number of descriptors which identify topics dealt with in the research reports, in general only one most generally or widely used descriptor has been selected arbitrarily to define major categories and topics. In some cases a single descriptor may include one or more closely related aspects or attributes. The following list includes descriptors which either have commonly used synonyms or which may indicate a related function.

Abundance; incidence; occurrence; percentage; persistence; presence
Activation; alerting
Adaptation; habituation
Aging; geriatric
Alert; alerting; awake; arousal; vigilance
Alpha patterns (article defines more than one parameter)
Amplitude; voltage
Analysis of physical data; techniques for data analysis; measurement techniques; recording techniques
ANS; autonomic nervous system
Anticipation; expectancy; preparatory interval
Arousal; alert; alerting
Attention; vigilance
Awake; wakefulness; alert
Awareness; consciousness
Biorhythms; biological rhythms; diurnal variation
Bispectrum analysis; spectral analysis
Blocking; desynchronization
Brain mechanisms; brain physiology
Cerebral dominance; hemispheric dominance
Childhood disorders (autism, mongolism, neurologic problems)
Cognition; intelligence; mental tasks
Consciousness; awareness
Cortical areas; topography; spatial maps
Data analysis; techniques for data analysis; data reduction; statistical analysis; EEG analysis; computer analysis; data organization
Data collection; techniques for data collection; methods; procedures; measurements
Desynchronization; alpha blocking
Diurnal variation; biological rhythms
Discrimination tasks (perceptual or motor or cognitive)
Dreams; REM; REM sleep

Drugs (all types)
EEG patterns (means more than alpha was considered)
Emotion; mood; motivation; anticipation
Enhancement; production; augmented; synchronization
ESP; parapsychology
Expectancy; anticipation; preparatory interval
Frequency analysis; period analysis
Geriatrics; aging
Habituation; adaptation
Hallucinogens; hallocinogenic drugs (includes LSD, mescaline, psilocybin, etc.)
Hemispheric dominance; cerebral dominance
Imagery; mental imagery
Incidence; abundance
Intellectual performance; intelligence; cognition; cognitive style; mental tasks
Measurements; data collection
Mental imagery; imagery
Occurrence; abundance
Percentage; abundance
Period analysis; frequency analysis
Persistence; abundance
Personality; behavioral traits
Phase; propagation time; conduction time (as distinguished from phase of wave period)
Photic flicker; photic stimulation; photic driving
Preparatory interval; anticipation; expectancy
Presence; abundance
Memory; recall; recognition
Reaction time (motor response to nerve, visual or auditory stimulation)
Recall; recognition
Recognition; recall
REM; REM sleep; dreams
Rhythmicity; repetition rate; regularity
Sensory deprivation; sensory isolation
Spatial orientation; field dependency
Spectral analysis; bispectrum analysis
Topography; cortical areas; spatial maps
Variation; variability; constancy
Vigilance; attention
Voltage; amplitude
Wakefulness; awake; alert

DESCRIPTOR INDEX

342